OSCE Questions and Model Papers in

Obstetrics and Gynaecology

with Answers for Undergraduate and Postgraduate Students

Illustrations by:
Kathyana Samarakoon
Dr. Prashan Edirisingha
Sagara Chandralal

OSCE Questions and Model Papers in
Obstetrics and Gynaecology

with Answers for Undergraduate and Postgraduate Students

Eranthi Samarakoon
MBBS, MD (Sri Lanka), FRCOG (UK)
Senior Lecturer in Obstetrics and Gynaecology
Faculty of Medicine, University of Peradeniya
Consultant Obstetrician and Gynaecologist
Teaching Hospital, Peradeniya
Sri Lanka

Chathura Ratnayake
MBBS, MD (Sri Lanka), FRCOG (UK)
Senior Lecturer in Obstetrics and Gynaecology
Faculty of Medicine, University of Peradeniya
Consultant Obstetrician and Gynaecologist
Teaching Hospital, Peradeniya
Sri Lanka

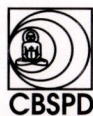

CBSPD

CBS Publishers & Distributors Pvt Ltd

New Delhi • Bengaluru • Chennai • Kochi • Kolkata • Lucknow • Mumbai
Hyderabad • Jharkhand • Nagpur • Patna • Pune • Uttarakhand

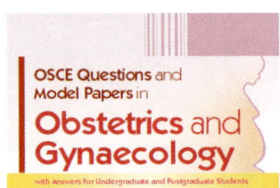

ISBN: 978-93-88178-81-5

Copyright © Authors and Publisher

First Edition: 2019

Reprint: 2022, 2023

Published by Satish Kumar Jain and produced by Varun Jain for

CBS Publishers & Distributors Pvt Ltd

4819/XI Prahlad Street, 24 Ansari Road, Daryaganj, New Delhi 110 002, India.

Ph: 011-23289259, 23266861   Website: www.cbspd.com
                               e-mail: delhi@cbspd.com

Corporate Office: 204 FIE, Industrial Area, Patparganj, Delhi 110 092, India
Ph: 011-4934 4934   Fax: 011-4934 4935   e-mail: publishing@cbspd.com;
                                                    publicity@cbspd.com

Branches

- **Bengaluru:** Seema House 2975, 17th Cross, KR Road, Banasankari 2nd Stage, Bengaluru 560 070, Karnataka, India
  Ph: +91-80-26771678/79   Fax: +91-80-26771680   e-mail: bangalore@cbspd.com
- **Chennai:** 7, Subbaraya Street, Shenoy Nagar, Chennai 600 030, Tamil Nadu, India
  Ph: +91-44-26680620, 26681266   Fax: +91-44-42032115   e-mail: chennai@cbspd.com
- **Kochi:** 42/1325, 1326, Power House Road, Opp KSEB, Power House, Ernakulum Kochi 682 018, Kerala, India
  Ph: +91-484-4059061-65,67   Fax: +91-484-4059065   e-mail: kochi@cbspd.com
- **Kolkata:** 147, Hind Ceramics Compound, 1st Floor, Nilgunj Road, Belghoria, Kolkata-700056, West Bengal, India
  Ph: +033-25633055, 033-25633056   e-mail: kolkata@cbspd.com
- **Lucknow:** Basement, Khushnuma Complex, 7 Meerabai Marg (Behind Jawahar Bhawan),Lucknow-226001, UP, India
  Ph: +91-522-4000032   e-mail: tiwari.lucknow@cbspd.com
- **Mumbai:** PWD Shed, Gala no 25/26, Ramchandra Bhatt Marg, Next to JJ Hospital Gate no. 2, Opp. Union Bank of India Noorbaug, Mumbai-400009, Maharashtra, India
  Ph: 022-66661880/89   e-mail: mumbai@cbspd.com

Representatives

• Hyderabad	0-9885175004	• Jharkhand	0-9811541605	• Nagpur	0-9421945513
• Patna	0-9334159340	• Pune	0-9923910676	• Uttarakhand	0-9716462459

Printed at HT Media Ltd, Greater Noida, UP, India

to
Late Mrs Chintha Wijemanne
(beloved mother of Dr Eranthi Samarakoon)

Mr and Mrs RM Wijeratne
(beloved parents of Dr Chatura Rathnayaka)

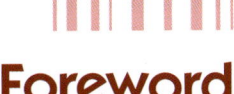

Foreword

Objective Structured Clinical Examination (OSCE) forms an important component of the undergraduate and postgraduate medical examinations in many countries of the world. Students have an undue fear regarding this method of assessment because it is based on practical aspects and there are very few books and model questions available for this relatively new coponent. The OSCE has replaced the clinical component in the MRCOG (UK) and in many other postgraduate and undergraduate examinations globally.

Dr Eranthi Samarakoon and Dr Chatura Ratnayaka who are senior teachers and active clinicians with a vast experience in teaching and examining undergraduate and postgraduate students are aware of the fear and anxiety of candidates facing an OSCE examination. This has inspired them to spend their valuable time to author this book which provides a practical guideline to face the examination with confidence. Though the main focus of this book is on undergraduates, it is also suitable for postgraduate students preparing for the Doctor of Medicine in Obstetrics and Gynaecology (Sri Lanka) and MRCOG part 3 examinations.

An unique feature of this book is the inclusion of 30 chapters containing practically based OSCE questions from almost the entire syllabus in obstetrics and gynaecology and 15 model papers. It covers all aspects of obstetrics and gynaecology required to answer OSCE questions. It is not merely a collection of questions. The answers have been formulated in a structured, orderly sequence to enhance the analytical and practical skills of the students.

The model papers simulate a true examination setting, and are intended for students, to understand the type and process of the OSCE examination and to test their knowledge and skills prior to the final examination.

All the practical details required for the final MBBS examination have been included. Hence, it will be of value not only for the OSCE component, but also for the clinical examination.

Images and photographs have been included as students are expected to identify these. There are questions from all the 14 tasks included in the MRCOG part 3 examination. When formulating these questions attention has been paid to the surgical skills and teaching modules for postgraduate students. Advanced surgical procedures have been included for postgraduate students.

The authors have used their vast experience as clinicians and senior teachers to formulate the questions in a manner which would be accepted globally. The principles of patient management given in this book are in accordance with the clinical guidelines of the Royal College of Obstetricians and Gynaecologists and the

NICE Guidelines (National Institute for Health and Care Excellence, UK) with minimal deviations to suit the practice in developing Asian Countries.

This is the only book on the subject written by Sri Lankan authors. I am sure that this book will be well accepted by undergraduate and postgraduate students in Sri Lanka and abroad.

Prof AS Abeyagunawardana
MBBS (SL), MD (Col), DCH (Col), MRCP(UK), FRCPCH (UK)
Senior Professor and Head,
Department of Paediatrics,
Dean, Faculty of Medicine
University of Peradeniya, Sri Lanka

Objective Structured Clinical Examination (OSCE) forms an important component of the undergraduate and postgraduate curriculum of medical schools in many countries of the world. The students find this relatively new method of assessment difficult, especially as it is based on practical aspects and because there are very few books and model questions available for them. The OSCE component has replaced the clinical examination in the MRCOG (UK) examination and in many other postgraduate and undergraduate examinations globally.

This book is intended for medical students preparing for the final MBBS examination and for postgraduate students preparing for the Doctor of Medicine in Obstetrics and Gynaecology, Part 2 and MRCOG, Part 3 Examinations. It has 420 pages, 30 chapters, 15 model papers, 350 questions with answers and 300 images.

The book has 30 chapters and 15 model papers. These chapters contain practically based OSCE questions from almost the entire syllabus in obstetrics and gynaecology. It contains a comprehensive collection of questions which are given for undergraduate and postgraduate examinations.

Questions have been included from almost every practical procedure which is carried out in the antenatal and gynaecology wards, clinics and the labour ward. There are questions regarding common surgical procedures. The answers are given in the appropriate order followed in performing these procedures, enabling the students to practice carrying out these procedures, as students are sometimes expected to demonstrate simple procedures to the examiners. Images and photographs have been included as students are expected to identify these. There are theory questions from the practical aspects of clinical obstetrics and gynaecology, as these form a major component of undergraduate and postgraduate OSCE examinations.

History taking, communication skills, surgical skills and teaching modules have been included for the benefit of undergraduate and postgraduate students. There are questions from all the 14 tasks included in the MRCOG, part 3 OSCE examination, which has replaced the clinical component. Some of the questions are long in keeping with the structured viva type OSCE questions asked at MD and MRCOG examinations. However, shortened versions of similar questions are asked from undergraduates.

When formulating these questions attention has been paid to the surgical skills and teaching modules for postgraduate students. Advanced surgical procedures have been included for postgraduate students. Questions which are more suitable for postgraduate students have been indicated.

The latter part of the book has 15 examination papers, each with 10 questions and detailed answers. These papers are similar to those given at the final examination in medical schools globally. These simulate a true examination setting, and are mainly intended for undergraduates, to understand the type and process of the OSCE examination and to test their knowledge and skills prior to the final examination. Areas which have not been covered in the chapters have been covered in the examination papers. The papers contain mainly new questions. Only a very few important questions have been taken from the chapters, but they too have been modified. These papers will be of help for the postgraduates too, as a wide range of questions have been included.

This book can be used to revise the subject quickly prior to the examination as the entire syllabus has been covered in a concise manner. Since it is in the form of questions and answers, it is thought provoking and will enhance the analytical skills of the students. All the practical details required for the Final MBBS examination have been included. Hence, it will be of value not only for the OSCE component, but also for the clinical examination.

Since there are a large number of diverse questions, lecturers can use it as a guide to set up OSCE stations for examinations. It can also be used as an aid to conduct mock examinations and practice sessions.

The principles of patient management given in this book are internationally accepted ones. They are in accordance with the clinical guidelines of the Royal College of Obstetricians and Gynaecologists and the NICE Guidelines (National Institute for Health and Care Excellence, UK) with minimal deviations to suit the practice in developing Asian Countries. Therefore, it will be useful for undergraduate and postgraduate students in many countries around the world.

We have used our vast experience as clinicians and senior teachers to formulate the questions in a manner which would be accepted globally.

There are very few books on OSCE questions in obstetrics and gynaecology. This is the only book which deals with all the aspects of the OSCE examination. Practical, surgical, history taking, clinical management, problem analysis, teaching and counselling skills have been included. Other books available in the market do not cover all aspects of the OSCE examination and do not give detailed answers.

Unlike other similar books in the market, this book is methodically arranged into 30 chapters and 15 model papers and covers all aspects of obstetrics and gynaecology required to answer OSCE questions. It is not merely a collection of questions.

This is the only book on the subject written by Sri Lankan authors.

Finally we are sure that this book will be helpful for undergraduates and postgraduates to face their examinations with confidence.

Eranthi Samarakoon
Chathura Ratnayake

Acknowledgements

We are thankful to Prof. AS Abeyagunawardana, for encouraging us to compile this manuscript and writing the Foreword.

We would like to acknowledge the guidance we received from the academic staff members of the Department of Obstetrics and Gynaecology, Faculty of Medicine, University of Peradeniya. A special word of thanks is extended to Dr MC Gihan for providing the cardiotocograph tracings.

We wish to thank Prof. Badra Hewawitharana, Consultant Radiologist for providing most of the ultrasound images. We also wish to thank consultant radiologists, Dr Ganganatha Rodrigo, Dr Jeewani Udupihilla and Dr Kumari Pussepitiya for providing ultrasound images.

We are thankful to Kathyana Samarakoon, Dr Prashan Edirisingha and Sagara Chandralal for carrying out the illustrations.

We wish to thank our consultant pathologists, Dr Manel Rathnayaka and Dr Sulochana Wijetunga for providing us with advice and images.

We thank Dr Senaka Kandegedara, Consultant Oncologist, for advising us regarding latest treatment procedures for gynaecological malignancies.

We are very grateful to Engr. Dr Sampath Deegalle for technical assistance and checking the manuscript for plagiarism. We appreciate the technical assistance and software provided by Engineer Mr. Asanka Amarasinghe. We thank Mr. Gamini Gunasekara for providing the photographs.

We very much appreciate the assistance of Mr. Kamal Hemantha, the Computer Applications Assistant of our Department, who did the preliminary formatting and type setting. He worked tirelessly to make this endeavour a success.

Finally we wish to thank all the academic staff members of the Faculty of Medicine, who helped us in numerous ways.

Eranthi Samarakoon
Chathura Ratnayake

Contents

Abbreviations

ABST	Antibiotic sensitivity test
AC	Abdominal circumference
ACTH	Adrenocorticotropic hormone
AFP	Alpha fetoprotein
AGC	Abnormal glandular cells
AIS	Adenocarcinoma *in situ*
APTT	Activated partial thromboplastin time
AUB	Abnormal uterine bleeding
BMI	Body mass index
BP	Blood pressure
BPD	Biparietal diameter
BPM	Beats per minute
Bpm	Beats per minute
BSS	Blood sugar series
cART	Combined anti-retroviral therapy
cffDNA	Cell free fetal DNA
CFTR	Cystic fibrosis transmembrane conductance regulator
Cm	Centimeters
CMV	Cytomegalovirus
CNS	Central nervous system
CRL	Crown rump length
CTG	Cardiotocograph
CTPA	Computerized tomography pulmonary angiogram
CVS	Chorionic villous sampling
DBP	Diastolic blood pressure
DES	Diethylstilbestrol
DIC	Disseminated intravascular coagulation
DM	Diabetes mellitus
DMPA	Depot medroxyprogesterone acetate
DV	Ductus venosus
DVT	Deep vein thrombosis
ECG	Electrocardiogram
ECV	External cephalic version
EEG	Electroencephalogram
EFW	Estimated fetal weight
ELISA	Enzyme-linked immunosorbent assay
ERPM	Examination required to practice medicine
FBS	Fasting blood sugar
FFP	Fresh frozen plasma
FGR	Fetal growth restriction
FIGO	International Federation of Gynecology and Obstetrics
FMH	Fetomaternal haemorrhage

FSH	Follicular stimulating hormone
FVS	Fetal varicella syndrome.
G	Gauge
GBS	Group B streptococcus
GDM	Gestational diabetes mellitus
GnRH	Gonadotropin releasing hormone
gr	Grams
GTD	Gestational trophoblastic disease
GTN	Gestational trophoblastic neoplasia
hCG	Human chorionic gonadotropin
HELLP	Hemolysis, elevated liver enzymes, low platelet count
HG	Hyperemesis gravidarum
HIV	Human immunodeficiency virus
HMB	Heavy menstrual bleeding
HPV	Human papilloma virus
HRT	Hormone replacement therapy
HSIL	High grade squamous intraepithelial lesion
HSV	Herpes simplex virus
IAP	Intrapartum antibiotic prophylaxis
IAT	Indirect antibody titer
ICSI	Intracytoplasmic sperm injection
ICU	Intensive care unit
IDA	Iron deficiency anaemia
IgG	Immunoglobulin G
IgM	Immunoglobulin M
IM	Intramuscular
INR	International normalization ratio
IU	International units
IUCD	Intrauterine contraceptive device
IV	Intravenous
Kg	Kilograms
LDH	Lactate dehydrogenase
LH	Luteinizing hormone
LMWH	Low molecular weight heparin
LNGIUS	Levonorgestrel releasing intrauterine system
LSCS	Lower segment cesarean section
LSIL	Low grade squamous intraepithelial lesion
MCA PSV	Middle cerebral artery peak systolic velocity
mcg	Micrograms
MCH	Mean corpuscular haemoglobin
MCHC	Mean corpuscular haemoglobin concentration
MCV	Mean corpuscular volume
Mg	Milligrams
Mm	Millimetres
mmHg	Millimetres of mercury
MoM	Multiples of the median
NESTROFT	Naked eye single tube red cell osmotic fragility test
NSAIDS	Nonsteroidal anti-inflammatory drugs
OCP	Oral contraceptive pills
OGTT	Oral glucose tolerance test
PAPPA	Pregnancy associated plasma protein-A
PCOS	Polycystic ovarian syndrome
PCR	Polymerase chain reaction

PE	Pulmonary embolism
PGE2	Prostaglandin E2
PI	Pulsatility index
PID	Pelvic inflammatory disease
POA	Period of amenorrhaea
PPBS	Postprandial blood sugar
PPH	Postpartum haemorrhage
PT	Prothrombin time
PTT	Partial thromboplastin time
RCOG	Royal College of Obstetricians and Gynecologists
Rh	Rhesus
RMI	Risk of malignancy index
SCJ	Squamocolumnar junction
SFH	Symphysis fundal height
SGA	Small for gestational age
SLCOG	Sri Lanka College of Obstetricians and Gynaecologists
SLE	Systemic lupus erythematosus
STI	Sexually transmitted infections
TSH	Thyroid stimulating hormone
TTTS	Twin to twin transfusion syndrome
TVUS/ TVS	Transvaginal ultrasound scan
U	Units
USS	Ultrasound scan
VBAC	Vaginal birth after caesarean section
VDRL test	Venereal disease research laboratory(VDRL) test
VTE	Venous thromboembolism
VZIG	Varicella zoster immunoglobulin
VZV	Varicella zoster virus
ZDV	Zidovudine

Chapter 1

Normal and Abnormal Labour

1.1 List 10 parameters which are monitored and recorded in the partogram during labour.
1.2 List the information which is recorded in the uppermost section of the partogram.
1.3 What are the parameters which indicate the progress of labour?

Answer 1.1

- Fetal heart rate.
- The duration of contractions and the interval between contractions
- Cervical dilatation
- Moulding of the skull bones and caput formation
- Abdominal and vaginal descent of the head
- Position of the fetal head
- Colour of the liquor
- Maternal pulse
- Temperature
- Blood pressure
- CTG findings
- Oxytocin drip rate

Answer 1.2

- Name
- Age
- BHT number
- Parity and gravidity
- Period of amenorrhoea
- Blood group
- Date and time of admission to the labour ward
- Special problems
- Special instructions

Answer 1.3

- Cervical dilatation
- Descent of the head.

QUESTION 2

2.1 **What are the parameters of fetal well-being which are monitored in the partogram?**

2.2 **Describe the method of monitoring the above parameters.**

2.3 **List 3 indications for continuous fetal heart rate monitoring.**

2.4 **What are the parameters of maternal well-being which are recorded in the partogram?**

2.5 **Describe the method of monitoring the above parameters.**

Answer 2.1

- Fetal heart rate
- CTG findings
- The colour of the liquor

Answer 2.2

The fetal heart rate: The fetal heart rate is auscultated using a hand held Doppler machine for 1 minute. This is done soon after a contraction to detect type 2 decelerations. It is difficult to auscultate accurately during contractions and also the type 1 decelerations which occur during contractions are not regarded as pathological. The fetal heart rate is recorded graphically in the partogram.

The frequency of auscultation is:
- From onset of labour to cervical dilation of 4 cm (during the latent phase)—every 30 minutes
- From cervical dilation of 4 to 10 cm—every 15 minutes
- From cervical dilation of 10 cm to onset of pushing (during the passive phase of the second stage)—every 10 minutes
- From onset of pushing to delivery of the baby (active phase of the second stage)—every 5 minutes.

CTG Recording

A CTG is usually performed if an abnormality is detected during intermittent auscultation. Continuous CTG monitoring is done in high risk patients.

The Colour of the Liquor

Perineal pads are inspected for the colour of the liquor half hourly after the membranes are ruptured and is recorded as clear (C) meconium (M) stained or blood stained. It is advisable to rupture the membranes early (at cervical dilatation of 4–5 cm) to allow observation of liquor and to augment labour.

Answer 2.3

- The presence of significant meconium.
- Fresh vaginal bleeding that develops in labour.

- Confirmed delay in the first or second stage of labour.
- Oxytocin use (*refer* Chapter 15, question 7 for all the indications for continuous fetal heart rate monitoring)

Answer 2.4

Maternal pulse, blood pressure and temperature are recorded.

Answer 2.5

Maternal pulse is recorded hourly, but may be recorded simultaneously with the fetal heart rate to differentiate between the two.
- The temperature is recorded once in 4 hours.
- The blood pressure is recorded 4 hourly. It is recorded half hourly in patients with PIH.

QUESTION 3

3.1 **What are the parameters of progress of labour which are recorded in the partogram?**
3.2 **Describe how these are monitored and recorded in the partogram.**
3.3 **Describe how the frequency and duration of contractions are monitored and recorded in the partogram.**

Answer 3.1

- Cervical dilatation
- Descent of the head.

Answer 3.2

The cervical dilatation is assessed by performing a vaginal examination 4 hourly and is graphically recorded.

Descent of the head
- Abdominal descent of the head is assessed by performing an abdominal examination once in 4 hours.
- It is assessed according to the number of fifths palpable per abdomen. The appropriate number of squares is marked in the partogram.
- The vaginal descent of the head is assessed by performing a vaginal examination once in 4 hours, simultaneous with the abdominal examination. It is assessed by the distance of the head to the ischial spines as –3, –2, –1, 0, +1 and +2. The appropriate number of squares is marked in the partogram.

Answer 3.3

- The duration of contractions and the contraction free interval is recorded and documented according to the key given in the second page of the partogram.
- The interval from the beginning of one contraction to the beginning of the next contraction is calculated and the number of contractions per 10 minutes can be calculated.

QUESTION 4

Is the progress of labour normal or abnormal in this partograph recording of a primiparous woman? Give reasons for your answer.

National Partogram

H. 1255

Name: Age: BHT. No:

Gravida: Parity: Blood Group: Date and Time:

Special Problems: Special Instructions:

Time of V/E																									
Hours	1	2	3	4	5	6	7	8	9	10	11	12	13	14	15	16	17	18	19	20	21	22	23	24	

Fetal Heart Record in 1st Stage: ≥180, 170, 160, 150, 140, 130, 120, 110, 100, <100

CTG

Contraction free interval + duration of contraction: 1, 2, 3, 4, 5

Oxy dose ml-h/ dpm

Cervical Dilatation / Abdo Descent: 10, 09, 08, 07, 06, 05, 04, 03, 02, 01, 0

Descent Vaginally: -3, -2, -1, 0, +1, +2

Liquor

Position

Caput

Moulding

Pulse

BP

Temp

Action

2nd Stage Fetal Heart Rate Record   Time: Fully dilated:..................... Commenced pushing:. .... (Mark ▼▼)

Time															
≥180															
170															
160															
150															
140															
130															
120															
110															
100															
<100															

Answer 4

The progress of labour is normal because:

- The latent phase has taken 4 hours from 2 cm.
- The cervix has dilated at the rate of 1 cm/hour in the active phase.
- The head has descended normally and it is fully engaged at the beginning of the second stage.
- There is no caput.
- Moulding is normal and is grade 1.
- The position of the head is occipito anterior.
- The frequency of contractions is adequate and the frequency has gradually increased up to 4–5 contractions/10 minutes at the end of the first stage.

QUESTION 5

5.1 **List 5 parameters which are recorded in a partograph which indicate the possibility of obstructed labour.**

5.2 **How will you treat obstructed labour in the first stage?**

5.3 **How will you treat obstructed labour in the second stage in a woman with a cephalic presentation?**

5.4 **How will you treat obstructed labour in a woman with an occipito-posterior position in the second stage?**

Answer 5.1

- Failure of cervical dilatation to progress in the presence of strong uterine contractions.
- Presence of a large caput (++).
- Severe moulding with overlapping of skull bones (+++).
- Failure of the head to descend during the first stage and presence of more than one fifth of the head palpable per abdomen at the beginning of the second stage.
- Failure of the head to descend during the second stage.

Answer 5.2

Perform a caesarean section.

Answer 5.3

The safest option is to perform a caesarean section because it is dangerous to apply instruments in the presence of obstructed labour, as there could be an undiagnosed brow presentation, mento-posterior face presentation, occipito-posterior position or cephalo-pelvic disproportion. The case should be assessed by a consultant. Instrumental delivery can be considered, if the above complications are carefully excluded and all the criteria for safe application of instruments are satisfied. However, the procedure should be carried out in the operating theatre with all preparations kept ready for caesarean section (trial of instrumental delivery).

Answer 5.4

If the pelvis is adequate and no part of the head is palpable per abdomen the obstruction could be relieved by rotation of the head to the occipito-anterior position. Therefore, Kielland's forceps delivery or vacuum delivery can be tried. However, the procedure should be carried out in the operating theatre with all preparations kept ready for caesarean section.

QUESTION 6

List the mistakes which have been made while maintaining the partogram and mention your corrections.

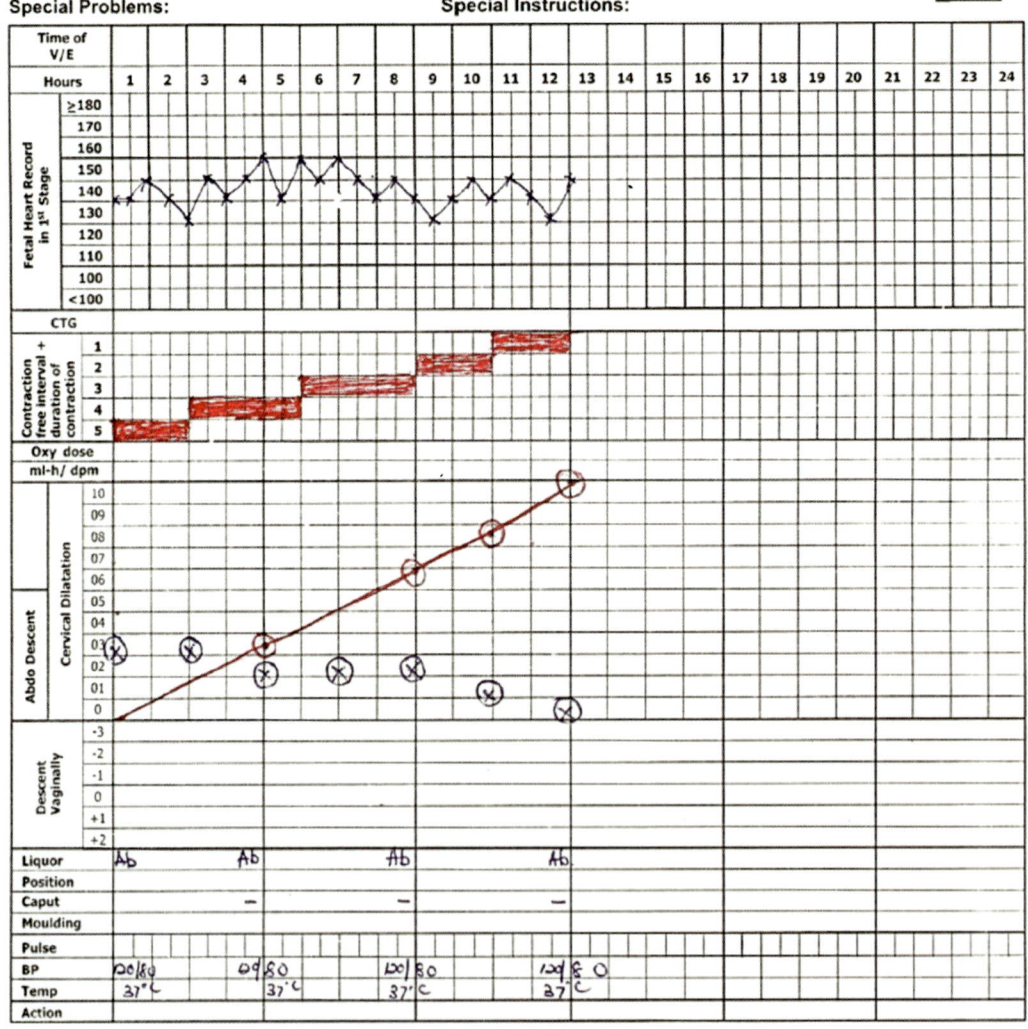

National Partogram   H. 1255

Name: Kusamawathie   Age: 30 yrs   BHT. No:

Gravida: G₁   Parity: P₁   Blood Group: O €Jve   Date and Time: 15/10/17

Special Problems: Special Instructions:

2nd **Stage Fetal Heart Rate Record Time: Fully dilated:..7..A.M....... Commenced pushing:. .8..AM........ (Mark ↓↓)**

Time	7 A M													8 A M																												
≥180																																										
170																																										
160																																										
150	X	X			X							X		X																												
140			X			X		X		X	X		X																													
130							X																																			
120																																										
110																																										
100																																										
<100																																										

Answer

- The name has been written without initials or a surname. It is important to write the full name to identify the patient as there may be two patients with similar names.
- The BHT number is not mentioned. The BHT number is important to identify the patient and to trace her ticket at a later date.
- The time of admission is not mentioned. The time is important to assess the duration of labour and to determine whether labour is becoming prolonged.
- The patient is Rhesus negative, but this has not been highlighted in the special problems.
- The need to take cord blood has not been mentioned in the special instructions.
- The fetal heart rate has been recorded half hourly during the active phase of the first stage, whereas it should be recorded every 15 minutes.
- The duration of contractions have not been marked. It should be marked according to the code mentioned in the partogram. Even though uterine hyperstimulation has occurred after cervical dilatation of 8 cm no intervention has been carried out.
- Vaginal examination has been performed once in 2 hours from 6–10 cm dilatation. Vaginal examination should be performed once in 4 hours during the first stage.
- Abdominal descent of the head has been recorded 2 hourly. It should be recorded once in 4 hours.
- Vaginal descent of the head has not been recorded at the time of the vaginal examination. It should be recorded 4 hourly during the first stage and hourly during the second stage.
- Amniotomy has not been performed. Amniotomy should be performed at a cervical dilatation of 5–6 cm.
- The position of the fetal head and moulding has not been recorded. These parameters should be recorded once in 4 hours during the vaginal examination.
- The fetal heart rate has been recorded once in 10 minutes after the woman commenced pushing. It should be recorded once in 5 minutes during this stage.
- The partogram has been maintained in a haphazard manner. Documentation should be done neatly and methodically in the standard manner.

QUESTION 7

The image given below is the partograph recording of a secondpara.

National Partogram

H. 1255

Name: Age: BHT. No:

Gravida: Parity: Blood Group: Date and Time:

Special Problems: Special Instructions:

7.1   Describe 4 important observations which have been recorded.

7.2   Name the abnormality of cervical dilatation.

7.3   What could be the cause of the abnormality in this patient?

7.4   List two other conditions which could cause this abnormality.

7.5   Mention how you could prevent this complication.

7.6   How will you treat this woman?

7.7   What are the maternal and fetal risks?

Answer 7.1

• The fetal position is occipito-posterior

• The frequency of contractions has followed the normal pattern with gradual increase in the frequency up to cervical dilatation of 8 cm. She is getting 4–5

contractions per 10 minutes which is regarded as adequate in the latter part of the active phase of the first stage. However, the frequency of contractions has increased after this point indicating uterine hyperstimulation.
- The cervical dilatation has progressed normally at first but dilatation has begun to arrest at 7 cm, in spite of strong uterine contractions lasting for 40–60 seconds, with a frequency of 4–5 per 10 minutes. It has deviated to the right from the alert line between 6 and 7 cm and has crossed the action line at 8 cm.
- The head has failed to descend with three fifths of the head still palpable above the pelvic brim. Vaginal descent of the head is static at station-2.

Answer 7.2

Secondary arrest.

Answer 7.3

Occipito-posterior position. The pelvis could be narrow and android in type.

Answer 7.4

- Brow presentation
- Mento-posterior face presentation

Answer 7.5

- The pelvis should be assessed before the onset of labour by the following methods.
  - Inquire regarding a history of prolonged labour or difficult instrumental deliveries in the first pregnancy and the birth weight of the previous baby.
  - Carry out clinical and ultrasonic evaluation of the fetal weight.
  - Measure the height of the woman
  - Clinical pelvic assessment should be performed before onset of labour, if cephalo-pelvic disproportion is suspected.
- Perform a careful vaginal examination early in labour (at 3–4 cm cervical dilatation) to exclude mento-posterior face and brow presentation and occipito-posterior position. If a mento-posterior face presentation or a brow presentation is found a caesarean section should be performed before obstruction occurs.
- If an occipito-posterior position is found, the pelvis should be assessed carefully to exclude an android pelvis and if the pelvis is adequate good contractions should be provided with timely use of an oxytocin infusion.

Answer 7.6

Perform a caesarean section immediately.

Answer 7.7

- Fetal hypoxia, fetal distress and fetal death.
- Obstructed labour
- Uterine rupture
- Sepsis

QUESTION 8

National Partogram

H. 1255

Name: Age: BHT. No:

Gravida: Parity: Blood Group: Date and Time:

Special Problems: Special Instructions:

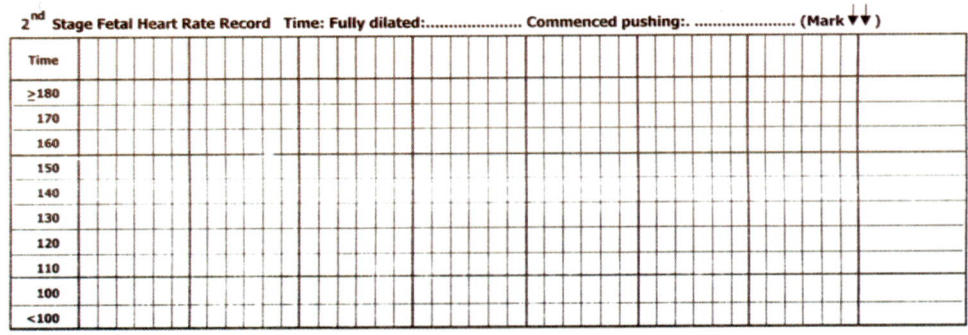

2nd Stage Fetal Heart Rate Record   Time: Fully dilated:.................... Commenced pushing:. .... (Mark ▼▼)

The image given on previous page is the partograph recording of a secondpara.

8.1   Describe 4 important observations which have been recorded.

8.2   Name the abnormality of cervical dilatation.

8.3   What is the main reason for this abnormality?

8.4   State 4 other conditions which could cause this abnormality.

8.5   What is the best treatment option for this woman? Give your reasons.

8.6   What are the indications for performing a caesarean section for this condition?

8.7   What precautions should be taken to prevent the occurrence of this complication?

8.8   What is your management if the reason for the delay is an occipito-posterior position?

Answer 8.1

- The fetal heart rate is within the normal range with good beat to beat variation and accelerations.
- The frequency of contractions is inadequate and static with two-three contractions per 10 minutes. For labour to progress normally there should be 4 contractions per 10 minutes in the latter part of the first stage.
- Labour has been slow from the beginning. The rate of cervical dilatation is about 2 cm in 4 hours during the active phase. The cervical dilatation has deviated to the right from the alert line at 5 cm and has crossed the action line at 7 cm.
- The head has descended and is engaged.

Answer 8.2

Primary dysfunctional labour.

Answer 8.3

Inadequate uterine contractions.

Answer 8.4

- Occipito-posterior position
- Mento-anterior face presentation
- Uterine over distension due to twin pregnancy
- Uterine over-distension due to polyhydramnios

Answer 8.5

The only abnormality seen in this partograph is the slow rate of cervical dilatation. The fetal heart rate is within the normal range. The descent of the head is satisfactory. However, a careful vaginal examination should be performed to exclude brow and mento-posterior face presentation, occipito-posterior position and cephalo-pelvic disproportion.

The woman should be reassured and explained regarding the available management options. An amniotomy should be performed and an oxytocin infusion should be commenced. The patient should be well hydrated. Adequate pain relief should be provided preferably with epidural analgesia. Continuous fetal heart rate monitoring should be commenced and the progress should be assessed by performing a vaginal examination in 2 hours.

Answer 8.6

- Fetal distress.
- Failure to progress 2 hours after augmentation.
- Presence of a previous caesarean section or a myomectomy scar.
- Cephalo-pelvic disproportion.
- Breech presentation.
- Occurrence of a malpresentation such as brow or mento-posterior face presentation.

Answer 8.7

- The frequency of contractions should be assessed half hourly.
- The progress of labour should be carefully assessed with 4 hourly abdominal and vaginal examinations.
- An early amniotomy should be performed at a cervical dilatation of 4–5 cm and an oxytocin infusion should be commenced after 2 hours if the progress is not satisfactory, in the absence of a scarred uterus, malpresentation, cephalo-pelvic disproportion or fetal distress.

Answer 8.8

Labour can be augmented as above with amniotomy and an oxytocin infusion in the absence of cephalo-pelvic disproportion.

QUESTION 9

9.1 **What is the accepted increase in the frequency of contractions throughout labour?**

9.2 **What are the parameters of progress of labour during the first stage?**

9.3 **What are the parameters of progress of labour during the second stage?**

Answer 9.1

- In the latent phase of the first stage, the frequency of contractions should be 1–2 per 10 minutes.
- In the early part of the active phase of the first stage frequency of contractions should be 2–3 per 10 minutes, while in the latter part it should be 4–5 per 10 minutes, with each contraction lasting from 45 seconds –1 minute.
- In the second stage, the frequency of contractions should be 5 per 10 minutes, with each contraction lasting for nearly 1 minute.

Answer 9.2

The parameters of progress during the first stage are dilatation of the cervix and abdominal and vaginal descent of the head, recorded by abdominal and vaginal examinations performed 4 hourly.

Answer 9.3

The parameter of progress during the second stage is the vaginal descent of the head, recorded by vaginal examination performed hourly.

QUESTION 10

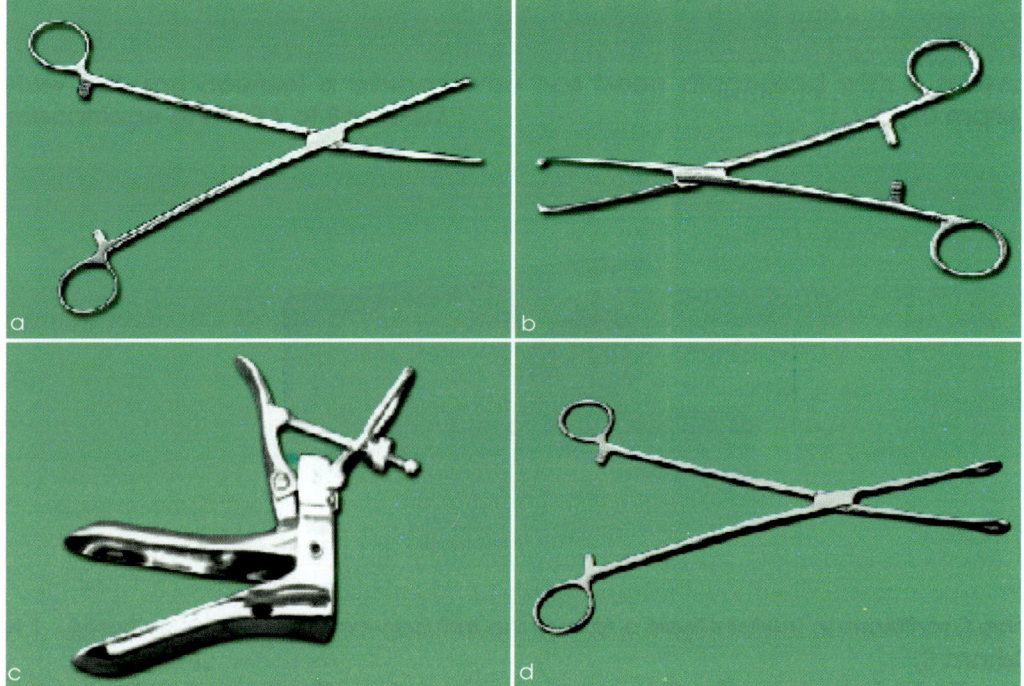

10.1 Pick and name the instrument/s needed to perform an amniotomy.
10.2 Describe in detail the method of performing an amniotomy.
10.3 How can you confirm amniotomy if liquor is not visualized.

Answer 10.1

a. Long artery forceps

Answer 10.2

- Amniotomy is performed in the labour ward under strict aseptic precautions.
- Place the patient in the dorsal position.
- Scrub and wear sterile gloves.
- Clean the vulva with an antiseptic solution.
- Insert 2 fingers of the right hand into the vagina and reach the cervical os.
- Assess the cervical dilatation, the presenting part and the level of the presenting part.
- Exclude cord presentation. Sweep the fingers around the head to exclude the presence of the cord in the vicinity.
- Amniotomy is performed at a cervical dilatation of 5 cm, if the presentation is vertex and the head is well applied to the presenting part. Amniotomy is delayed in breech presentation and in the presence of a high head, because of the risk of cord prolapse.
- Hold a blunt long artery forceps in the left hand and guide it along the right hand into the cervical os.

- Grab the membranes with the forceps and pull to break the membranes.
- Keep the fingers in the os and release the liquor slowly.
- Remove the fingers when the liquor is drained and the head has descended.
- Do not remove an excessive amount of liquor.
- Exclude cord prolapse.
- Auscultate the fetal heart sounds.

Answer 10.3

If amniotomy has occurred there will be hair in the artery forceps.

QUESTION 11

11.1 Mention 2 advantages of amniotomy.

11.2 List 4 risks of amniotomy.

11.3 What precautions will you take to prevent the complications you have mentioned?

Answer 11.1

It augments labour and reduces the risk of amniotic fluid embolism. Oxytocin should not be commenced without performing an amniotomy because of the risk of amniotic fluid embolism. Colour of the liquor can be seen. Meconium and blood staining can be excluded.

Answer 11.2

- Cord prolapse
- Sepsis
- Tissue trauma
- Placental abruption, if a large volume of liquor is released suddenly.

Answer 11.3

- Cord prolapse is prevented by:
  - Performing a vaginal examination to exclude cord presentation.
  - Sweeping around the presenting part to exclude the presence of the cord in the vicinity.
  - Releasing the liquor gradually by keeping the fingers in the os till the head descends
  - Delaying amniotomy till the presenting part is well descended and well applied to the cervix
- Sepsis is prevented by:
  - Performing the procedure in the labour room under strict aseptic precautions.
  - Minimizing the amniotomy delivery interval by commencing an oxytocin infusion, if the contractions are not adequate.
- Tissue trauma is prevented by using a blunt artery forceps for the procedure.
- Placental abruption is prevented by releasing the liquor in the bag of forewaters gradually. Release of an excessive amount of liquor should be avoided.

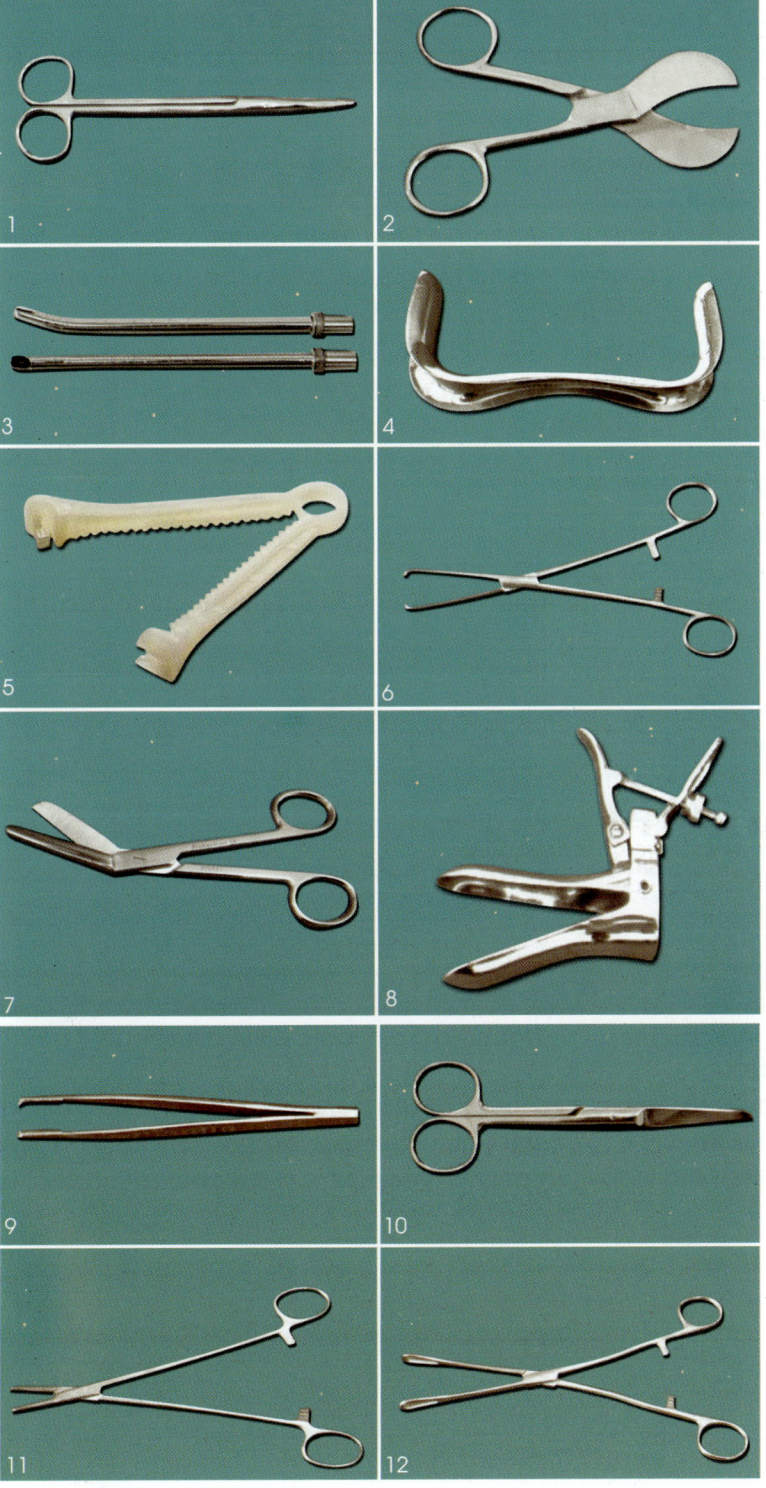

12.1 Select and name the instruments which are required to conduct a normal vaginal delivery.

12.2 Mention the use of each instrument you have selected.

12.3 List the other equipment/material required to conduct a normal vaginal delivery.

Answers 12.1 and 12.2

2. Cord scissor is used to cut the baby's cord
5. Cord clamp is used to clamp the baby's cord.
7. Episiotomy scissor is used to perform an episiotomy.
9. Catch forceps is used to hold the tissues while suturing the episiotomy.
10. Dressing scissor is used to cut thread.
11. Needle holder is used to hold the needle while suturing the episiotomy.
12. Sponge holding forceps is used to hold gauze swabs to clean the blood while suturing the episiotomy.

Answer 12.3

- Four sterile cloth towels
- One 2 cc syringe to give oxytocin
- One 10 cc syringe to infiltrate lignocaine to the perineum to perform and suture the episiotomy.
- Gauze swabs and gauze towels
- Perineal pads
- Oxytocin 5 units
- 10cc of 1% lignocaine
- A large tray to place the placenta
- Infant resuscitaire cum warmer
- A supply of oxygen
- A good light

QUESTION 13

13.1 List 4 indications for performing a clinical pelvic assessment before the onset of labour.

13.2 List the steps you would follow when performing a clinical pelvic assessment.

13.3 What is the POA at which you would perform a clinical pelvic assessment?

13.4 Which of the following pelvic types is most suitable for normal labour?

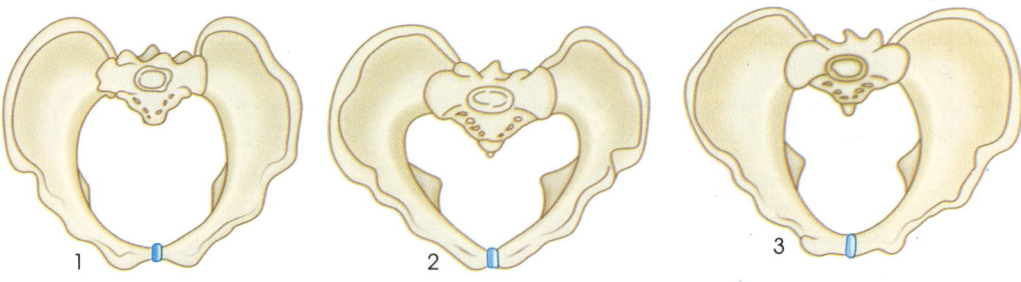

Answer 13.1

Routine clinical pelvic assessment is done before deciding to allow a vaginal delivery in a woman with:

- Breech presentation.
- Previous caesarean section.
- Occipito-posterior position.
- A non-engaged head at term in the first pregnancy.

Answer 13.2

- This is performed in the clinic or in the ward.
- A vaginal examination is performed after placing the patient in the dorsal position.
- The pelvis is assessed at the inlet, mid-cavity and the outlet.
- The inlet is adequate if the sacral promontory is not felt. If the promontary is felt the diagonal conjugate should be measured (refer paper 15 question 1).
- Next the fingers are passed along the sacrum. In an adequate gynaecoid pelvis the sacrum is concave. If the sacrum is flat the space in the mid-cavity may be inadequate.
- Next the ischial spines and the sacrospinous ligaments are felt. The mid-cavity is adequate if the ischial spines are not prominent and the sacrospinous ligaments accommodate three fingers.
- The sub-pubic angle and the inter-tuberous diameter are measured to assess the outlet. If the outlet is adequate the sub-pubic angle should admit 3 fingers and the inter-tuberous diameter should accommodate 4 knuckles. However, the outlet can be enlarged by performing an episiotomy as the posterior boundary is not bony.

Answer 13.3

It is performed after 38 weeks by which time the fetal growth is complete.

Answer 13.4

Number 1-Gynaecoid pelvis.

QUESTION 14

14.1 List 2 clinical situations in which this chart should be used for monitoring purposes.

14.2 List 5 ways in which the above chart has reduced the clinical risk in obstetric patients.

14.3 Name 2 categories of officers other than doctors who could maintain the above chart.

Modified Early Warning Signs Chart

H No: PH 1237

Name: ....

BHT: ....

Ward No: ....

Date and Time ....

* If any two parameters Yellow or one parameter Orange, **inform immediately**

		0	15	30	45	60	75	90	105	120	
Restless or Drowsy											
Alert & Oriented											

Temperature

°F	°C
105.8	41
104	40
102	39
100.4	38
98.6	37
96.8	36
<95	<35

| Respiratory Rate | >30 | 21-30 | 11-20 | <10 |

| Pulse Rate | 130 120 110 100 90 80 70 60 50 40 |

| Systolic BP | 200 190 180 170 160 150 140 130 120 110 100 90 80 70 60 50 |

| Diastolic BP | 130 120 110 100 90 80 70 60 50 |

| Urine output | <30ml | >30ml |

| Bleeding | Yes | No |

| Postpartum monitoring | |

| Uterus | Soft | Hard |

| Level of Fundus | Rising | Same |

Answer 14.1

It should be used to monitor women after:

- Caesarean section
- Normal delivery
- Instrumental delivery

Answer 14.2

- This chart should be attached to the BHT of all postpartum patients.
- It is a standard, universal method of observation and has replaced the haphazardly maintained observation charts.
- It is mandatory to monitor all the parameters at given frequent intervals.
- The level of risk is clearly visible as it is indicated in different colours. Deterioration can be identified early.
- Situations which need medical attention are clearly indicated by different colours.
- It can be maintained even in a primary care unit and the patient can be transferred early as the clinical risk is clearly indicated.

Answer 14.3

It can be maintained by nurses and midwives.

QUESTION 15

15.1 What are the parameters which are monitored in the modified early warning chart in a woman during the first 2 hours after partus and what is the frequency of monitoring?
15.2 How do you assess the level of the risk?
15.3 When should a medical officer be informed?

Answer 15.1

Parameters which are monitored at 15 minute intervals include:

- Maternal pulse rate.
- Systolic and diastolic blood pressure
- Respiratory rate.
- Tone of the uterus and the level of the fundus
- Visual estimation of the blood loss.
- The level of alertness
  The urine output is charted every 30 minutes.
  The temperature should be checked before the patient leaves the labour ward.
  It is mandatory to monitor the above parameters during the first 2 hours, while the patient is in the labour ward.
  Further monitoring may be needed in high risk patients.

Answer 15.2

- The chart contains green, yellow and orange areas.
- If the observed value is recorded in a green area it is within the normal range.
- If it is recorded in a yellow area the risk is moderate.
- If it is recorded in an orange area the risk is high.

Answer 15.3

- A medical officer should be informed if any parameter is recorded in an orange area or if 2 parameters are recorded in a yellow area.
- If the observations are recorded only in green areas usual frequency of observation could be continued.

Chapter 2

Management of the Third Stage and Postpartum Haemorrhage

QUESTION 1

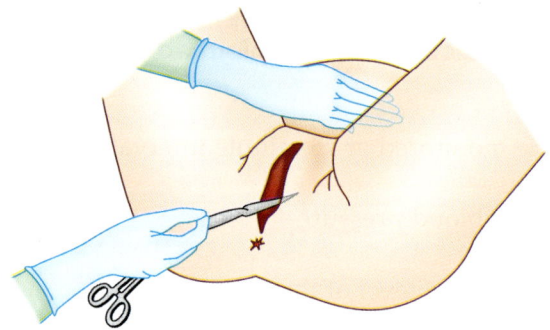

1.1 What is this procedure?
1.2 What precautions are taken to prevent inversion of the uterus during this procedure?
1.3 List 5 steps in the active management of the third stage.
1.4 When will you perform manual removal of the placenta?

Answer 1.1

Application of controlled cord traction to deliver the placenta.

Answer 1.2

- The procedure is commenced only if the uterus is well contracted.
- It is better to wait for signs of placental separation.
- The uterus is pushed up with the ulnar border of the left hand.
- Gentle traction is applied on the cord.

Answer 1.3

- Administer 5 units of oxytocin with the delivery of the anterior shoulder.
- Clamp the cord close to the introitus after 2 minutes of birth and separate the baby.

- Confirm contraction of the uterus by abdominal palpation.
- Wait for signs of placental separation.
- Apply controlled cord traction and gently deliver the placenta. The uterus is pushed up with the ulnar border of the left hand and gentle traction is applied on the cord with the right hand.
- Inspect the placenta and membranes for completeness.

Answer 1.4

Manual removal is performed if the placenta is not delivered after 30 minutes.

QUESTION 2

A primipara develops postpartum haemorrhage soon after an uncomplicated vaginal delivery.

2.1   Mention 3 important steps in the initial management.
2.2   How will you determine the cause of the haemorrhage?
2.3   What is the first step in the management of atonic PPH if there is no retained placental tissue?
2.4   Mention four drugs (with their dose and mode of administration) which are used to stop bleeding in atonic postpartum haemorrhage.

Answer 2.1

- Insert two 14 gauge cannulae and commence intravenous crystalloids. Give oxygen by face mask and keep the patient warm.
- Crossmatch 5 units of blood.
- Call for help and inform senior staff members.
- Estimate the blood loss by assessing the pulse rate, blood pressure and the colour of the patient. Perform a vaginal examination to assess the volume of clots and blood in the vagina.

Answer 2.2

- Palpate the abdomen to determine whether the uterus is well contracted and hard or soft and atonic.
- If the uterus is soft the bleeding is due to uterine atony.
- In atonic PPH inspect the placenta and membranes to determine whether they are complete. If there is any doubt about their completeness perform an USS.
- If the uterus is hard bleeding is due to trauma to the genital tract.
- Inspect the genital tract to determine the site of the injury.
- Exclude the possibility of coagulopathy.

Answer 2.3

- Treat with oxytocic drugs and massage the uterus continuously.
- Replace the lost blood volume.

Answer 2.4

- Administer oxytocin 5 units as an intravenous bolus. This can be repeated once. Commence an intravenous infusion of 30–40 units of oxytocin in one pint of normal saline.

- Ergometrine 0.5 mg is administered intravenously. This can be repeated once.
- Misoprostol 800 µg is inserted into the rectum.
- Administer an intramuscular injection of 0.25 mg of carboprost. Can be repeated once in 15 minutes up to a maximum of 8 doses. Carboprost 0.5 mg can be administered as an intramyometrial injection (carboprost is contraindicated in those with bronchial asthma).

Reference for Questions 1 and 2: Munro Kerr's Operative Obstetrics, 12th edition, Chapter 20.

QUESTION 3

3.1   What is the next step in the management if treatment with oxytocic drugs fail to control bleeding in a woman with atonic postpartum haemorrhage?

3.2   Describe how you would teach a junior doctor the procedure mentioned in 3.1 using an improvised device. *(Teaching and surgical skills module for postgraduate students, but undergraduates also can be questioned on the basic method.)*

3.3   Draw a diagram to show how this device is placed in the uterus.

Answer 3.1

Insert a condom catheter-balloon tamponade.

Answer 3.2

Bleeding can be controlled by the technique of balloon tamponade using a condom catheter.

- The equipment required include a Foley catheter, a condom, silk suture material, two Sim's speculums, a sponge holding forceps, a long artery forceps, a gauze pack, normal saline drip and a good light.
- A condom is tied firmly (with black silk) at 2 points to the end of a 16 gauge Foley catheter. Check for leakage by inserting a little saline.
- The procedure is explained to the patient and she is reassured.
- Informed consent is obtained.
- The patient is placed in the lithotomy position.
- The cervix is exposed by retracting the anterior and posterior vaginal walls using two Sim's speculums.
- The anterior lip of the cervix is held with a sponge holding forceps.
- The condom is inserted completely into the uterus using a long artery forceps.
- The bulb of the catheter is inflated.
- The catheter is connected to a normal saline drip and the condom is filled with 250–500 ml of solution. The condom will expand like a balloon and compress the placental bed, thereby preventing bleeding from the uterine sinuses in the placental bed.
- The cervical os is packed with gauze to prevent the catheter from slipping down.
- The height of the fundus should be marked and the fundal height, pulse, vaginal bleeding and the blood pressure should be checked every 10–15 minutes. The urine output should be measured hourly.
- She should preferably be nursed in an ICU.
- If there is any doubt whether blood is collecting above the balloon an USS should be performed.

- An oxytocin infusion is continued.
- Broad spectrum antibiotics should be given.
- The balloon can be kept in situ (up to 24 hours) till the patient's condition is stable.

Answer 3.3

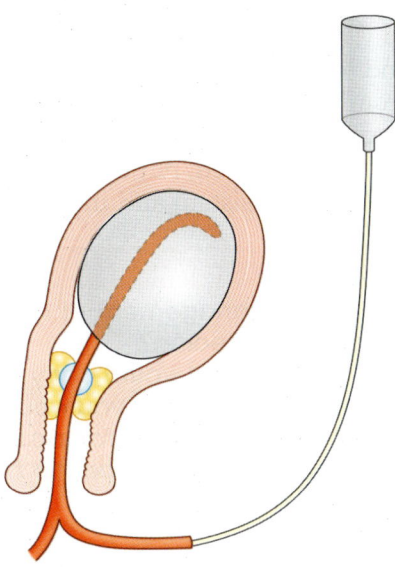

4.1 What is the next step in the management of atonic PPH after normal delivery, if balloon tamponade fails to control bleeding?

4.2 Draw a diagram to show how you would carry out this procedure.

4.3 Using your drawing explain in detail how you would carry out this procedure. *(Teaching and surgical skills module for postgraduate students, but undergraduates also can be questioned on the basic method).*

Answer 4.1

Perform a laparotomy under general anaesthesia and insert Hayman's vertical sutures (Hayman's modification of B-Lynch suture).

Answer 4.2

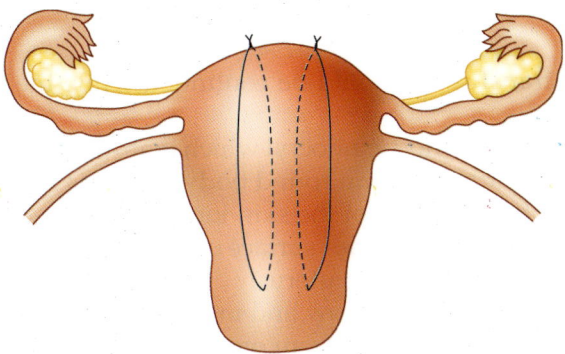

Answer 4.3

- Adequate blood transfusion should be continued while the procedure is being carried out. Informed consent should be obtained. Bladder should be catheterized.
- Perform a laparotomy. General anaesthesia is used if the patient is not already under epidural anaesthesia.
- Open the peritoneum of the lower uterine segment and reflect the bladder away from the operating field. The uterus should be taken out of the skin incision
- Use a straight needle and no. 1 monocryl which is absorbed in 21 days.
- The suture is passed from anterior to posterior approximately 3 cm below the site of a lower segment caesarean section incision.
- At least 2 sutures should be performed, but up to 5 sutures can be inserted.
- The uterus is compressed by an assistant and the sutures are tied at the fundus.

QUESTION 5

5.1 **What is the next step in the management of PPH at caesarean section if oxytocic drugs fail to control bleeding?**

5.2 **Draw a diagram's to show how you would carry out this procedure.**

5.3 **Using your drawings explain in detail how you would carry out this procedure (Teaching and surgical skills module for postgraduate students, but undergraduates also can be questioned on the basic method).**

Answer 5.1

Insert a B-Lynch suture.

Answer 5.2

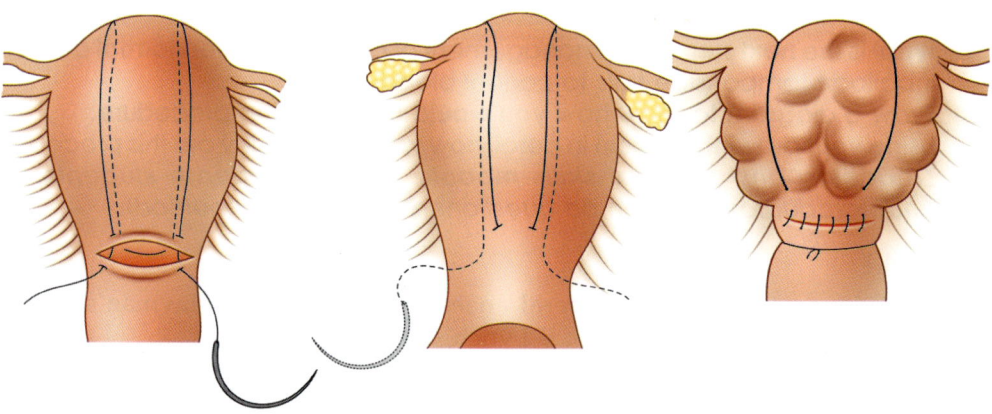

Answer 5.3

- Adequate blood transfusion should be continued while the procedure is being carried out.
- The best suture material is no.1 monocryl which is absorbed in 21 days. The length should be 90 cm. A curved 17 mm round body needle is ideal.
- The uterus should be taken out of the skin incision.
- The first drawing shows the anterior surface of the uterus and the second drawing shows the posterior surface of the uterus.
- The first stitch is inserted 3 cm below and medial to the lateral edge of the lower flap of the lower segment incision from outside to inside.

- The end of the thread is held with an artery forceps.
- The needle is next guided through the uterine cavity and is inserted from inside to outside at a point 3 cm above the upper edge of the uterine incision.
- The thread is passed over the fundus to the posterior surface of the uterus.
- The needle is next inserted at the level of the uterosacral ligaments from outside into the cavity.
- The needle is again passed out into the posterior surface roughly at the opposite lateral margin of the uterine incision.
- The thread is passed over the fundus to the anterior surface.
- The needle is passed from outside to inside at a point 3 cm above the anterior flap of the uterine scar at the lateral margin of the uterine incision.
- Finally the needle is passed from inside to outside at a point 3 cm below the lower flap.
- The threads which are looped over the fundus are placed about 4 cm from the lateral borders of the uterus
- The both ends of the thread are held together tautly with an artery forceps.
- The third diagram shows the anterior surface of the uterus
- The uterus is compressed by an assistant.
- The ends of the B-Lynch suture are tied together tightly to compress the uterus.
- The uterine incision is closed
- The patient should be observed for bleeding.
- This procedure can be combined with internal iliac artery ligation.
- The abdomen is closed once the bleeding has stopped.

Reference for Questions 4 and 5: Munro Kerr's Operative Obstetrics, 12th edition, pages 257–259.

QUESTION 6

6.1 **What are the next steps before resorting to hysterectomy if bleeding is not controlled after inserting a B-Lynch suture?**

6.2 **Describe how you would perform internal iliac artery ligation to control postpartum haemorrhage *(teaching and surgical skills module for postgraduate students, but undergraduates also can be questioned on the basic method).***

6.3 **Draw a diagram to show the relationship of the vein and the ureter to the artery.**

Answer 6.1

- Bilateral uterine artery ligation
- Bilateral internal iliac artery ligation

Answer 6.2

- Adequate blood transfusion should be continued while the procedure is being carried out.
- The uterus should be lifted out of the abdominal incision.
- Clamp and divide the round ligament at the midpoint.
- Enter the retroperitoneal space by lifting and snipping the peritoneum of the posterior leaf of the broad ligament at the level of the infundibulo-pelvic ligament.

- The retroperitoneal space can be bluntly dissected using a moist gauze swab placed on a long artery forceps.
- The bifurcation of the common iliac artery, the internal iliac artery and the external iliac artery can be seen and the arterial pulsations can be palpated.
- The ureter can be seen crossing the bifurcation of the common iliac artery. It can be identified as a cord like structure with peristalsis.
- Identify the ureter and gently push it further medially.
- The internal iliac artery is the more medial vessel seen between the external iliac artery and the ureter. It can be differentiated from the vein by its colour and the pulsations.
- Identify the internal iliac artery. It could be gently lifted with a babcock forceps.
- It is ligated 3–4 cm away from the bifurcation.
- A right angled clamp is passed under the artery from lateral to medial to avoid damage to the adjacent veins which is the greatest danger of this procedure.
- The artery is ligated using a double strand of absorbable suture material which is fed into the right angled clamp.
- Repeat the procedure on the opposite side.
- The dorsalis pedis pulse should be felt and saturation should be checked with a pulse oxymeter.
- Bleeding should subside before the abdomen is closed after placing a drain.
- The woman should be closely monitored in an ICU.

Answer 6.3

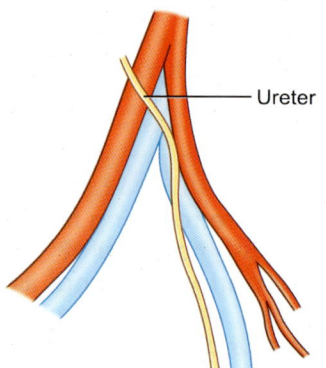

Ureter

Reference for Question 6: Munro Kerr's Operative Obstetrics, 12th edition, pages 263–264.

QUESTION 7

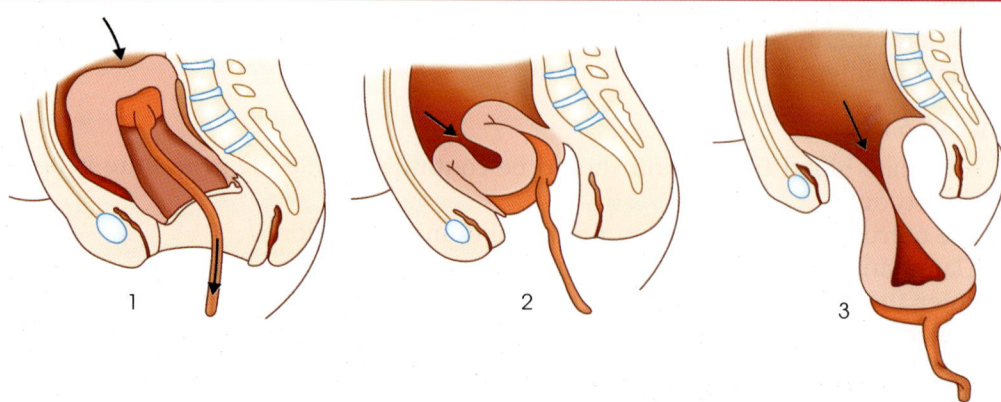

1   2   3

7.1 Name the condition which has occurred in each of these diagrams.
7.2 Mention 2 causes of death in a woman with this condition.
7.3 Mention 3 predisposing factors.
7.4 What precautions should you take to prevent its occurrence?

Answer 7.1

The drawings show the 3 stages of uterine inversion.
1. Dimpling of the fundus
2. Partial inversion of the uterus
3. Complete inversion of the uterus

Answer 7.2

- Neurogenic shock
- Postpartum haemorrhage

Answer 7.3

- Mismanagement of the third stage
  - Applying traction on the cord before the placenta is separated and the uterus is well contracted.
  - Failure to apply the technique of controlled cord traction to deliver the placenta.
  - Failure to give oxytocin with the delivery of the anterior shoulder
- Presence of a morbidly adherent placenta.
- Presence of an abnormally short umbilical cord.
- Manual removal of the placenta
  - The fundus can invert if the placenta is delivered through the cervix, while still adherent at the fundus
- Increase in intra-abdominal pressure due to coughing or vomiting while the uterus is relaxed.

Answer 7.4

- Give 5 units of oxytocin with the delivery of the anterior shoulder.
- Wait for signs of placental separation and uterine contraction before attempting to deliver the placenta.
- Apply gentle traction on the cord while pushing the uterus up with the ulnar border of the left hand placed above the symphysis pubis-controlled cord traction. The procedure should not be continued if the placenta is not delivered easily.

QUESTION 8

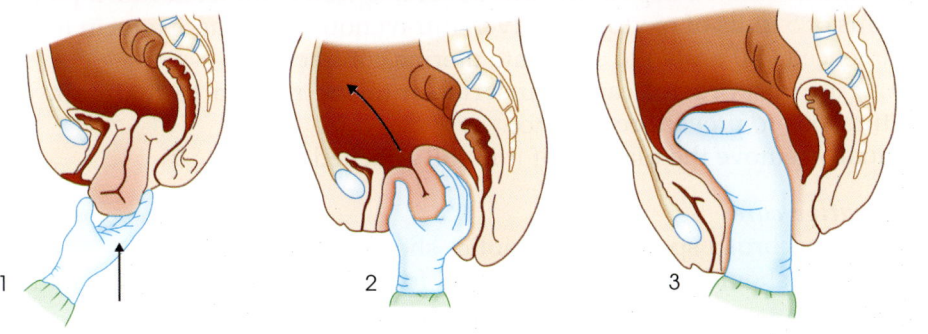

8.1   Name this procedure.
8.2   Where is it performed?
8.3   Mention 2 prerequisites for this procedure.
8.4   Describe in detail how you would perform this procedure? (*Teaching and surgical skills module for postgraduate students, but undergraduates also can be questioned on the basic method.*)
8.5   What is the next step in the management if this procedure is not successful?

Answer 8.1

Manual replacement of an uterine inversion.

Answer 8.2

- It can be done in the labour ward soon after the inversion has occurred.
- If there is a delay, it has to be done under anaesthesia in the operating theatre.

Answer 8.3

- It should be performed soon after occurrence of an uterine inversion.
- Oedema of the tissues should be minimal.

Answer 8.4

- Call for help.
- Informed verbal consent should be obtained quickly.
- Manual reduction should be performed as soon as possible to minimize oedema, venous congestion and contraction of the uterus.
- It can be performed in the labour ward, only immediately after an inversion occurs. Within a few minutes oedema, venous congestion and contraction of the uterus makes the procedure impossible and painful.
- The procedure should be performed only if the operator is present in the labour ward at the time the inversion occurs.
- Instruct an assistant to insert two 14 gauge cannulae and commence a rapid infusion of crystalloids. Give oxygen by face mask.
- The placenta should not be removed if it is still attached.
- The procedure is facilitated by giving intravenous ritodrine or glyceryl trinitrate if available in the labour ward.
- The fundus is held in the cupped palm (first picture).
- The uterus is inserted into the vagina and squeezed through the cervix using the fingers and the thumb. Fundus should be pushed in last (second picture).
- The left hand is placed on the abdomen to feel the uterine fundus.
- The hand should be kept in the uterus till it is well contracted (third picture).
- A bolus of 5 units of oxytocin is given intravenously and an oxytocin infusion is commenced (30 units) to stimulate uterine contractions.
- 800 µg of misoprostol can be inserted into the rectum to maintain uterine contractions to prevent recurrence.
- Manually remove the placenta if it is still attached.

Postoperative care
- Intravenous broad spectrum antibiotics should be commenced
- The patient should be closely monitored for vital signs and bleeding in the ICU.

- The procedure should be carefully documented,
- The patient should be debriefed the next day.

Answer 8.5

Attempt manual replacement under general anaesthesia and if it fails, perform O' Sullivan hydrostatic method of replacing an uterine inversion.

QUESTION 9

Describe the steps of O' Sullivan hydrostatic method of replacing an uterine inversion. (Teaching and surgical skills module for postgraduate students, but undergraduates also can be questioned on the basic method.)

Answer

- It is performed under general anaesthesia preferably using halothane or isoflurane.
- Insert two 14 gauge cannulae and commence a rapid infusion of crystalloids.
- Five pints of blood should be cross matched.
- The placenta should not be removed if it is still attached. Lacerations of the vagina and the cervix   should be excluded.
- The vulva should be cleaned with an antiseptic solution and sterile towels should be placed.
- The bladder should be emptied.
- The vagina is filled with 3–5 liters of warm saline at 37°C using intravenous tubing. Saline bottles are placed at a height to maintain pressure. Pressure is applied on the saline bags.
- The tube is guided into the posterior fornix with one hand which also cups the fundus and exerts pressure.
- When the vagina is filled with normal saline and the fornices are distended, the cervical ring is stretched allowing replacement of the uterine fundus.
- Saline is prevented from leaking out by the wrist of the vaginal hand and by holding the labia together by an assistant.
- The tubing can be connected to a plastic vacuum extractor cup or an anaesthetist mask which can be inserted into the vagina for better sealing.
- Tocolysis may be necessary if difficulty is encountered.
- The left hand is placed on the abdomen to feel the uterine fundus.
- Once the uterus is replaced keep the clenched fist in the uterus until it is contracted.
- Give an intravenous bolus of 5 units of oxytocin and commence an oxytocin infusion after the uterus is replaced. Insert 800 μg of misoprostol into the rectum.
- Manually remove the placenta if it is still attached.
- Carry out postoperative care as in question 8.4

Reference for Questions 7–9: Munro Kerr's Operative Obstetrics, 12th edition, Chapter 22.

QUESTION 10

A woman develops bleeding soon after a vaginal delivery. Placenta and membranes were expelled soon after delivery and were found to be complete. The uterus remains well contracted.
10.1 What is the likely cause of bleeding?

10.2 List 5 predisposing factors.
10.3 List 4 steps in your immediate management.
10.4 What is your definitive management?

Answer 10.1

The bleeding is due to trauma to the genital tract

Answer 10.2

- Precipitate labour
- Unattended delivery
- Face to pubes delivery
- Delivery of a baby larger than 4 kg
- Instrumental delivery

Answer 10.3

- Insert two 14 gauge cannulae and commence intravenous crystalloids.
- Crossmatch 5 units of blood and commence blood transfusion..
- Keep the patient warm and give oxygen by face mask.
- Call for help and inform senior staff members.
- Estimate the blood loss by assessing the pulse rate, blood pressure and the colour of the patient. Perform a vaginal examination to assess the volume of clots and blood in the vagina.

Answer 10.4

The genital tract should be inspected for tears and any injuries should be sutured.

QUESTION 11

A woman develops bleeding soon after a vaginal delivery. Placenta and membranes were expelled soon after delivery and were found to be complete. The uterus remains well contracted. Genital tract trauma is suspected.

Describe how you would inspect the genital tract for injuries and carry out suturing of any injuries you have found.

Answer

- Preliminary preparation
  - This is carried out in the labour ward or the theatre.
  - The patient should be reassured and informed consent should be obtained.
  - If the woman is not under epidural analgesia a general anaesthetic can be given.
  - It could even be carried out under pethidine 75 mg administered intramuscularly, especially at a peripheral hospital.
  - Two Sim's speculums, 4 Green-Armytage forceps, a sponge holder, plenty of gauze swabs and towels, No. 00 and No. 0 polyglactin sutures, needle holder, catch forceps and a good light are necessary.
  - An assistant should be present.
  - Insert two intravenous cannulae and commence crystalloid infusion.
  - Crossmatch 5 units of blood and commence blood transfusion.
  - The patient is placed in the lithotomy position.

- The obstetrician should scrub and wear sterile gown and gloves.
- The vulva should be cleaned with antiseptic solution and sterile drapes should be placed.
- The bladder should be emptied if required.
- Inspecting the cervix for tears
    - A Sim's speculum is inserted into the vagina.
    - The blood is mopped by the assistant.
    - The anterior lip of the cervix is found and is held with a Green-Armytage forceps.
    - The posterior lip can be exposed by applying gentle traction on the forceps. A Green-Armytage forceps is applied on the posterior lip.
    - Gentle traction on both forceps will expose the two angles. Two pairs of Green-Armytage forceps are applied on the angles.
    - The cervix is inspected between these forceps.
    - If any significant tears are found they are sutured with No. 00 polyglactin using continuous sutures, commencing at the apex. Small tears which are not bleeding do not need suturing.
    - If there is oozing after the tear is sutured place a Green-Armytage forceps on the tear for a few hours.
- Inspecting the vaginal walls for tears
    - Next remove the forceps and gently push the cervix away from the operating field. It is useful to insert a gauze towel into the uppermost part of the vagina. This will also help to keep the operating field free of blood.
    - Next insert 2 Sim's speculums deep into the vagina to retract the vaginal walls. First inspect the lateral walls from each fornix downwards, by gently sliding down the speculums.
    - Inspect the anterior and posterior walls in the same manner.
    - Suture any tears using the same method as when suturing the vaginal mucosa in an episiotomy (*see* Chapter 3).
    - Reaching the apex of a deep tear.
        - o Apply the first suture at the highest accessible point.
        - o Keep the ends of the thread long.
        - o Apply gentle traction on the thread and insert the next stitch at a higher level.
        - o Repeat the procedure till the apex is reached.
- Inspecting the vestibule and the perineum
    - Next inspect the vestibule.
    - Any tears which are bleeding profusely are sutured with No. 000 polyglactin using a very fine needle. Small tears will stop bleeding when the patient's legs are crossed and a perineal pad is placed.
    - An urinary catheter should be inserted if the tear is close to the urethral orifice.
    - Next suture the muscles of the perineal body and the perineal skin in the same manner as in an episiotomy (*see* Chapter 3)
    - If third or fourth degree tears are present suturing should be carried out under general/epidural anaesthesia (*see* Chapter 3)

Reference for Questions 10 and 11: Munro Kerr's Operative Obstetrics, 12th edition, Chapter 23.

QUESTION 12

12.1 What is the indication to perform manual removal of the placenta?

12.2 Where is it performed in Sri Lanka?

12.3 What is the anaesthesia used for the procedure in Sri Lanka?

12.4 Describe the procedure in detail once the patient is anaesthetized, preliminaries are completed and placed in the lithotomy position and cleaned and draped.

12.5 What is your management if a plane of cleavage is not found between the placenta and the myometrium at the beginning of the procedure or during the procedure at a peripheral hospital.

Answer 12.1

Failure to deliver the placenta after 30 minutes of delivery of the baby when the active management of the third stage is practised.

Answer 12.2

It should be performed by medical officers in primary care hospitals as the time taken for transfer to a tertiary care unit can cause haemorrhage, shock and infection. It can be performed in the labour ward.

Answer 12.3

Intramuscular injection of 75 mg of pethidine.

Answer 12.4

- Catheterize the bladder.
- Intravenous broad spectrum antibiotics should be given.
- Clamp and cut the cord close to the introitus.
- Insert the right hand into the uterus. Follow the cord to reach the placental edge.
- Find a plane of cleavage between the placenta and the myometrium.
- Place the left hand on the fundus of the uterus and stabilize it.
- Commence separating the placenta along the plane of cleavage.
- Direct your fingers towards the lumen of the uterus.
- Once the entire placenta is separated bring it out.
- Inspect to see whether the placenta and membranes are complete.
- You may insert your hand once more to ensure that the cavity is empty.
- An intravenous bolus of 10 units of oxytocin should be given and an oxytocin infusion should be commenced. 800 µg of misoprostol should be inserted into the rectum.
- The genital tract should be inspected for tears and the episiotomy should be sutured.
- The patient should be kept in the labour room and should be monitored every 15 minutes for 2 hours according to the modified early warning chart, every 30 minutes for 2 hours and once a hour for 12 hours in the postnatal ward.
- Intravenous broad spectrum antibiotics should be given for 48 hours and oral antibiotics for 5 days.
- The woman should be discharged after 4 days with instructions to attend a tertiary care unit for the next delivery as recurrence could occur.

Answer 12.5

If a plane of cleavage is not found at the beginning, the possibility of a morbidly adherent placenta should be considered. The procedure should be abandoned in a peripheral hospital. The woman should be transferred to a tertiary care unit. An intravenous bolus of 10 units of oxytocin should be given and an oxytocin infusion should be commenced. Intravenous antibiotics should be given. The tertiary care unit should be informed and the patient should be accompanied by a nurse or a doctor.

If a plane of cleavage is not found during the procedure, remove as much as possible. An intravenous bolus of 10 units of oxytocin should be given and an oxytocin infusion should be commenced. Intravenous broad spectrum antibiotics should be commenced. The nearest tertiary care unit should be contacted and she should be transferred as soon as possible accompanied by a doctor. The risk of bleeding and collapse is greater than in the former situation. Placenta should be removed under general anaesthesia by a consultant obstetrician.

Episiotomy and Perineal Tears

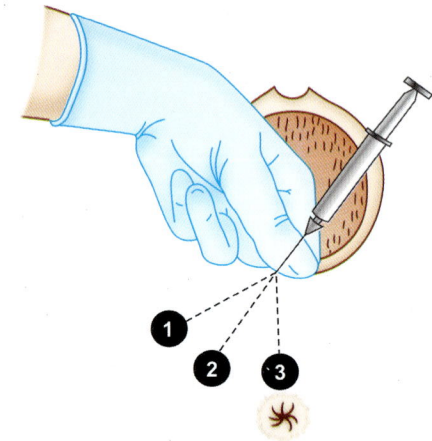

1.1 Which of the above episiotomy incisions do you wish to perform? What is the name of the episiotomy you have selected?

1.2 What are the (a) advantages and (b) disadvantages of your incision?

1.3 When should the incision be performed in: (a) Cephalic presentation, (b) Breech presentation

1.4 What is the ideal suture material?

1.5 What is the anaesthesia used to perform and suture an episiotomy?

1.6 List the instruments and the other material required (a) to perform an episiotomy (b) to suture an episiotomy.

Answer 1.1

2. Mediolateral episiotomy

Answer 1.2

a. If an extension occurs it will not damage the anal sphincter or the anal canal.

b. It cuts through the perineal muscles and gaping of the incision is more than in a midline episiotomy. It is more vascular than a midline episiotomy.

Answer 1.3
a. At the crowning of the head
b. When the breech has climbed up the perineum

Answer 1.4
No. 0 polyglycolic acid absorbable suture material is used.

Answer 1.5
If the patient is not under epidural analgesia perineal infiltration of 5–10 cc of 1% lignocaine is used to provide analgesia for this procedure.

Answer 1.6
a. • 1% lignocaine
   • A 10 cc syringe
   • A pair of curved scissors
b. • No 0 vicryl sutures
   • A round bodied and a cutting needle and 1% lignocaine
   • Catch forceps
   • Needle holder
   • Sponge holding forceps
   • Sterile gauze towels and gauze swabs
   • Perineal pad
   • Antiseptic solution

QUESTION 2
2.1 From where will you begin suturing an episiotomy?
2.2 What is the method you would adopt to reach the apex of a deep episiotomy/tear?
2.3 List the tissue planes you have to suture.
2.4 List 5 conditions where it is essential to perform an episiotomy

Answer 2.1
Suturing is commenced at a point just above the apex of the mucosal cut.

Answer 2.2
• Insert the first stitch at the highest accessible point.
• Leave the end of the thread long.
• The next stich can be applied at a higher point by applying traction on the thread.
• The apex of the tear can be reached by applying several sutures in this manner.

Answer 2.3
The tissue planes which are sutured include:
• The vaginal mucosa
• The perineal muscles
• The perineal skin

Answer 2.4

It is essential to perform an episiotomy during delivery of a:
- Twin pregnancy
- Breech presentation
- Occipito-posterior position
- Large baby
- Woman with precipitate labour
- Primipara

  It is also performed during instrumental deliveries.

QUESTION 3

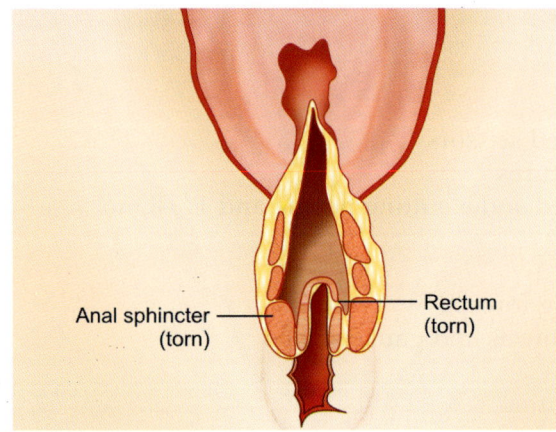

3.1 Identify the above injury. Give reasons for your diagnosis.
3.2 List 5 causes for the above injury.
3.3 What are the most appropriate anaesthetic agents which should be given to suture the above injury?
3.4 List 3 important aspects of immediate postoperative management.
3.5 How can you prevent obstetric perineal injuries?

Answer 3.1

Fourth degree perineal tear.

The vaginal mucosa, the perineal muscles, the external and internal anal sphincters and the anal mucosa are torn.

Answer 3.2

- Failure to support the perineum at the time of delivery.
- Instrumental delivery.
- Face to pubes delivery.
- Delivery of a baby larger than 4 kg.
- Precipitate/unattended delivery.

Answer 3.3

Epidural, spinal or general anaesthesia

Answer 3.4

- Pain should be relieved.
  - Usually paracetamol and NSAIDs such as diclofenac sodium suppositories are adequate. Intramuscular pethidine may be needed in the immediate postoperative period.
- Antibiotics should be given
  - A broad spectrum antibiotic combination such as co-amoxyclav and metronidazole is ideal. The first dose is given intravenously at the time of the repair. Oral antibiotics are given for 5–7 days.
- Stools are kept soft by administration of lactulose for 10 days.

Answer 3.5

- The perineum should be supported at the time of the delivery by an assistant.
- A timely episiotomy should be performed.
- The patient should be carefully assessed for instrumental deliveries and the proper technique should be practised.
- A caesarean section should be performed for large babies.

QUESTION 4

Describe in detail the method of repairing a third degree perineal tear. (Teaching and surgical skills module for postgraduate students, but undergraduates also can be questioned on the basic method.)

Answer

- Reassurance and explanation is essential. Informed consent should be obtained.
- It is performed under regional or general anaesthesia in the operating theatre.
- It should be performed by an appropriately trained senior consultant or by a trainee under supervision.
- The internal anal sphincter should be identified between the anal wall and the external anal sphincter. It is whitish in colour. It is held with Allis forceps and approximated with interrupted mattress sutures with overlapping.
- For repair of a full thickness external anal sphincter tear, either an overlapping or an end-to end approximation method can be used. For partial thickness (all 3a and some 3b) tears, an end-to-end technique should be used. 2 or 3 mattress sutures are used in the end-to-end method.
- Figure of eight sutures should be avoided as it may impair the blood supply. 2-0 polyglactin suture material is used. The suture length should be 90 cm.
- Surgical knots should be buried beneath the superficial perineal muscles to minimise the risk of knot and suture migration to the skin.
- The vaginal mucosa is sutured with continuous non-interlocking sutures from the apex of the tear up to the fourchette.
- The perineal muscles are approximated with continuous or interrupted sutures.
- The skin is closed with sub-cuticular or interrupted mattress sutures.
- A rectal examination should be performed after the repair to ensure that sutures have not been inadvertently inserted through the anorectal mucosa. If a suture is identified it should be removed.

- For immediate postoperative care refer answer to question 3.4.
- Debriefing should be carried out the next day.
- She should be reviewed in 6 weeks. Endoanal ultrasound scan should be performed by a trained person to determine the integrity of the anal sphincters.
- If fecal incontinence or anal pain is present she should be referred to an anorectal surgeon.
- The next delivery should be preferably by caesarean section.

QUESTION 5

5.1 Which techniques should be used to repair the anorectal mucosa in a fourth degree tear?
5.2 How do you debrief the woman?

Answer 5.1

It should be sutured in two layers with continuous sutures. 3–0 polyglactin suture material is ideal. It is better to get help from the surgical team.

Answer 5.2

- Debriefing is done 48–72 hours after the event.
- It is preferably carried out by the senior obstetrician.
- The partner should preferably be present.
- Explain regarding:
  - The birth.
  - The course of events and the reason for the complications.
  - Reasoning behind decisions made.
  - The operative procedure.
  - The postoperative course to date.
  - Postoperative care (*refer* answer to question 3.5).
  - Further treatment and special care.
  - The need for delivery by caesarean section during the next pregnancy
  - The possibility of developing difficulties in bowel control
- Examine the operation site/wound.
- Inquire regarding pain and bowel movements and offer relief.
- Allow the woman an opportunity to ask questions about the procedure and what to expect in the future.
- Determine the appropriate clinic follow up and arrange for appropriate referrals to the GP, local hospital, and dietician or to the anorectal surgeon if necessary.
- The interview and the referrals should be clearly documented.

QUESTION 6

6.1 Pick the instruments required to perform and suture an episiotomy
6.2 Describe in detail the method of performing an episiotomy.

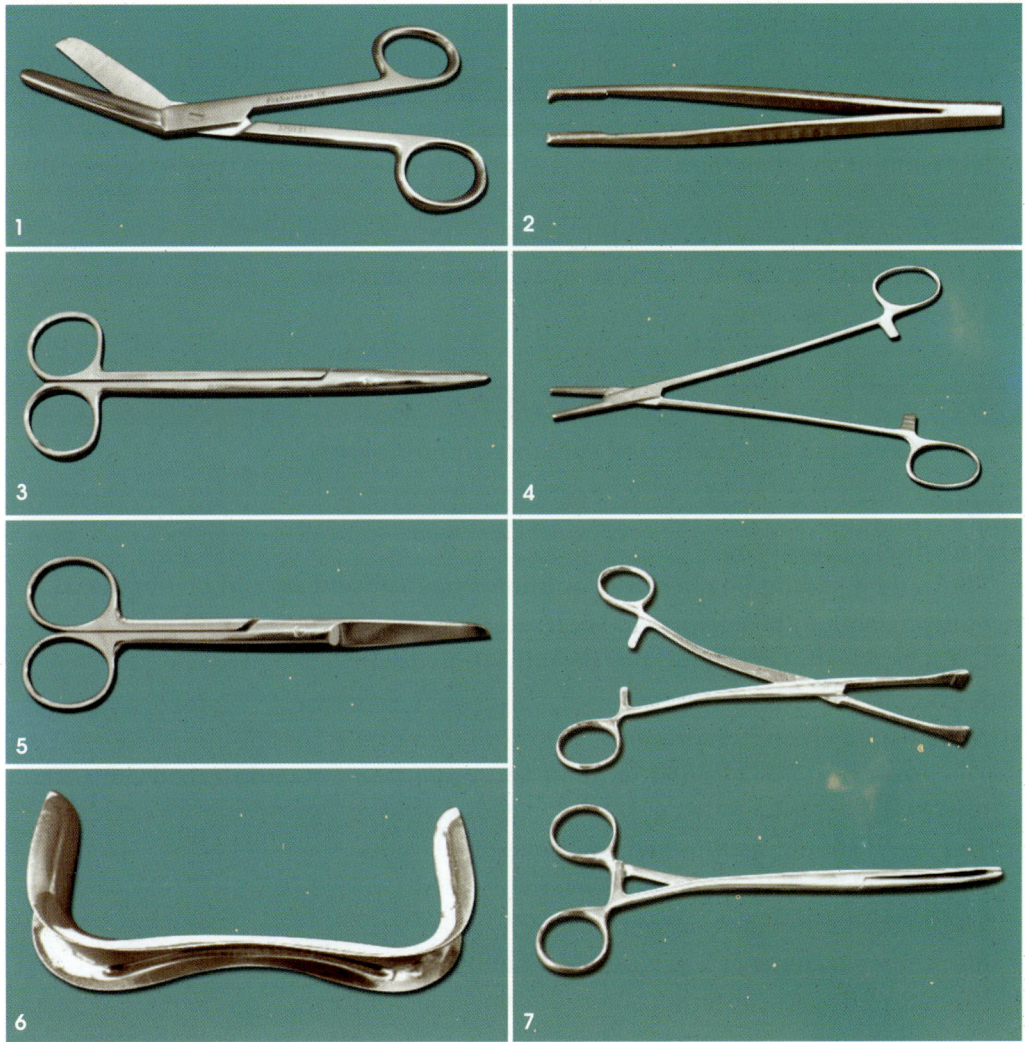

Answer 6.1

1, 2, 4, 5

Answer 6.2

- The patient should be reassured and informed consent should be obtained.
- When the head has descended to the pelvic floor place the woman in the dorsal position.
- Clean the perineum with an antiseptic solution.
- Infiltrate 5 cc of 1% lignocaine along the planned incision.
- The episiotomy is performed when the head is crowned or when the breech has climbed up the perineum.
- It is performed when the perineum is stretched at the height of a contraction.

- A medio-lateral episiotomy is performed.
- Two fingers of the left hand are inserted into the vagina between the fetus and the vaginal wall to prevent injury to the fetus. Special care should be taken to prevent genital injury in a breech presentation.
- It is better if an episiotomy scissor is available. However, any type of scissor may be used.
- The incision is commenced in the midline at the fourchette.
- It is extended for about 1 inch at an angle of 45 degrees.
- Observe for bleeding.

QUESTION 7

Describe in detail the method of suturing an episiotomy.

Answer

The method of suturing:
- The patient should be reassured and informed consent should be obtained.
- Suturing should be performed soon after the third stage is completed.
- Confirm that the perineum has been infiltrated with 1% lignocaine.
- A good light is necessary.
- An assistant should be present.
- The area should be cleaned with an antiseptic solution and draped with sterile towels.
- The blood should be mopped by an assistant.
- No. 0 polyglycolic acid suture material is used.
- The vaginal mucosa is sutured first.
- Suturing is commenced at a point just above the apex of the cut.
- It is sutured with continuous non-interlocking sutures.
- Only the edges of the mucosa are included. If thick bites are taken the vagina can be shortened.
- The suturing is continued up to the fourchette.
- The needle is passed through the skin at the edge of the fourchette into the muscle layer.
- The muscles of the perineal body are sutured with continuous non-interlocking sutures.
- If the cut is deep two layers of sutures may be needed for the perineal muscles.
- The needle is brought out at the inferior end of the incision just under the skin.
- The perineal skin is sutured with sub-cuticular sutures. Interrupted mattress sutures also can be used. A rectal examination should be performed after the repair to ensure that sutures have not been inadvertently inserted through the anorectal mucosa. If a suture is identified it should be removed.
- The area should be cleaned with an antiseptic solution.
- A perineal pad is placed.

QUESTION 8

How will you manage an infected episiotomy wound?

Answer

- A swab should be sent for culture and antibiotic sensitivity test.
- Broad spectrum antibiotics should be commenced and changed once the sensitivity test is available
- Mild infections can be treated with antibiotics and sitz baths in warm dilute salt solutions.
- If there is a swelling indicating the presence of underlying pus, the wound should be opened and irrigated daily with normal saline. Sitz baths should be carried out.
- Pain can be relieved with mild analgesics.
- Resuturing is done when the acute infection subsides and granulation tissue has formed.
- Resuturing is performed under regional/local analgesia. Careful debridement of the wound is done.
- Non-absorbable nylon sutures are used.

Reference for chapter 3: Munro Kerr's Operative Obstetrics, 12th edition, Chapter 23.

Malpresentations

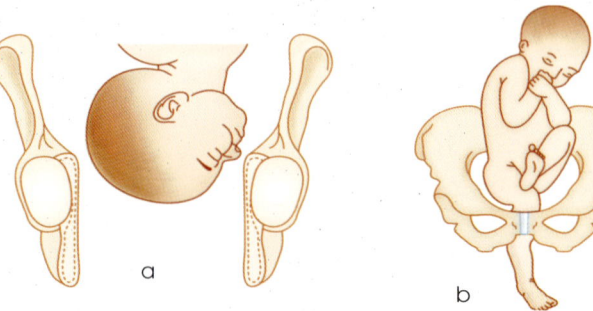

1   2   3   4

1.1 Name the above diameters of the fetal skull and the presentations and positions.

1.2 Name the presentations shown below. What is the mode of delivery in each of them?

a

b

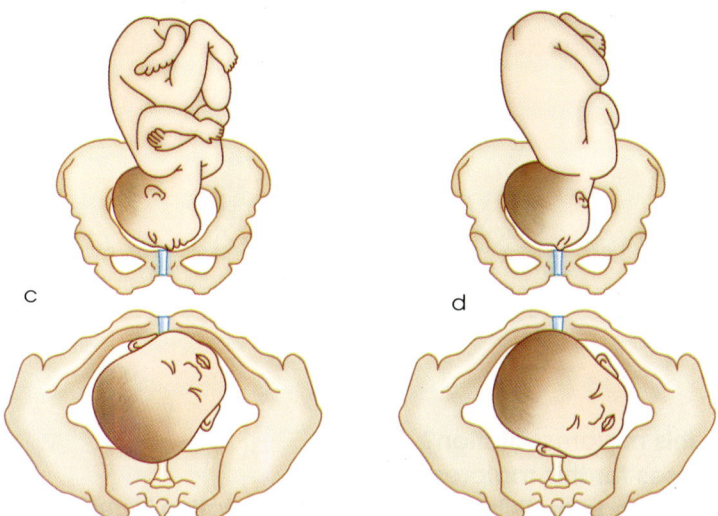

c   d

1.3 What is the best management option if there is prolonged first stage in: a, c and d?

1.4 What is the best management option if there is prolonged second stage in: a, c and d?

Answer 1.1

1. Suboccipito-bregmatic diameter—vertex presentation with occipito-anterior position
2. Occipito-frontal diameter—occipito-posterior position
3. Mento-vertical diameter—brow presentation
4. Submento-bregmatic diameter—mento-anterior face presentation

Answer 1.2

a. Brow presentation. Should be delivered by emergency caesarean section.
b. Footling breech presentation. Should be delivered by emergency caesarean section.
c. Mento-anterior face presentation. Can be delivered vaginally.
d. Mento-posterior face presentation. Should be delivered by emergency caesarean section.

Answer 1.3

a. Perform an emergency caesarean section.
c. Perform an amniotomy and commence an oxytocin infusion if the pelvis is adequate and there is no fetal distress.
d. Perform an emergency caesarean section.

Answer 1.4

a. Perform an emergency caesarean section.
c. Apply obstetric forceps if the head is at or below the ischial spines and the pelvis is adequate.
d. Perform an emergency caesarean section.

QUESTION 2

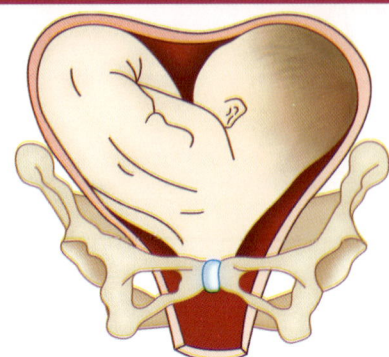

2.1   **What is this malpresentation?**
2.2   **List 3 causes for this malpresentation.**
2.3   **What is the mode of delivery if this malpresentation is detected in the second stage of labour and the fetus is dead?**
2.4   **What is the best management option if this malpresentation is detected at 40 weeks, before the onset of labour in a multiparous woman without any other complications?**
2.5   **What is the best management option if this malpresentation is detected at a cervical dilatation of 5 cm in a multiparous woman without any other complications?**
2.6   **What are the complications of this malpresentation?**

Answer 2.1

Transverse lie of the fetus with shoulder presentation.

Answer 2.2

- Placenta previa
- Lower segment fibroids
- Twin pregnancy
- Polyhydramnios
- Fetal abnormalities

Answer 2.3

Perform an emergency caesarean section.

Answer 2.4

Perform an external cephalic version or a stabilising induction at the onset of labour.

Answer 2.5

If the contractions are infrequent ECV can be performed in-between contractions or caesarean section may be a safer option.

Answer 2.6

- Pre-labour rupture of membranes
- Hand prolapse

- Cord prolapse
- Fetal death
- Obstructed labour
- Uterine rupture in multiparous women
- Sepsis

References for Questions 1 and 2
- *SBA Questions in Obstetrics 1st Edition, Chapter 5.*
- *Obstetrics by Ten Teachers,19th Edition, pages 95–101.*

QUESTION 3

3.1   What is meant by assisted breech delivery?

3.2   What is meant by breech extraction?

3.3   Give an indication for breech extraction.

3.4   A multiparous woman in the second stage of labour with a breech presentation, develops recurrent type two decelerations with a baseline fetal heart rate of 100 bpm. The breech is at the level of the ischial spines. What is the best management option? Give your reasons.

3.5   A multiparous woman is in the first stage of labour with a breech presentation. The cervical dilatation is 5 cm at 8 am and 7 cm at 1 pm. She is getting 2 contractions per 10 minutes. The estimated fetal weight is 2.8 kg and the pelvis is adequate. The membranes are intact. What is the best management option? Give your reasons.

3.6   A multiparous woman is in the first stage of labour with a breech presentation. The cervical dilatation is 5 cm. The foot is felt at the level of the internal os. The estimated fetal weight is 2.8 kg and the pelvis is adequate. The membranes are absent. The cord is not felt. What is the best management option? Give your reasons.

Answer 3.1

During assisted breech delivery the delivery is completed by the voluntary efforts of the patient. The operator will only assist. The principle of assisted breech delivery is masterly inactivity by the operator.

Answer 3.2

It is a procedure where the operator commences the delivery by bringing down one leg by inserting a hand into the uterus. The delivery is completed by traction applied by the operator and voluntary efforts of the mother.

Answer 3.3

Breech extraction is performed only in the case of fetal distress or any other emergency requiring quick delivery during the second stage, in the second of twins presenting by the breech.

Answer 3.4

Perform a lower segment caesarean section immediately. Breech extraction is contraindicated in a singleton pregnancy.

Answer 3.5

Perform a lower segment caesarean section immediately. Augmentation with oxytocin is contraindicated as undiagnosed CPD can result in head entrapment.

Answer 3.6

Perform a lower segment caesarean section immediately. Vaginal delivery is not allowed for footling breech presentation because of the risk of cord prolapse and head entrapment.

QUESTION 4

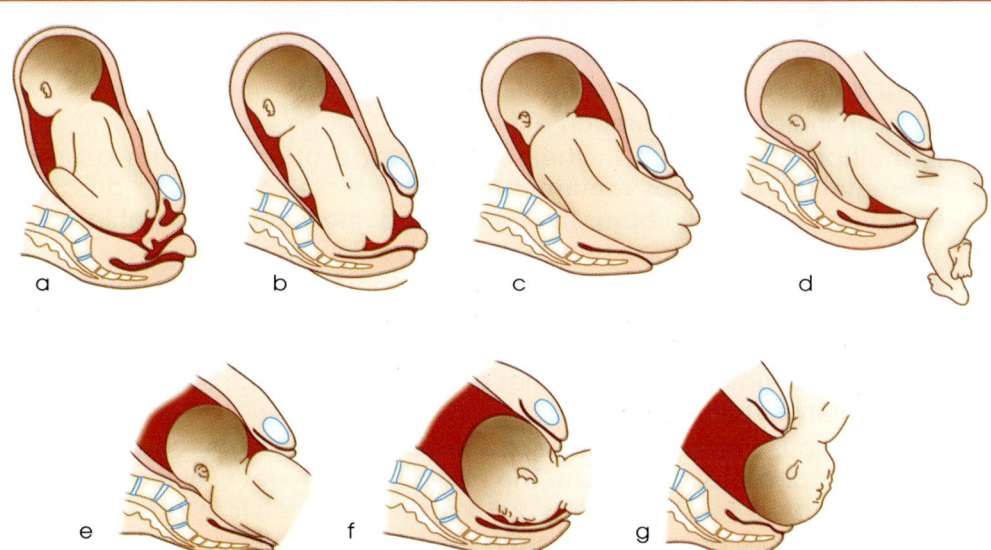

a   b   c   d

e   f   g

The stages of vaginal breech delivery are given above. State the procedures which should be carried out by the operator at each stage.

Answer

a. • Place the patient in the lateral position.
   • Prevent the patient from bearing down.
b. • Place the patient in the lithotomy position.
   • Encourage the patient to bear down.
c. • Perform an episiotomy.
   • Allow the buttocks to deliver.
   • Perform Pinard's manoeuver if the legs are extended.
d. • The buttocks should be anterior.
   • Wrap the baby in a sterile towel.
   • Hold the baby by the pelvis.
   • Pull down a loop of the cord.
e. • Commence delivery of the shoulders.
   • Perform Loveset's manoeuver if the arms are extended.
   • Ease out the arms with the fingers if they are flexed.

f. • Allow the baby to hang down so that the weight of the baby will facilitate the descent of the head.
  • Commence delivery of the head when the inferior hair line is seen.

g. • Complete the delivery of the head by the Burns Marshall manoeuvre.

QUESTION 5

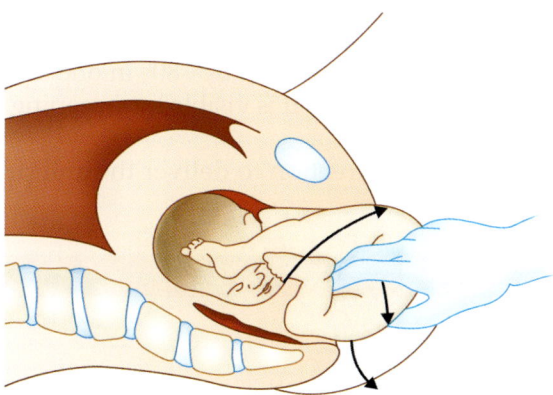

5.1 **What is this manoeuvre?**
5.2 **What is the indication for it?**

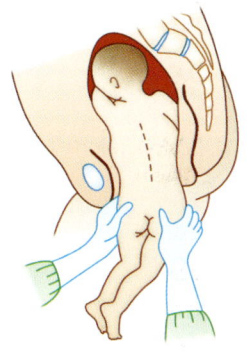 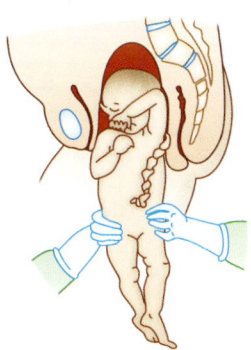 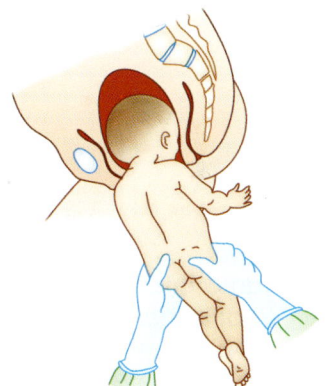

5.3 **Name this manoeuvre.**
5.4 **What is the indication to perform it?**
5.5 **Briefly describe the procedure.**

Answer 5.1
Pinard's manoeuvre

Answer 5.2
It is performed to deliver extended legs.

Answer 5.3
Loveset's technique.

Answer 5.4

It is performed to deliver extended arms.

Answer 5.5

- Delivery of the arms is commenced when the inferior angle of the scapula is visible.
- Loveset's technique is performed if the arms are extended.
- The trunk is held by the pelvis and is gently drawn down and the body is lifted to cause upward and lateral flexion.
- The baby is held by the pelvis and rotated by 180° in one direction to deliver the posterior arm. Ease out the arm when it is visible by sweeping the humerus across the fetal chest.
- Rotate by 180° in the opposite direction to deliver the anterior arm. Ease out the arm when it is visible.

QUESTION 6

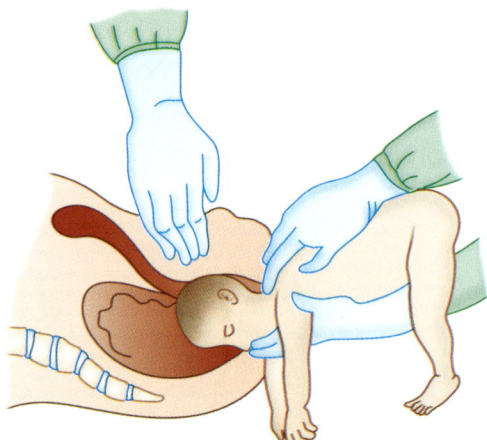

6.1 Name this manoeuvre.
6.2 What is the indication for it?

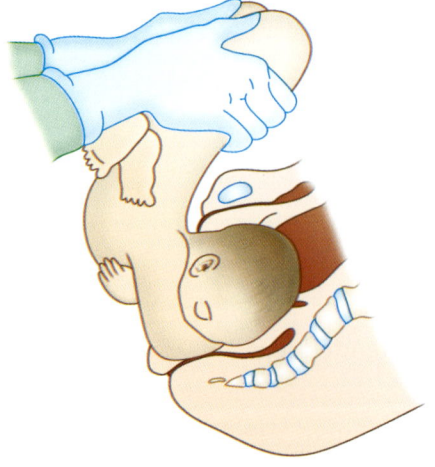

6.3   Name this manoeuvre. What is the indication for it?
6.4   What are the disadvantages of this method?
6.5   State another method to deliver the after-coming head.
6.6   What are the methods which are recommended to deliver the after-coming head safely?

Answer 6.1

Mauriceau-Smellie-Veit manoeuvre

Answer 6.2

It is performed to deliver the head at breech delivery, if the delivery is occurring rapidly and there is no time to apply forceps or in the absence of assistance to apply forceps.

Answer 6.3

Burns Marshall technique to deliver the after-coming head.

Answer 6.4

- It can cause injuries to the cervical spine.
- The delivery of the head cannot be well controlled. Therefore sudden decompression at the time of delivery can cause tentorial tears

Answer 6.5

Application of obstetric forceps.

Answer 6.6

- Application of obstetric forceps.
- Mauriceau-Smellie-Veit manoeuvre

QUESTION 7

Describe in detail how you would perform an assisted breech delivery. (Teaching and surgical skills module for postgraduates, but undergraduates should know the basic method.)

Answer

- The delivery should be carried out by a senior experienced member of the medical staff. An assistant should be present.
- The paediatrician should be present.
- Confirm full dilatation of the cervix and assess the station of the breech by performing a vaginal examination.
- Allow the breech to descend and prevent the patient from pushing during the passive phase of the second stage.
- Once the breech has descended and the woman gets bearing down sensation place her in the lithotomy position at the edge of the bed.
- Clean and drape the patient. Empty the bladder, if necessary.
- The patient is advised to push with the contractions.
- The principle of 'masterly inactivity' is followed. The entire effort is by the mother and the operator will only assist.

- When the breech is distending the introitus and the anterior buttock and the anus are seen, a wide medio-lateral episiotomy is given. This should be done at the height of a contraction taking care not to damage the fetal genitalia.
- Legs will deliver spontaneously if they are flexed.
- If legs are extended Pinard's manoeuvre is done. Three fingers are placed on the thigh of the anterolateral leg, above the knee to slightly abduct and flex the hip followed by flexion of the knee. The procedure is repeated on the other side.
- Buttocks should always be anterior. Otherwise gentle rotation is carried out.
- The baby is wrapped in a sterile towel and gently held by the pelvis, but traction should not be applied.
- A loop of the cord is pulled down to ensure that it is not too short and to prevent cord compression.
- Delivery of the arms is commenced when the inferior angle of the scapula is seen.
- If the arms are flexed they can be eased out.
- Loveset's manoeuvre is used to deliver extended arms.
  - The trunk is held by the pelvis and is gently drawn down and the body is lifted to cause upward and lateral flexion.
  - The baby is held by the pelvis and rotated by 180° in one direction to deliver the posterior arm. Ease out the arm when it is visible by sweeping the humerus across the fetal chest.
  - Rotate by 180° in the opposite direction to deliver the anterior arm. Ease out the arm when it is visible.
- The baby is allowed to hang down from the edge of the bed and the mother is encouraged to push.
- Delivery of the head is commenced when the hairline is seen.
- The head is preferably delivered with forceps.
  - Although Piper forceps were designed for this purpose Simpson's forceps or Kielland's forceps can be used.
  - The operator should ideally kneel to see under the trunk.
  - An assistant should hold the infant's body and arms in a horizontal plane.
  - The forceps are assembled and applied in the normal way (*refer* to Chapter 6).
  - During the initial descent the body of the fetus should be in the horizontal plane.
  - Once the mouth and chin are visible the body of the fetus and the forceps are rotated upwards.
- Mauriceau-Smellie-Veit manoeuvre is used to deliver the head if the delivery is occurring rapidly and there is no time to apply forceps or in the absence of an assistant to apply forceps.
  - The operator's forearm is placed under the baby with a foot placed on either side.
  - The forefinger and the middle finger are placed on the maxilla beside the nose and the head is gently flexed.
  - Flexion may be attempted at the lower jaw if the maxilla is out of reach, but care must be taken as dislocation can occur.
  - The other hand is placed on the fetal back with the middle finger pushing up the occiput to cause flexion.

- The other fingers are placed on the fetal shoulders on either side.
- This manoeuvre will splint and protect the cervical spine while promoting flexion.
- Gentle traction is applied in a downward and backward direction to complete the delivery.
- This manoeuvre is used to control and slow down the delivery.
- If traction is required it is safer to use forceps.
- A paediatrician should be present and all arrangements should be made to resuscitate the baby. The baby should be examined for neural, skeletal and internal injuries.
- The third stage is managed actively. 5 units of oxytocin is given after the delivery of the baby. Controlled cord traction is applied to deliver the placenta.
- The genital tract is inspected for tears. The episiotomy is sutured.

References for Questions 3 to 7:
- *Munro Kerr's Operative Obstetrics, 12th edition, Chapter 16*
- *SBA Questions in Obstetrics 1st Edition, Chapter 5*
- *The management of breech presentation, RCOG Green—top Guideline 20b (Nov. 2014)*

QUESTION 8

A 28-year-old primipara attends the antenatal clinic at a period of amenorrhoea of 36 weeks. She is found to have a single fetus in breech presentation.
8.1 What is the first step in the management?
8.2 If she has no other complications what is the next step in the management?
8.3 What is the period of amenorrhoea at which an ECV can be performed?
8.4 Describe how you would teach a registrar to perform an ECV. (Teaching and surgical skills module for postgraduates, but undergraduates should know the basic method).

Answer 8.1

Perform an USS to:
- Confirm the malpresentation
- Confirm dates
- Localize the placenta
- Assess the liquor volume
- Exclude twins
- Exclude fetal abnormalities
- Exclude uterine abnormalities

Answer 8.2

Perform an ECV

Answer 8.3

ECV can be performed after 36 weeks in a primipara and after 37 weeks in a multipara. There is no upper limit of the POA and the procedure can be performed till the onset of labour.

Answer 8.4

- The procedure is explained to the patient and informed consent is obtained.
- She should avoid heavy meals for six hours, but light snacks can be taken till 2 hours before the procedure.
- It is better to admit the patient before performing ECV.
- An USS is performed to exclude the complications (such as placenta previa, poly and oligohydramnios, twins, fetal abnormalities and uterine abnormalities) and to determine the type of breech.
- Perform a CTG for 20 minutes.
- The procedure should be performed without causing pain. This will prevent complications.
- The patient should be told that she will feel the pressure, but there should be no pain.
- Ultrasound jelly should be removed from the abdomen and talcum powder should be sprinkled.
- It is usually performed without tocolysis or anaesthesia. Tocolysis with beta adrenergic drugs are used only in cases which fail due to increased uterine tone.
- The first step is to dislodge and elevate the breech from the pelvis. This requires sustained pressure from both hands.
- While the right hand is elevating the breech the left hand should grasp the head from behind and begin to turn it in the direction the baby is facing. Sustained pressure is required for success, but undue force should not be exerted.
- With the hands working together pressure is applied on both fetal poles.
- Once the version is complete a cardiotocograph is performed for 30 minutes.
- An USS is performed to confirm the presentation.
- A Kleihauer test should be performed in rhesus negative women and the appropriate dose of anti-D should be given.
- A CTG is performed after 2 hours and the woman is discharged if the fetal heart rate is normal and she has no pain, dribbling or bleeding.

Reference for Question 8: *External cephalic version and reducing the incidence of breech presentation, RCOG Green-top Guideline 20a (1/12/2006).*

QUESTION 9

9.1   **What are the causes of cervical entrapment of the head during breech delivery?**
9.2   **How will you manage cervical entrapment?**
9.3   **What precautions will you take to prevent this complication?**

Answer 9.1

Entrapment of the head is caused by:
- Attempting delivery before confirming that the cervix is fully dilated..
- Prematurity because the small body can descend through a partly dilated cervix.
- Footling breech. The foot can descend to the pelvic floor before full dilatation of the cervix and cause bearing down sensation, resulting in partial descent and entrapment of the head.

Answer 9.2

- If it is detected before the head has descended enough to compress the umbilical cord, delivery should be delayed for a few minutes, to allow full dilatation, as dilatation progresses rapidly at this stage.

- If the head is enclosed by the cervix, cord compression will occur and the delivery should be expedited by incising the cervix at 4 and 7 o'clock positions with a pair of long scissors. Care should be taken to prevent extension of the incision as the uterine vessels can be damaged.

Answer 9.3

- The patient should be advised not to bear down till full dilatation is confirmed and the breech has descended.
- It is safer to perform a caesarean section for premature breeches.
- Footling breech presentation should be detected by performing a vaginal examination during early labour. Emergency caesarean section is mandatory for footling breech presentation.

Reference for Question 9: Munro Kerr's Operative Obstetrics, 12th edition, Chapter 16, pages 165–166.

QUESTION 10

Describe the method of diagnosing the following malpresentations.
10.1 Brow presentation
10.2 Mento-anterior face presentation
10.3 Mento-posterior face presentation

Answer 10.1

- Brow presentation appears as a cephalic presentation with a non-engaged head before the onset of labour. It can be suspected if the head is not engaged at the onset of labour.
- It is diagnosed by vaginal examination during early labour when the cervix is dilated to about 4–5 cm.
- The anterior fontanelle, frontal suture, frontal bones, forehead supraorbital ridges and the bridge of the nose can be palpated. The diagnosis is confirmed by palpation of the supraorbital ridges and the bridge of the nose.

Answer 10.2

- Face presentation appears as a cephalic presentation before the onset of labour.
- It is diagnosed by vaginal examination when the cervix is dilated to about 4–5 cm. A soft presenting part with orbital ridges, mouth, nose and malar bones is felt. It can be differentiated from a breech, by palpating the nose and the mouth with gum margins. The mouth can be differentiated from the anus by the presence of gum margins. Face presentation has a triangular configuration of the mouth to the malar eminences compared to breech presentation where the anus and the ischial tuberosities are in one line.
- The chin will be anterior in a mento-anterior face presentation.

Answer 10.3

If the chin is felt posteriorly with the above physical signs a mento-posterior face presentation is diagnosed.

References for Question 10:
- *SBA Questions in obstetrics, Chapter 5*
- *Obstetrics by Ten Teachers, 19th Edition, Chapter 14, pages 209–210.*

Occipito-Posterior Position

1.1   What is this fetal position?

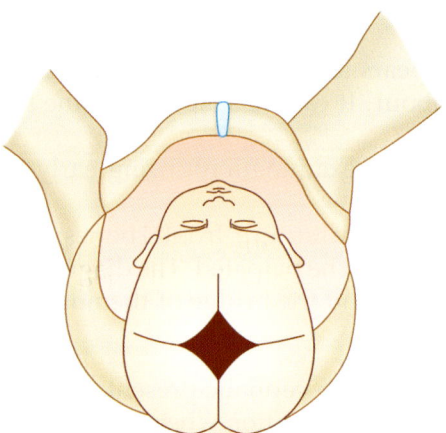

1.2   How do you diagnose this abnormality?
1.3   What is the presenting diameter?
1.4   What is the outcome of labour in a woman with this abnormality?

Answer 1.1

Occipito-posterior position

Answer 1.2

Consider occipito-posterior position, if the following physical signs are present.
- Non-engaged fetal head at term.
- Flattening of the abdomen below the umbilicus.
- The fetal back will be felt in the mother's flank and the limbs in the midline.
- Fetal heart sounds will be heard in the midline and in the flank

However, it can be confirmed only by performing a vaginal examination after onset of labour, when the cervix is dilated to 4–5 cm. In an occipitoposterior position the anterior fontanelle will be felt.

Answer 1.3

Occipito-frontal diameter measuring 11.5 cm.

Answer 1.4

- Progress will be slow.
- If the pelvis is adequate and good contractions are provided, rotation to the occipitoanterior position will occur, resulting in normal vaginal delivery.
- In an anthropoid pelvis with a large anteroposterior diameter, delivery can occur in the occipitoposterior position.
- Labour can become obstructed at the brim or in the midcavity in an android pelvis with narrow diameters.
- Delay can occur in the second stage, due to persistence of the occipitoposterior position or partial rotation to the transverse position especially in an android pelvis. If the spines are prominent arrest can occur (deep transverse arrest).

QUESTION 2

Name the following pelvic types. What is the outcome of labour in a woman with an occipitoposterior position in each of these pelvic types?

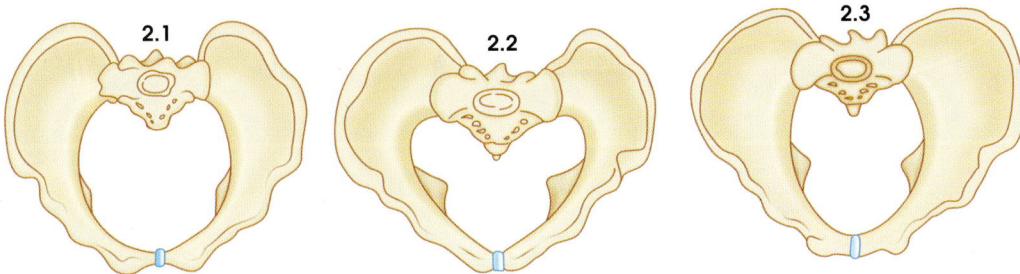

Answer 2.1

- Gynaecoid pelvis.
- The fetal head will undergo rotation to the occipitoanterior position and normal vaginal delivery will occur. Augmentation with oxytocin may be necessary if labour is slow, as good uterine contractions are required for rotation to occur.

Answer 2.2

- Android pelvis.
- Obstruction can occur at the brim or in the mid-cavity. Deep transverse arrest can occur at the level of the ischial spines during the second stage as the spines are prominent.

Answer 2.3

- Anthropoid pelvis.
- Delivery can occur in the occipitoposterior position, as it has a large antero-posterior diameter.

QUESTION 3

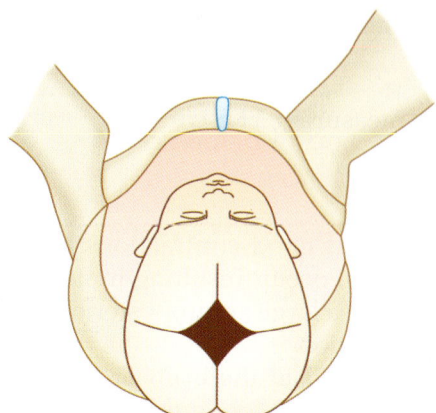

3.1 What are the methods available to manage prolonged first stage of labour, in a woman with the above abnormality?

3.2 Which of the following instruments can be used to complete the delivery, if the malposition persists, causing delay in the second stage?

3.3 State 4 criteria which should be satisfied to apply these instruments.

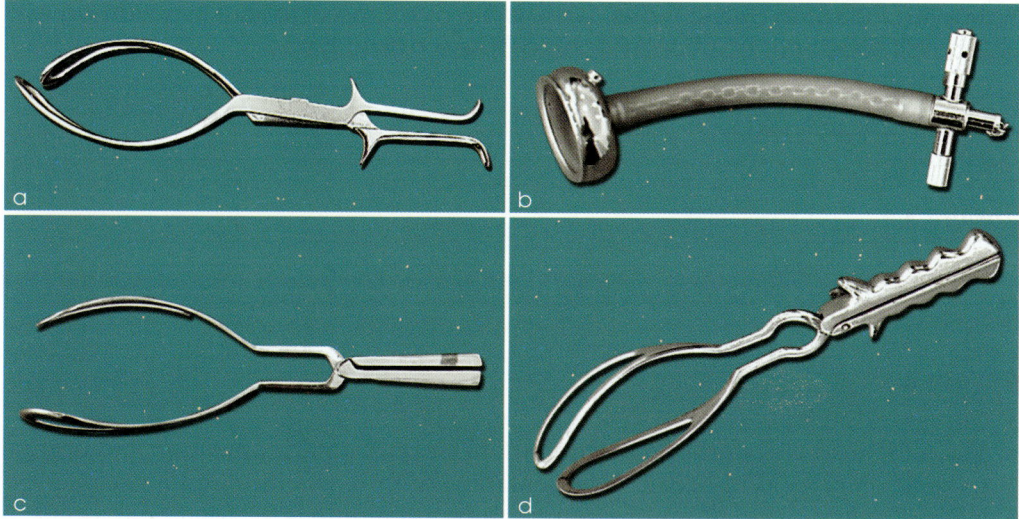

Answer 3.1

If labour is prolonged only due to the malposition and inadequate contractions in the absence of a scarred uterus, cephalopelvic disproportion (CPD) or fetal distress, labour can be augmented with amniotomy followed by an oxytocin infusion. Adequate pain relief should be provided with epidural analgesia.

Continuous fetal heart rate monitoring should be carried out. Progress should be reviewed after 2 hours. A caesarean section should be performed if CPD is suspected.

Answer 3.2

a and b

Answer 3.3

- The pelvis should be adequate.
- Cervix should be fully dilated.
- The head should be at or below the level of the ischial spines.
- The patient should be suitably anaesthetized. Vacuum extraction can be performed under pudendal block, while epidural or spinal analgesia is required for application of Kielland's forceps.

QUESTION 4

4.1 What is this abnormality?

4.2 What is the cause for its occurrence?

4.3 In which pelvic type is it most likely to occur?

4.4 How can you diagnose this condition?

4.5 What is the best management option?

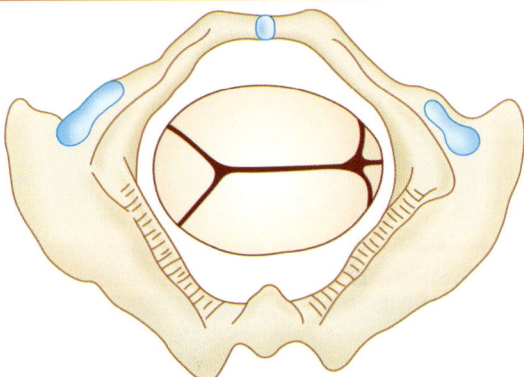

Answer 4.1

Deep transverse arrest

Answer 4.2

It occurs during the second stage of labour due to partial rotation of an occipito-posterior position into the transverse diameter and arrest at the level of the ischial spines.

Answer 4.3

It is most likely to occur in an android pelvis with prominent ischial spines.

Answer 4.4

- The second stage will be prolonged in the presence of strong uterine contractions.
- The head will be at or just above the level of the ischial spines.
- The sagittal suture will be in the transverse plane with the anterior and posterior fontanelles on either side. However, diagnosis may be difficult in the presence of a large caput and moulding.

Answer 4.5

- The safest management option in most cases is to perform a caesarean section.
- Kielland's forceps delivery or vacuum extraction can be tried, if the spines are not prominent and the head is at or below the level of the spines.

References for Questions 1 to 4:
- *SBA Questions in obstetrics, Chapter 5*
- *Munro Kerr's Operative Obstetrics, 12th edition, pp 103–111*

Instrumental Delivery

QUESTION 1

a b

1.1 **Name the two instruments.**
1.2 **List the criteria which should be satisfied to apply obstetric forceps.**
1.3 **What are the indications for using a?**
1.4 **List 2 specific indications for using b.**

Answer 1.1

a. Simpson's forceps
b. Wrigley's forceps

Answer 1.2

- The cervix should be fully dilated.
- No part of the head should be palpable per abdomen.
- The head should be at or below the level of the ischial spines on vaginal examination.
- The pelvis should be adequate.
- The presentation and position should be suitable. Obstetric forceps can be applied for cephalic presentation with occipito-anterior position, face presentation with mento-anterior position and after-coming head of breech presentation.
- The patient should be anaesthetized with epidural analgesia or a pudendal block.
- The bladder should be empty.

Answer 1.3

- Prolonged labour or fetal distress or maternal distress during the second stage of labour, in the presence of an occpito-anterior position or mento-anterior face presentation.
- Delivery of the after-coming head of breech presentation.

Answer 1.4

- For lift out forceps deliveries when the head is 2 cm below the ischial spines.
- To deliver the fetal head at caesarean section.

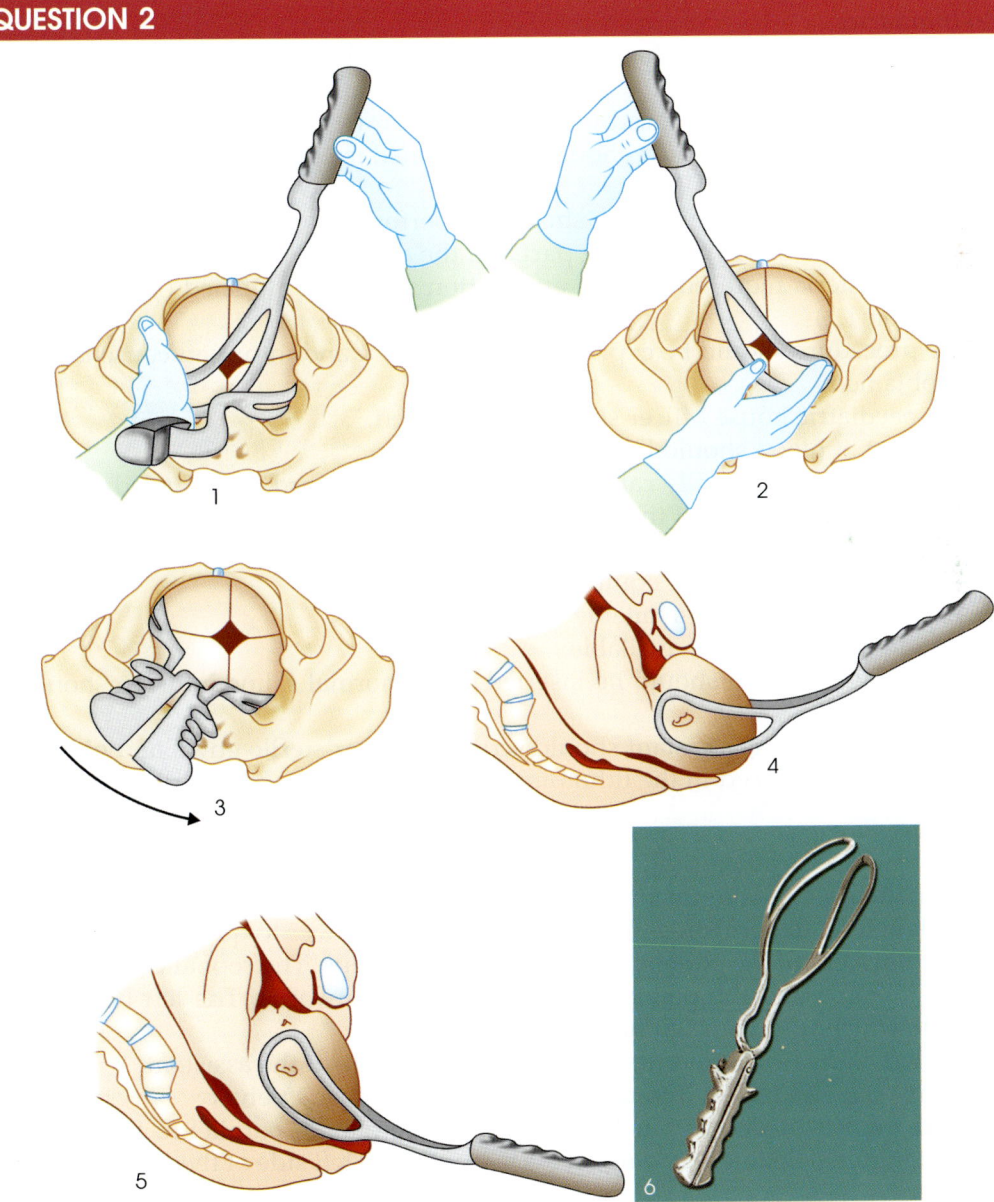

2.1 The above drawings show the steps involved in applying Simpson's forceps. Place them in the correct order in which the procedure is carried out.

2.2 Using the above drawings describe in detail how you would teach a junior doctor to carry out this procedure safely in a cephalic presentation. *(Teaching module for postgraduate students, but undergraduates also can be questioned on the basic method.)*

Answer 2.1

6, 2, 1, 3, 5 and 4

Answer 2.2

Preliminaries

- I would first question whether he has performed or witnessed this procedure before.
- The indication for the procedure should be clear (*refer* answer to question 1.3)
- An abdominal examination should be performed to confirm that the head is fully engaged.
- A careful vaginal examination should be performed to assess the presentation, position, level of the presenting part and the adequacy of the pelvis
- All the criteria required for safe application should be satisfied (*refer* answer to question 1.2)
- The procedure should be explained to the patient and informed consent should be obtained.
- The paediatric house officer should be informed.
- One pint of blood should be reserved.
- The procedure is usually carried out in the labour ward. It is carried out in the operating theater only if there is a possibility of failure and the need to resort to caesarean section.
- Forceps and all the other equipment should be ready.
- An assistant should be available.
- A good light should be available.
- A 14 gauge cannula should be inserted and a normal saline infusion should be commenced.
- The doctor and the assistant should scrub and wear sterile gown and gloves.
- The patient is placed in the lithotomy position and cleaned and draped.

The procedure

- The bladder is catheterised.
- The patient should be suitably anaesthetized, if she is not under epidural analgesia. Explain how to perform a pudendal block (*refer* answer to question 7).
- Stand in front of the patient and assemble the forceps. The cephalic curve should face inwards and the pelvic curve should face outwards. The left blade is the blade which is in your left hand (6)
- The left blade is inserted first. Hand the right blade to the assistant.
- Insert your right hand into the left side of the mother's pelvis.
- Hold the left blade in your left hand with the handle parallel to the mother's right inguinal ligament and insert it gently into the left side of the mother's pelvis (2)

- Apply the right blade in the same manner (1)
- Lock the blades without exerting undue force (3)
- Apply moderate traction with uterine contractions and mother's efforts, first in a downward and backward direction (5)
- Give an episiotomy when the head is crowned.
- Direct the pull in an upward and forward direction and gently complete the delivery (4)
- Carry out active management of the third stage.
- Inspect the genital tract for tears.
- Suture the episiotomy.

Postoperative management
- Monitor the vital parameters and observe for bleeding every 15 minutes for 2 hours according to the modified early warning signs chart, half hourly for 2 hours and hourly for 4 hours. The patient can be mobilised on the same day and discharged in 48 hours.
- Document the procedure and the postoperative management.
- Debrief the patient on the following day.

QUESTION 3

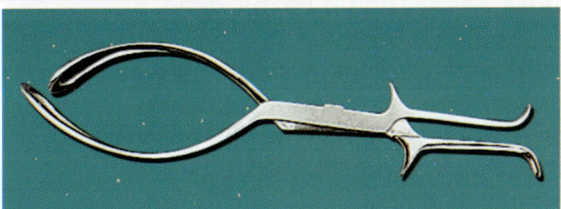

3.1 Name this forceps.
3.2 List 2 special characteristics of this forceps.
3.3 What are the indications to apply this instrument?
3.4 Mention two methods of anaesthesia which are suitable for application of the above forceps.

Answer 3.1
Kielland's forceps.

Answer 3.2
- It has a sliding lock to correct the asynclitism of the fetal head and a very shallow pelvic curve to help in the rotation of the head.
- It has two knobs which can be used to point towards the occiput.

Answer 3.3
- To rotate and deliver the head in occipito-posterior and occipito-transverse positions.
- To deliver the after-coming head of breech presentation.

Answer 3.4
- Epidural analgesia
- Spinal analgesia

QUESTION 4

Describe in detail how you would teach a junior doctor to apply Kielland's forceps safely. (*Teaching module for postgraduate students, but undergraduates also can be questioned on the basic method.*)

Answer

Preliminaries
- I would first question whether he has performed this procedure before.
- The indication for the procedure should be clear. It is carried out for prolonged labour or fetal distress or maternal distress during the second stage in the presence of an occipito-posterior or an occipito-transverse position.
- An abdominal examination should be performed to confirm that the head is fully engaged.
- A careful vaginal examination should be performed to assess the presentation, position, level of the presenting part and the adequacy of the pelvis.
- All the criteria required for safe application should be satisfied (*refer* answer to question 1.2)
- The procedure should be explained to the patient and informed consent should be obtained.
- The paediatric house officer should be informed.
- One pint of blood should be reserved.
- The procedure could be carried out in the labour ward or in the operating theatre.
- It is carried out under spinal or epidural analgesia. The analgesia provided by a pudendal block may not be adequate for the procedure.
- Forceps and all the other equipment should be ready.
- An assistant should be available.
- A good light should be available.
- A 14 gauge cannula should be inserted and a normal saline infusion should be commenced.
- The doctor and the assistant should scrub and wear sterile gown and gloves.
- The patient is placed in the lithotomy position and cleaned and draped.

The procedure
- Perform an abdominal examination to determine the position. The back points to the occiput. The head should be fully engaged.
- Assemble the forceps. The knob in the anterior blade should point to the occiput.
- Perform a vaginal examination and locate the ear.
- Apply the anterior blade over the face and guide it gently towards the anterior ear with the fingers.
- Apply the posterior blade directly into the sacral hollow.
- Lock the blades gently.
- Correct the asynclitism of the head by sliding the blades over each other. It may be necessary to dislodge the head by pushing the blades gently upwards after locking.
- The operator should kneel down and bring the shanks very close to the perineum so that the blades will be in a vertical position.
- Carry out rotation in-between contractions.

- Apply traction with the contractions in a downward and backward direction, once the rotation is complete.
- Perform an episiotomy once the head is crowned.
- Direct the pull in an upward and forward direction and gently complete the delivery.
- Inspect the genital tract for tears.

Postoperative management
- Monitor the vital parameters and observe for bleeding every 15 minutes for 2 hours according to the modified early warning signs chart, half hourly for 2 hours and hourly for 4 hours. The patient can be mobilised on the same day and discharged in 48 hours.
- Document the procedure and the postoperative management.
- Debrief the patient on the following day.

References for Questions 1 to 4: Munro Kerr's Operative Obstetrics, 12th edition, pages 97–113.

QUESTION 5

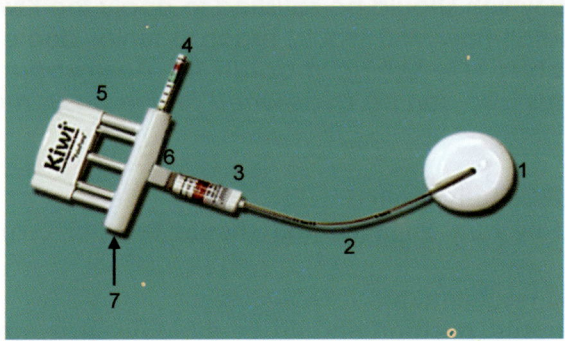

5.1 Name this instrument.
5.2 Name the parts.
5.3 List 4 conditions in which application of obstetric forceps is preferable to the use of this instrument.
5.4 What are the indications to apply this instrument?
5.5 List 2 conditions in which application of this instrument is preferable to obstetric forceps.

Answer 5.1

The Kiwi cup vacuum.

Answer 5.2

1. Cup
2. Suction/traction tube
3. Traction force indicator
4. Vacuum level indicator
5. Palm pump
6. Palm pump handle
7. Button to release the suction

Answer 5.3

- Face presentation
- Prematurity (less than 36 weeks)
- Cord prolapse
- Bleeding from the site of obtaining scalp blood
- Rupture of vasa praevia
- Delivery of the after-coming head of a breech presentation.

Answer 5.4

Prolonged second stage of labour or fetal distress or maternal distress during the second stage in the absence of the above contraindications.

Answer 5.5

- Occipito-posterior position
- Occipito-transverse position

QUESTION 6

6.1   **List the criteria which should be satisfied to apply the Kiwi cup vacuum.**
6.2   **Describe in detail how you would teach a junior doctor to carry out this procedure safely. *(Teaching module for postgraduate students, but undergraduates also can be questioned on the basic method.)***

Answer 6.1

- The cervix should be fully dilated.
- The head should be fully engaged and should be at or below the level of the ischial spines.
- The pelvis should be adequate.
- The presentation and position should be suitable. It is applied for cephalic presentation with occipito-anterior, occipito-posterior or occipito-transverse positions.
- The patient should be anaesthetized with epidural analgesia or a pudendal block.
- The bladder should be empty.

Answer 6.2

Preliminaries
- I would first question whether he has performed or witnessed this procedure before.
- The indication for the procedure should be clear (*refer* answers to questions 5.3, 5.4 and 5.5)
- An abdominal examination should be performed to confirm that the head is fully engaged.
- A careful vaginal examination should be performed to assess the presentation, position, level of the presenting part and the adequacy of the pelvis.
- All the criteria required for safe application should be satisfied (*refer* answer to question 6.1)
- The procedure should be explained to the patient and informed consent should be obtained.

- The paediatric house officer should be informed.
- One pint of blood should be reserved.
- The procedure is carried out in the labour ward.
- All the equipment required for an instrumental delivery should be ready.
- An assistant should be available.
- A good light should be available.
- A 14 gauge cannula should be inserted and a normal saline infusion should be commenced.
- The doctor and the assistant should scrub and wear sterile gown and gloves.
- The patient is placed in the lithotomy position and cleaned and draped.
- The bladder is catheterized.
- The patient should be suitably anaesthetized. If she is not under epidural analgesia perform a pudendal block (*refer* answer to question 7).

Location of the flexion point and measuring the insertion distance,
- Perform a vaginal examination to locate the flexion point.
- The posterior fontanelle is felt and the finger is passed along the sagittal suture towards the anterior fontanelle. The flexion point is located 3 cm from the anterior fontanelle.
- Next measure the distance from the flexion point to the perineum. This is done by placing the tip of the middle finger at the flexion point and measuring the distance to the back of the finger where it touches the posterior fouchette. This is known as the insertion distance.

Insertion of the cup
- The cup is held on the side maintaining the lowest profile.
- The thumb is placed on the groove at the back side of the cup and the index finger is placed on the edge of the cup.
- The labia are parted with the other hand and the cup is gently placed on the fetal head. The fingers are removed from the vagina to allow the stem of the cup to rest on the perineum.

Placing the cup on the flexion point
- Using the fingers manoeuvre the cup towards the flexion point.
- If the cup is placed on the flexion point, the distance of the stem at the point where it touches the posterior fouchette, should be equal to the distance measured previously.
- Otherwise push the cup posteriorly on the midline till the correct distance is reached.
- The stem of the Kiwi cup is marked at 6 and 11 cm.

Building the vacuum: Use the palm pump to build the vacuum up to 600 mm Hg (up to the top of the green area on the pressure gauge). Pass the fingers around the cup to prevent entrapment of maternal tissue.

Applying traction
- Traction is applied with the uterine contractions and maternal effort, in the axis of the maternal pelvis, first in a downward and backward direction.

- The cup is prevented from slipping by placing the index finger on the fetal scalp and the thumb on the back of the cup. The stem should be at 90 degrees to the cup when possible.
- The axis of traction will change with the descent of the head.
- When the head is crowned give an episiotomy, get an assistant to support the perineum and direct the traction in an upward direction. Deliver the head gently.
- Release the cup by pressing the cup release button on the back of the pump.
- Inspect the genital tract for tears and suture the episiotomy.

Postoperative management

- Monitor the vital parameters and observe for bleeding every 15 minutes for 2 hours according to the modified early warning signs chart, half hourly for 2 hours and hourly for 4 hours. The patient can be mobilised on the same day and discharged in 48 hours.
- Document the procedure and the postoperative management.
- Debrief the patient on the following day.

QUESTION 7

What are the anaesthetic methods which should be used for:
7.1 Wrigley's forceps delivery
7.2 Vacuum extraction
7.3 Simpson's forceps delivery
7.4 Kielland's forceps delivery
7.5 Breech delivery
7.6 Twin delivery
7.7 Describe how you would teach a junior doctor to perform a pudendal block.
     (Teaching module for postgraduate students, but undergraduates also can be questioned on the basic method.)

Answer 7.1

- Pudendal block
- Perineal infiltration

Answer 7.2

- Pudendal block
- Perineal infiltration

Answer 7.3

- Pudendal block
- Epidural analgesia

Answer 7.4

- Epidural analgesia
- Spinal analgesia

Answer 7.5

- Pudendal block
- Perineal infiltration

Answer 7.6

- Pudendal block
- Epidural analgesia

Answer 7.7

- The transvaginal route is less painful and more accurate than the transperineal route.
- A 20 cc syringe and a guarded needle are required.
- 10 ml of 1% lignocaine is used.
- The syringe is held in the right hand. The middle and the index fingers of the left hand are inserted into the vagina and are used to guide the needle towards the left ischial spine.
- The guarded needle is guided through the vagina to a point medial and just below the ischial spine.
- After aspiration 5 cc of lignocaine is injected.
- The opposite hands are used to carry out the injection on the right side.
- If a guarded needle is not available a spinal needle can be used. The tip of the needle should be carefully guarded between the fingers, but personal injury can occur when the injection is carried out.
- Transperineal injection is painful and is recommended only when the head is very low.
- The skin is pierced with a long spinal needle, after injecting a local anaesthetic, at a point midway between the ischial tuberosity and the anus.
- The needle is guided towards the injection point by the index finger placed in the vagina.

Reference for Question 7: Munro Kerr's Operative Obstetrics, 12th edition, Chapter 27.

Shoulder Dystocia

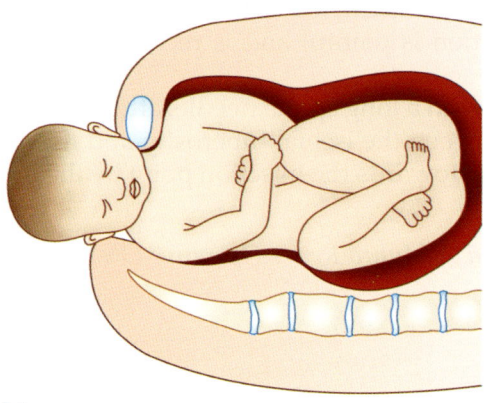

1.1   Name this obstetric emergency.
1.2   List 5 predisposing factors.
1.3   Name the following procedures which are carried out to complete the delivery in the above emergency situation.

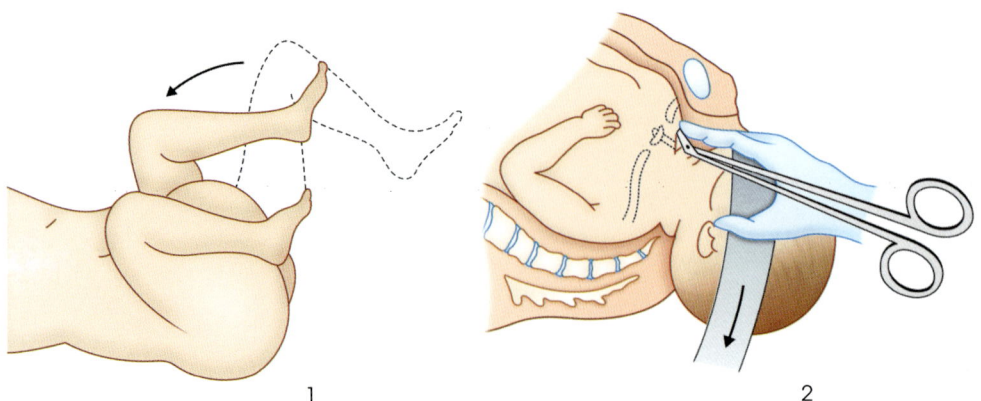

1   2

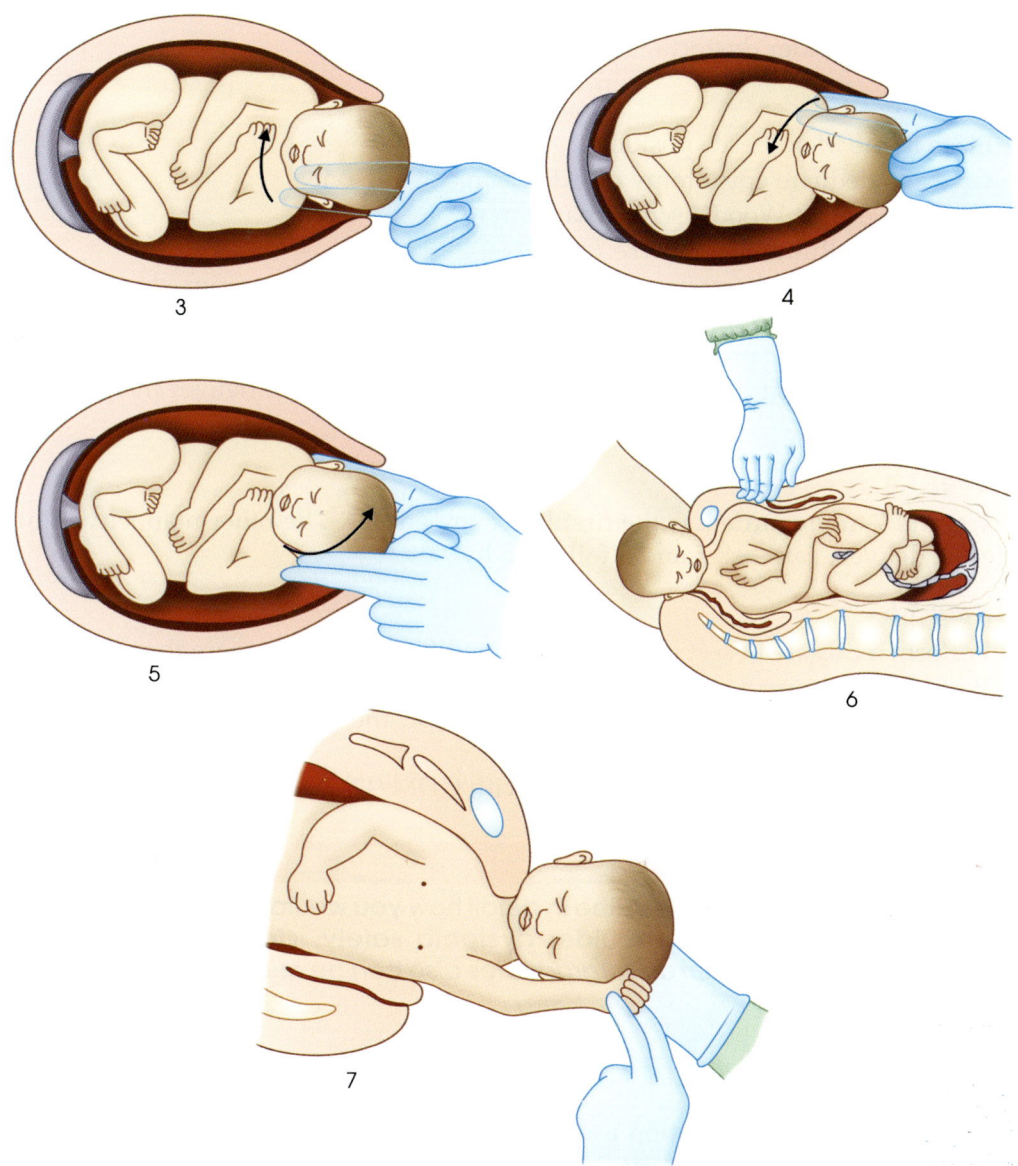

3

4

5

6

7

1.4 Arrange the procedures in the order in which they are carried out.

1.5 How do you prevent the occurrence of this complication?

Answer 1.1

Shoulder dystocia

Answer 1.2

- Fetal weight more than 4 kg
- Diabetes mellitus
- Maternal obesity
- Prolonged first stage of labour

- Prolonged second stage of labour
- Previous shoulder dystocia

Answer 1.3

1. Place in the McRobert's position.
2. Give an adequate episiotomy or extend an existing one.
3. Perform reverse Wood's screw manoeuvre.
4. Perform the Rubin manoeuvre.
5. Perform the Wood's screw manoeuvre and rotate the posterior shoulder and deliver the posterior arm first.
6. Apply suprapubic pressure.
7. Insert the hand into the posterior aspect of the vagina and deliver the posterior arm first.

Answer 1.4

1, 2, 6 and 7 are regarded as the first line manoeuvres. The other manoeuvres are tried, if delivery fails—4, 5 and 3 followed by 7.

Answer 1.5

- Perform a caesarean section if the estimated fetal weight is more than 4 kg.
- Perform a caesarean section in cases of previous shoulder dystocia unless if the weight of the baby is estimated to be less than the previous one and less than 4 kg.
- Induce labour at 39 weeks in women with GDM/DM.

QUESTION 2

Using the above diagrams describe in detail how you would teach a junior doctor to deliver a woman with shoulder dystocia safely. (Teaching module for postgraduate students, but undergraduates also can be questioned on the basic method.)

Answer

Preliminaries
- Reassurance and explanation is essential.
- Advise the patient not to bear down.
- Call for help. A senior obstetrician, a paediatrician and an anaesthetist should ideally be available.
- Remove pillows and place the patient flat in the supine position.
- Remove the lower part of the bed and place the patient at the edge of the bed.
- Empty the bladder.
- The delivery should be completed in 5 minutes.

The method of delivery
- Give an episiotomy or extend an existing one (2)
- Place in McRobert's position (1). This will increase the anteroposterior diameter of the pelvis by straightening the sacrum relative to the lumbar spine.

- Get two assistants to hold the legs on either side. The legs should be abducted at the hips and hyperflexed onto the mother's chest. Apply gentle axial traction on the fetal head for 30 seconds and attempt to complete the delivery.
- Get an assistant to apply suprapubic pressure (6) continuously or in a rocking manner. If the side of the fetal back is known pressure should be applied from behind the fetal back. This manoeuvre will adduct the shoulders and rotate them into the wider oblique diameter of the pelvis. Apply gentle axial traction on the fetal head for 30 seconds and attempt to complete the delivery.
- Delivery of the posterior arm:
  - If the above methods fail to deliver the baby delivery of the posterior arm should be tried first (7)
  - The hand should be inserted into the pelvis. It is best to insert the hand posteriorly as there is more room in the sacral hollow.
    - o Hold the posterior arm by the wrist sweep, it across the chest and deliver the arm. This could be tried, if the arms are flexed across the chest.
    - o If the arms are extended it should be flexed by applying pressure on the cubital fossa.
- Rotational manoeuvres. These manoeuvres are tried, if delivery of the posterior arm is not successful. The aim of these are to move the shoulders from the narrow AP diameter into the wider oblique or transverse diameter of the pelvis. It will also reduce the bisacromial diameter by adducting the shoulders.
  - The Rubin manoeuvre (4)
    - o Place the fingers on the anterior scapula and apply pressure on the posterior aspect of the anterior shoulder. This manoeuvre will rotate and dislodge the shoulder. Maintain suprapubic pressure and lateral traction to facilitate the delivery
  - If this fails to deliver the baby, perform the Wood's screw manoeuvre (5)
    - o While maintaining pressure on the anterior shoulder in the above manner, apply pressure with the fingers of the other hand on the anterior aspect of the posterior shoulder, to rotate in the direction shown by the arrows and dislodge the shoulders to facilitate the delivery. Suprapubic pressure is maintained and lateral traction is applied to facilitate the delivery.
  - If this fails to deliver the baby perform the reverse Wood's screw manoeuvre (3)
    - o Apply pressure on the anterior aspect of the anterior shoulder and on the posterior aspect of the posterior shoulder to rotate in the opposite direction. Try to dislodge the shoulders and deliver. Suprapubic pressure is maintained and lateral traction is applied to facilitate the delivery.

If all these fail, place the woman on all fours and perform all these manoeuvres. This will be difficult if the patient is under epidural analgesia.

If everything fails perform a symphysiotomy or a caesarean section after pushing in the head. The uterus retracts after delivery of the head. Therefore, tocolysis is required to replace the head. Document the procedure in the shoulder dystocia documentation form recommended by the RCOG. Debrief the patient on the next day.

References for Questions 1 and 2: *Munro Kerr's Operative Obstetrics, 12th edition, Chapter 12. RCOG Green-top Guideline No. 42.*

Twin Pregnancy

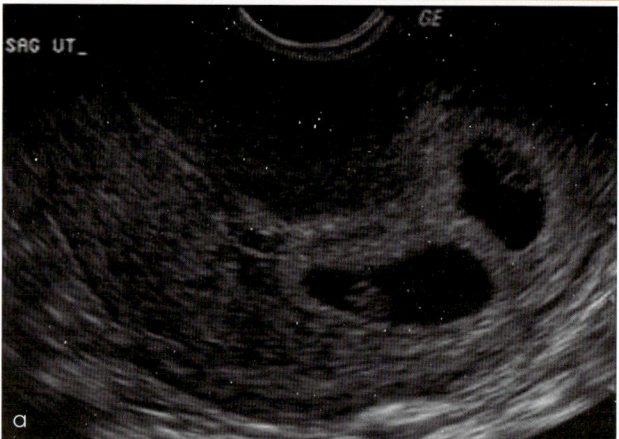

Reproduced with permission from: http://www.fetalultrasound.com.

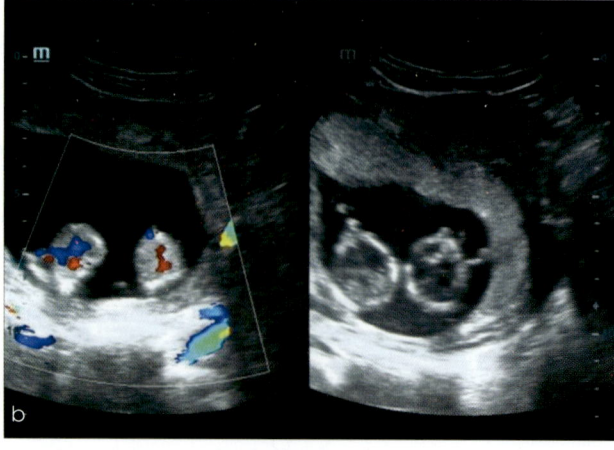

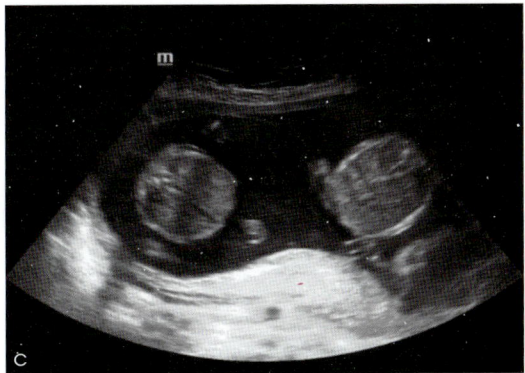

1.1 Name the type of twins in a, b and c.
1.2 List 3 complications which are specific to b and c.
1.3 State a complication which is specific for c.
1.4 At what period of amenorrhoea and how would you deliver a, b and c.

Answer 1.1

a. Dichorionic diamniotic (DCDA) twins
b. Monochorionic diamniotic (MCDA) twins
c. Monochorionic monoamniotic (MCMA) twins

Answer 1.2

• Twin to twin transfusion syndrome
• Fetal weight discordance
• Death of one twin will result in death or handicap of the other twin

Answer 1.3

Cord complications can occur because both fetuses are lying in one sac.

Answer 1.4

a. At 37–38 weeks by induction of labour. Caesarean section is done for obstetric indications only.
b. At 36–37 weeks by caesarean section.
c. At 32–33 weeks by caesarean section.

QUESTION 2

2.1 Name this complication.
2.2 In which twins can it occur?
2.3 List 3 criteria for diagnosing this complication.
2.4 How can you detect this complication early?
2.5 List 4 clinical abnormalities in the smaller twin.
2.6 What is the basic mechanism of this condition?
2.7 What is the treatment?

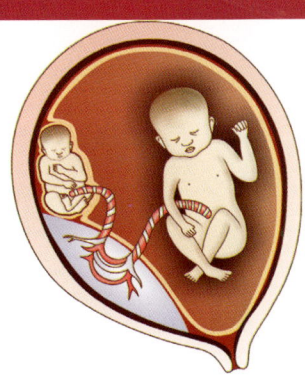

Answer 2.1

Twin to twin transfusion syndrome (TTTS).

Answer 2.2

It can occur in b and c.

Answer 2.3

- The presence of a MCMA or MCDA twin pregnancy.
- The presence of oligohydramnios (defined as a maximal vertical pocket of <2 cm) in one sac, and polyhydramnios (a maximal vertical pocket of >8 cm) in the other sac.
- Occurrence of fetal weight discordance.

Answer 2.4

Early diagnosis is carried out by performing serial ultrasound scans once in two weeks from 16 weeks onwards.

Answer 2.5

- Anaemia
- Oliguria
- Hypotension
- Growth restriction

Answer 2.6

In the case of monochorionic twins, after receiving oxygen and nutrients from the placenta, an artery from one of the twins may return not to the same twin, but to the other twin instead. This is due to arterio-venous anastomosis. Veno-venous and arterio-arterial anastomoses can also occur. These communications can occur in the surface vessels or in the deep vessels of the placenta.

Answer 2.7

Photocoagulation of the anastomosing blood vessels is performed using laser.

QUESTION 3

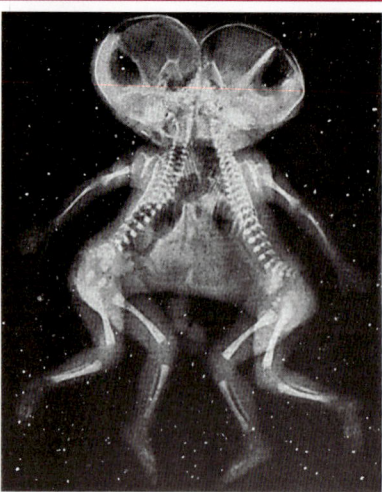

From Wikipedia commons

3.1 Name this complication.
3.2 In which type of twins can it occur?
3.3 State the reason for the occurrence of this complication.
3.4 List 3 possible outcomes.

Answer 3.1

Conjoined twins

Answer 3.2

It occurs in monozygotic twins

Answer 3.3

It occurs due to late division of the embryo after 12 days.

Answer 3.4

- Stillbirth can occur.
- They can die in the early neonatal period.
- Surgical separation may be possible in early childhood.

QUESTION 4

A woman has delivered the first twin without any complications.
4.1 List 5 steps in the management of the delivery of the second twin.
4.2 What is your management, if the second twin is in breech presentation?
4.3 What is your management, if the second twin is in the transverse lie?

Answer 4.1

- Perform an abdominal examination to determine the lie of the second twin.
- Perform a vaginal examination to confirm the lie and presentation and to exclude cord presentation.
- Commence continuous fetal heart rate monitoring.
- If the lie is longitudinal wait for a few minutes for the presenting part to descend and perform an amniotomy and release the liquor gradually to prevent cord prolapse.
- Commence an oxytocin infusion, if the contractions are inadequate.
- Deliver the second twin as soon as possible after the delivery of the first twin.

Answer 4.2

- Perform a vaginal examination to confirm the presentation and to exclude cord presentation.
- Commence continuous fetal heart rate monitoring
- Wait for a few minutes until the presenting part has descended and perform an amniotomy and release the liquor gradually to avoid cord prolapse.
- Commence an oxytocin drip, if the contractions are inadequate.
- Perform an assisted breech delivery.

Answer 4.3

Transverse lie of the second twin can be easily corrected by external cephalic version (ECV), if detected before membranes rupture, because there is enough space to carry out this procedure. However, ECV will not be successful if liquor has drained away and there are strong uterine contractions. Delivery by caesarean section is the safest option in this situation.

QUESTION 5

5.1 **List the complications which can occur during the delivery of the second twin.**

5.2 **What is your management if cord prolapse occurs with the second twin presenting by the vertex?**

5.3 **What is your management, if antepartum haemorrhage occurs with the second twin presenting by the breech? Describe the procedure briefly.**

5.4 **What are the indications for caesarean section after the delivery of the first twin?**

5.5 **How do you treat locked twins?**

Answer 5.1

- Transverse lie/hand prolapse of the second twin
- Fetal distress
- Cord prolapse
- Antepartum haemorrhage
- Delay in delivery of the second twin
- Locked twins

Answer 5.2

Deliver the fetus immediately by application of Simpson's forceps.

Answer 5.3

- Deliver the fetus immediately by performing breech extraction under epidural or general anaesthesia.
- If the groins are visible traction is applied with a finger in each groin. Traction should be applied during uterine contractions.
- If the groin is not visible the hand is inserted into the uterus and the ankle of the anterior leg is grasped and is gently brought down. The posterior leg is brought down in the same manner.
- Traction is applied on both legs concomitant with the uterine contractions and mother's bearing down efforts, till the pelvis is visible. Wrap the baby in a sterile towel.
- Continue the delivery in the normal manner of a breech delivery, but continuous gentle traction is applied. This is aided by the mother's expulsive efforts.
- However, the arms may be extended as traction has been applied.
- Loveset's manoeuvre is required to deliver the arms.
- Forceps are applied to deliver the head.

Answer 5.4

- Hand prolapse or persistence of transverse lie after rupture of membranes.
- Delay in delivery of the second twin with partial closure of the cervix.

Answer 5.5

The uterus should be relaxed with intravenous tocolytics. Under general anaesthesia try to disimpact the twins by elevating the first twin and pushing away the second twin.

If this is not successful perform a classical caesarean section.

QUESTION 6

6.1 **What is the best method to screen for Down's syndrome in twin pregnancy? Give your reasons.**

6.2 **Mention how you would confirm Down's syndrome at a POA of 15 weeks in monochorionic and dichorionic twins. Give your reasons.**

6.3 **Mention how you would screen for fetal structural abnormalities in monochorionic and dichorionic twins. Give your reasons.**

6.4 **List the indications for elective caesarean section in a twin pregnancy.**

Answer 6.1

An USS is performed for nuchal translucency at 11–13 weeks. Biochemical tests cannot be reliably used for this purpose as they are elevated in twin pregnancies.

Answer 6.2

Amniocentesis should be performed from both sacs in dichorionic twins, because they may be dizygotic and have different chromosomal compositions. Therefore, chromosomal abnormalities may affect only one twin.

Amniocentesis should be performed from one sac only, in monochorionic diamniotic twins, because they are monozygotic and have the same chromosomal compositions. Therefore, chromosomal abnormalities will affect both twins.

Answer 6.3

USS is performed in both fetuses at 20 weeks because structural abnormalities can affect one or both twins in both monochorionic and dichorionic twins.

Answer 6.4

- Monochorionic monoamniotic twins
- Monochorionic diamniotic twins
- Breech presentation in the first twin
- Transverse lie in the first twin
- Previous caesarean section or myomectomy scars
- Any other obstetric indications

References for Questions 1 to 6
- Munro Kerr's Operative Obstetrics, 12th edition, Chapter 17.
- Management of twin and triplet pregnancy in the antenatal period, NICE Guideline CG 129 (February 2011).
- Management of monochorionic twin pregnancy, RCOG Green-top Guideline No. 51 (December 2008).
- Obstetrics by Ten Teachers, 19th Edition, Chapter 14, pages 218–219.
- SBA Questions in Obstetrics, Chapter 14.

Rhesus Negative Mother

QUESTION 1

A Rhesus negative secondpara attends the antenatal clinic at a POA of 8 weeks. An antibody screen revealed an indirect antibody titer of 1:8.

1.1 List 3 steps in the initial management.
1.2 What are the critical levels of anti-D?
1.3 What are the critical levels of anti-C?
1.4 What are the critical levels of anti-K?

Answer 1.1

- The next step is to check the father's rhesus genotype
- If the father is heterozygous, the fetus may be rhesus positive or negative. Therefore, the next step is to check the fetal blood group by analysing cell free fetal DNA in the maternal blood. If the father is homozygous the fetus will be rhesus positive.
- If the fetus is rhesus positive antibody titers are performed monthly, until 24 weeks of gestation and once in two weeks thereafter.
- If the critical antibody levels are reached middle cerebral artery peak systolic velocity (MCAPSV) should be performed.
- If the fetus is rhesus negative further monitoring is not necessary.

Answer 1.2

- Direct antibody level: 15 IU /ml
- Indirect antibody titer: 1: 32
- Albumin titer: 1: 16

Answer 1.3

Direct antibody level greater than 20 IU/ml

Answer 1.4

Severe fetal anaemia can occur even with low titers of anti-K antibodies.

QUESTION 2

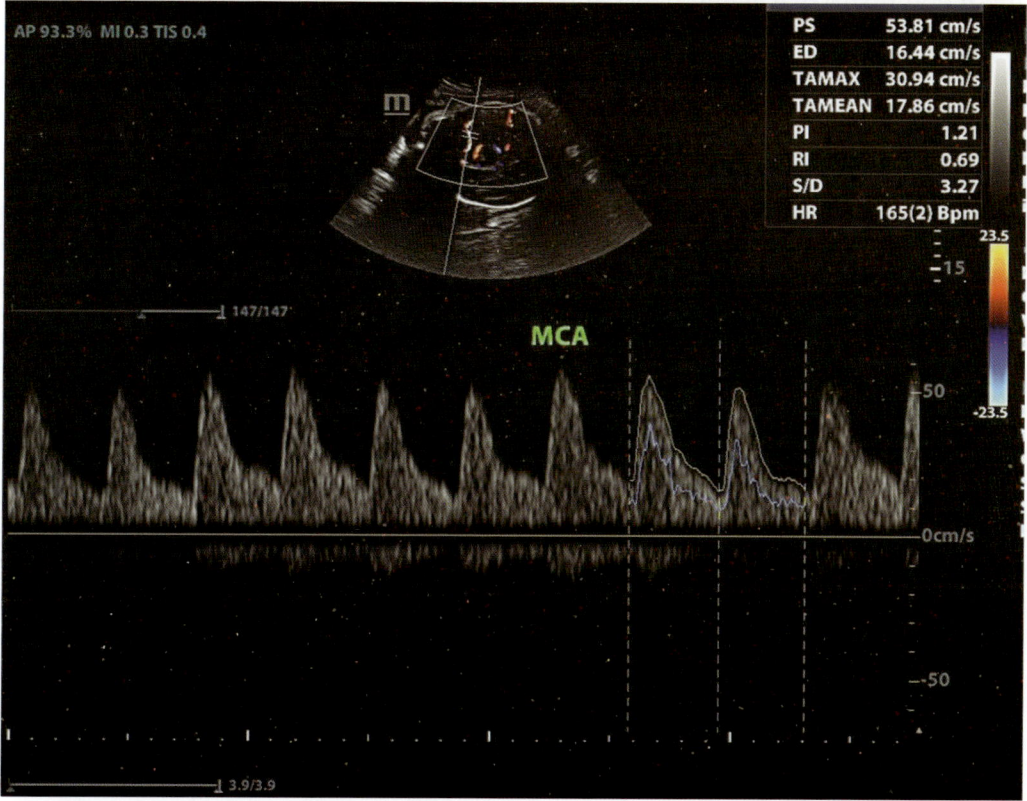

AP 93.3% MI 0.3 TIS 0.4

PS	53.81 cm/s
ED	16.44 cm/s
TAMAX	30.94 cm/s
TAMEAN	17.86 cm/s
PI	1.21
RI	0.69
S/D	3.27
HR	165(2) Bpm

MCA

147/147

3.9/3.9

2.1 What is this investigation?

2.2 The antibody level is found to be 15 IU/ml at 24 weeks. State 2 methods available for further assessment of the fetal condition.

2.3 Which of the two methods would you select?

2.4 Give reasons for your selection.

2.5 What is the critical value of the investigation you have selected, beyond which the fetus is regarded as seriously affected?

Answer 2.1

It is performed to measure the middle cerebral artery peak systolic velocity.

Answer 2.2

• Perform ultrasonographic assessment of the middle cerebral artery peak systolic velocity.

• Perform amniocentesis to assess the amniotic fluid bilirubin levels.

Answer 2.3

Ultrasonographic assessment of the middle cerebral artery peak systolic velocity is the best method for further assessment of the fetus.

Answer 2.4

It is a non-invasive test and hence can be repeated as frequently as indicated, while amniocentesis is an invasive test.

MCAPSV has a sensitivity of 100% and a false positive rate of 12%.

Answer 2.5

1.5 multiples of the median.

QUESTION 3

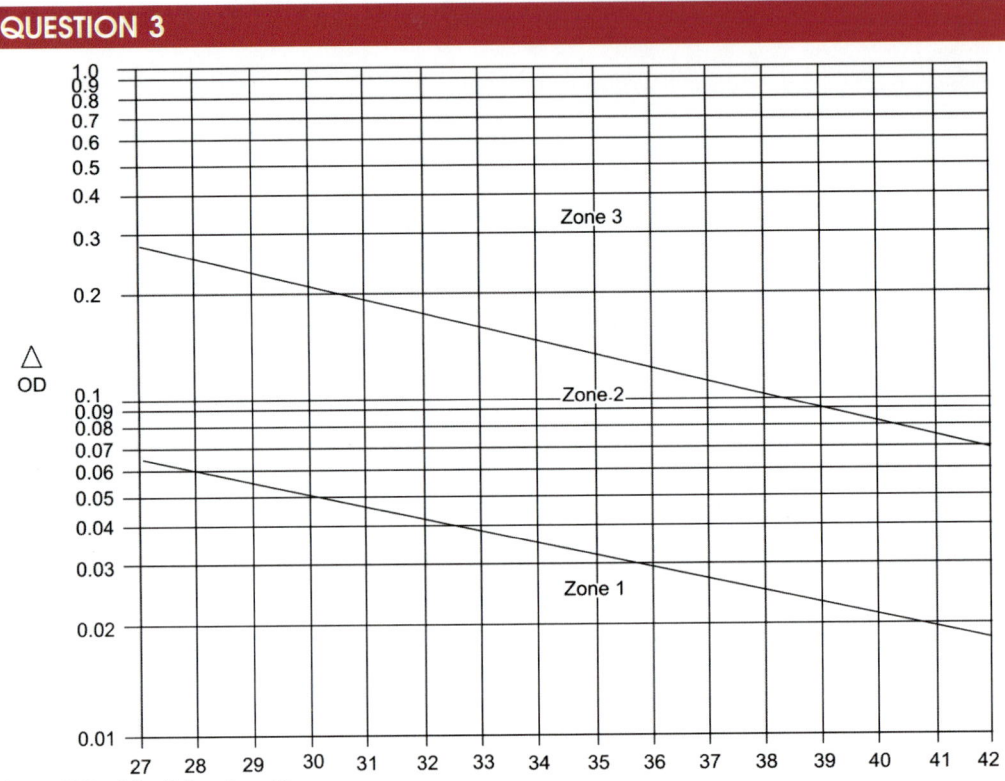

3.1 What is this chart?
3.2 What is the parameter which is charted?
3.3 What is the indication to chart the parameter you have mentioned?
3.4 What are the disadvantages of the procedure?
3.5 What is the point on this chart beyond which the fetus is regarded as seriously affected?

Answer 3.1

The Liley curve

Answer 3.2

Amniotic fluid bilirubin levels

Answer 3.3

Amniotic fluid bilirubin levels are charted if the maternal red cell antibody level exceeds the critical value in a sensitized woman.

Answer 3.4

Amniocentesis has to be performed to assess the amniotic fluid bilirubin levels. It is an invasive test and cannot be performed more often than once in two weeks. Also it can cause further iso-immunization, infection, trauma to the fetus and preterm labour.

Answer 3.5

Upper part of of zone 2.

QUESTION 4

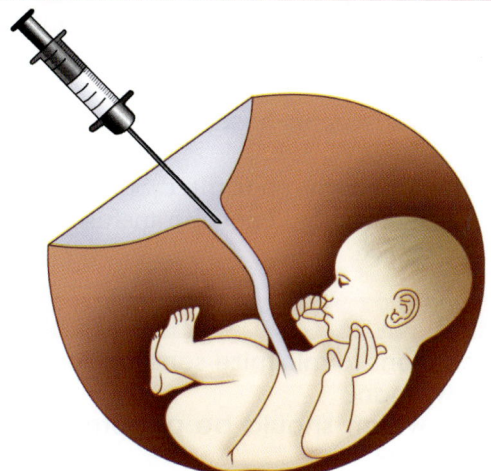

4.1 What is this procedure?

4.2 What is the parameter which is detected by this procedure in the management of rhesus isoimmunisation?

4.3 State 3 indications for this procedure in the management of rhesus isoimmunisation.

4.4 What is the level of the haematocrit at which intrauterine transfusion is indicated?

4.5 What is the range of the gestational ages at which intrauterine transfusion is indicated to treat fetal anaemia?

4.6 State the characteristics of a blood sample which is used for intrauterine transfusion.

Answer 4.1

Cordocentesis

Answer 4.2

Fetal haemoglobin level

Answer 4.3

- Middle cerebral artery peak systolic velocity of 1.5 multiples of the median.
- An amniotic fluid bilirubin level which falls into the upper middle zone of the Liley chart.
- Ultrasound evidence of fetal hydrops.

Answer 4.4

Below 30% (a fetal hemoglobin level which is two standard deviations below the mean value for the gestational age)

Answer 4.5

Between 18 and 34 weeks

Answer 4.6

The blood sample should:
- Be less than 5 days old.
- Be O Rhesus-negative or ABO identical with the fetus if the group is known. It should be negative for the antigens corresponding to the maternal red cell antibodies.
- Have a haemoglobin level of 22–24 g/dL (haematocrit of 70–85%).
- Be cytomegalovirus negative.
- Be irradiated to prevent graft-versus-host reaction and transfused within 24 hours of irradiation.
- Be processed through a leukocyte-poor filter. Some centres use maternal blood as the source of red cells. Blood should not be transfused at the storage temperature of 4°C.

QUESTION 5

5.1   What are the precautions to minimize sensitization at the time of delivery in a rhesus negative woman?
5.2   What are the tests which should be performed after delivery, before administration of anti-D?
5.3   How do you calculate the dose of anti-D?

Answer 5.1

- Clamp the cord soon after delivery.
- Avoid instrumental delivery and manual removal of the placenta.
- Pack the peritoneal cavity well and avoid manual removal of the placenta at caesarean section.

Answer 5.2

Cord blood is taken (after clamping the baby's side) for the following investigations.
- Blood group and rhesus factor
- Haemoglobin level
- Serum bilirubin level
- Direct Coomb's test
- Reticulocyte count

These tests are done to assess whether the baby is affected. Anti-D is given to the mother if the baby is rhesus positive, the direct Coomb's test is negative and there is no other evidence of haemolysis or anaemia. It is better if Kleihaur test is performed to measure the FMH.

Answer 5.3

- In all cases, it is best to measure the FMH by performing a Kleihauer test as soon as possible after the sensitizing event.

- 500 IU of anti-D will neutralize 4 ml of fetomaternal haemorrhage (FMH). For each ml above 4 ml a further 125 IU is required.
- The standard dose for sensitizing events before 20 weeks is 250 IU and after 20 weeks is 500 IU.
- The standard dose after delivery is 1500 IU (300 µg) and will neutralize 15 ml of fetomaternal haemorrhage.
- A larger FMH can occur in caesarean sections, forceps deliveries, manual removal of retained placenta, stillbirths and twin pregnancies. It is essential to perform a Kleihaur test in these situations.

QUESTION 6

6.1 What are the other antibodies (other than rhesus) in the maternal blood which can cause haemolytic disease of the fetus and the newborn (HDFN)?
6.2 How do you test for these antigens in the fetal blood?
6.3 What are the threshold levels of these antibodies which warrant further monitoring?
6.4 Once detected how frequently should antibody levels be tested?
6.5 How will you monitor when the upper threshold limits of antibodies are reached?

Answer 6.1

C, c, E, e and K

Answer 6.2

This can be done non-invasively by testing cell free fetal DNA in the maternal blood.

Answer 6.3

- An anti-c level of >7.5 IU/ml but <20 IU/ml indicate a moderate risk of HDFN and require referral to a fetal medicine unit.
- An anti-c level of >20 IU/ml indicates a high risk of HDFN and requires monitoring with MCA PSV.
- In the case of anti-K antibodies, severe fetal anaemia can occur even with low titers. Therefore, referral should take place once detected.
- The presence of anti-E potentiates the severity of fetal anaemia due to anti-c antibodies. Therefore, referral at lower levels/titers is indicated.

Answer 6.4

- Anti-K antibody titers are performed monthly, until 28 weeks of gestation and once in two weeks thereafter. The pregnancy can be continued to term if the antibody levels are below the critical titer.
- The other antibodies are re-tested at 28 weeks.
- The blood bank should be informed regarding the antibody levels to check the availability of compatible blood.

Answer 6.5

- Perform MCA PSV weekly.
- This should be done once anti-K antibodies are detected as fetal anaemia can occur with low levels.

- Intrauterine transfusion should be considered when the MCA PSV rises above 1.5 multiples of the median.

References for Questions 1 to 6

- *British Committee for Standards in Haematology (BCSH) guideline for the use of anti-D immunoglobulin for the prevention of haemolytic disease of the fetus and newborn (21/1/2014).*
- *Management of the Rhesus negative mother, Sri Lanka College of Obstetricians and Gynaecologists, National Guideline (2007).*
- *Obstetrics by Ten Teacher, 19th Edition, Chapter 8, page 104.*
- *The Management of Women with Red Cell Antibodies during Pregnancy, RCOG Green top Guideline 65.*
- *SBA Questions in Obstetrics, Chapter 12.*

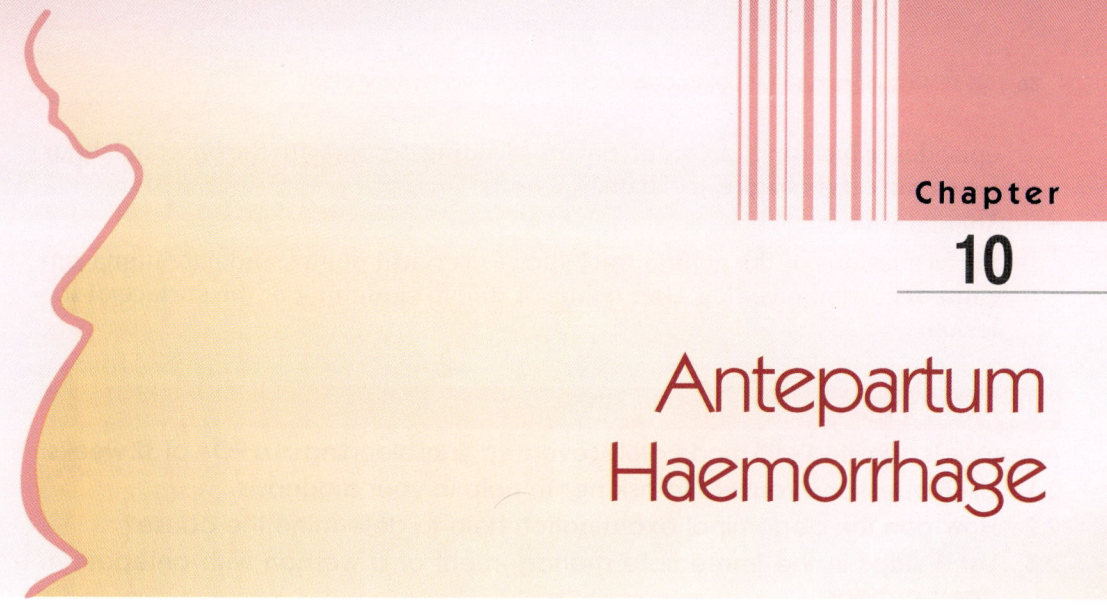

Antepartum Haemorrhage

QUESTION 1

1.1 List the causes of antepartum haemorrhage.
1.2 Which of the above causes carry a risk to the fetus? Explain your answer.
1.3 Which of the above causes carry the greatest risk to the mother? Explain your answer.
1.4 Which of the above can cause recurrent haemorrhage?

Answer 1.1

- Placenta previa
- Placental abruption
- Rupture of vasa previa
- Incidental causes

Answer 1.2

- Rupture of vasa previa:
  - Bleeding occurs due to rupture of fetal blood vessels on the membranes and fetal blood is lost. Exsanguination of the fetus can occur, if delivery is not performed immediately.
- Placental abruption
  - Fetus can die due to placental separation causing hypoxia.

Answer 1.3

Placental abruption
- The general condition of the woman may be worse than the external blood loss as concealed haemorrhage can occur.
- Disseminated intravascular coagulation and renal failure can occur.

Answer 1.4

- Placenta previa.
  - The lower part of the uterus stretches to form the lower segment. This can cause separation of a placenta situated in the lower segment and recurrent

episodes of bleeding can occur. Severe bleeding occurs with the onset of labour when the cervix begins to dilate.

- Incidental causes
  - Surface lesions of the genital tract such as cervical polyps and carcinoma can cause recurrent bleeding after coitus or due to sloughing of the surface of the lesion.

QUESTION 2

A woman is admitted with moderately severe vaginal bleeding at a POA of 32 weeks.

2.1 List 5 questions you would ask her to help in your diagnosis.
2.2 How can the abdominal examination help to determine the cause?
2.3 List 3 steps in the immediate management of a woman with antepartum haemorrhage.

Answer 2.1

- Did she experience pain?
- Is there a history of abdominal trauma?
- Were there previous recurrent episodes of bleeding?
- Did she have pregnancy induced hypertension?
- Was she informed about the placental site at previous ultrasound scans?
- Is she taking cocaine or any other drugs?

Answer 2.2

- In placenta previa and in incidental causes:
  - The uterus will be soft and non-tender and the fetal parts can be palpated easily. Braxton Hicks contractions or labour contractions can be palpated. Fetal heart sounds will be within the normal range. In placenta previa there will be a high presenting part or a malpresentation.
- In rupture of vasa previa:
  - The uterus will be soft and non-tender and the fetal parts can be palpated easily. Braxton Hick's contractions or labour contractions can be palpated. There will be severe fetal bradycardia.
- In placental abruption:
  - The uterus will be tense and tender. The head may be engaged. It will be difficult to palpate the fetal parts. Uterine contractions cannot be felt easily. Fetal heart sounds may be absent or there may be fetal distress.

Answer 2.3

- Insert two 14 gauge cannulae and commence an infusion of crystalloids.
- Send blood for cross matching and reserve 5 units of blood.
- Perform an USS to localize the placenta.
- Perform a CTG.

QUESTION 3

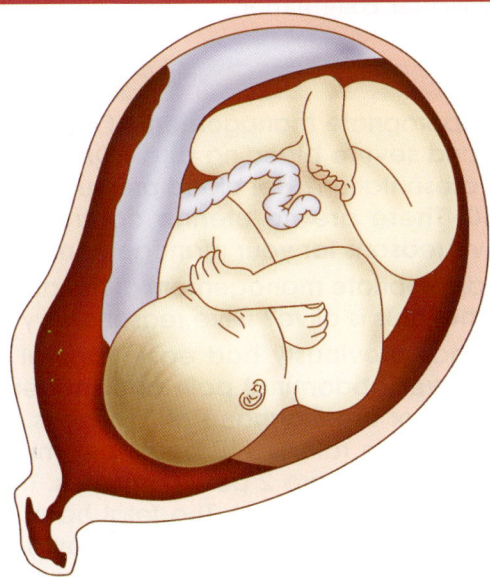

3.1 **What is the condition shown in this drawing?**
3.2 **List 5 causative factors.**
3.3 **Mention 5 clinical features of this condition.**
3.4 **Mention 4 complications of this condition.**

Answer 3.1

Placental abruption

Answer 3.2

- Pregnancy induced hypertension.
- Cocaine addiction
- Abdominal trauma
- Pregnancy following assisted reproduction
- Advanced maternal age
- Low BMI
- Smoking

Answer 3.3

- Sudden onset of bleeding with pain.
- Tachycardia and low blood pressure.
- Tenderness over the uterus.
- The head will be in the lower pole and may be engaged.
- The uterus will be tense and tender and it will be difficult to palpate the fetal parts.
- Fetal distress or fetal death.

Answer 3.4

- Fetal death
- Maternal haemodynamic compromise

- Renal failure
- Disseminated intravascular coagulation.

QUESTION 4

4.1 What is the most appropriate management of a woman who presents with abdominal pain and severe bleeding at a POA of 34 weeks with a dead fetus in cephalic presentation? Her blood pressure is 90/ 50 mmHg and the pulse rate is 130. There are no uterine contractions. Resuscitation is commenced. Give reasons for your management.

4.2 What is the most appropriate management of the above woman if her POA is 31 weeks and the fetus is alive? Give reasons for your management.

4.3 A thirdpara who has previously had easy vaginal deliveries, develops sudden onset of lower abdominal pain and moderately severe vaginal bleeding at a period of amenorrhoea of 37 weeks. The blood pressure is 100/60 mm Hg, the pulse rate is 110 beats per minute and the uterus is tender. Uterine contractions are 2 per 10 minutes. The fetus is in cephalic presentation. The head is engaged. The fetal heart rate is 130 beats per minute. Ultrasound scan excludes placenta praevia. The cervix is thin and dilated to 6 cm. What is the most appropriate management? Give reasons for your management.

Answer 4.1

Perform a caesarean section immediately.

This is a case of placental abruption because there is pain and sudden onset of bleeding with death of the fetus. Even though the fetus is dead, the woman is bleeding profusely with haemodynamic compromise. The only method to stop the bleeding is to empty the uterus as soon as possible. Even though the fetus is dead vaginal delivery is not possible because she is not in labour and hence induction of labour and delivery will take a long time, with a great risk for the mother.

Answer 4.2

Perform a caesarean section immediately.

Expectant management is not indicated because:
- The woman is bleeding profusely with haemodynamic compromise and the only method to stop the bleeding is to empty the uterus as soon as possible.
- It is a case of placental abruption and further abruption can occur causing fetal death.
- Further abruption and concealed haemorrhage can occur causing maternal and fetal death.
- Mother can develop complications such as DIC and renal failure.

Answer 4.3

Augment labour with amniotomy followed by oxytocin infusion. Commence continuous fetal heart rate monitoring. Carefully monitor the vital signs and observe for bleeding every 15 minutes. Perform a coagulation profile and maintain an intake output chart. Crossmatch five units of blood. The third stage should be managed actively and the woman should be observed for PPH.

This is a case of placental abruption. As the maternal and fetal conditions are not seriously compromised, the fetus is mature and she is in the active phase of the first stage, augmentation of labour (which is the most appropriate method of delivery for abruption) is a better option than caesarean section. Also she is a multipara who has previously had easy vaginal deliveries and quick delivery can be expected following augmentation.

QUESTION 5

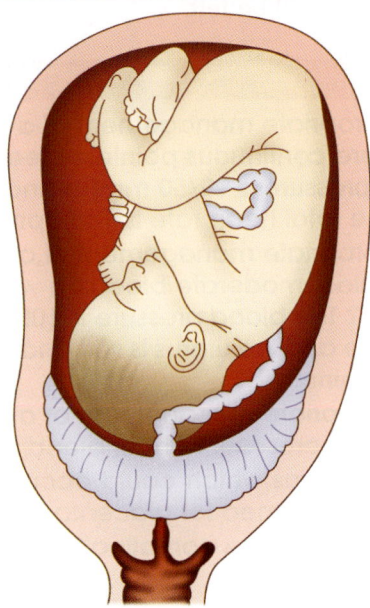

5.1 **What is the above condition?**
5.2 **What are the presenting symptoms?**
5.3 **Mention 5 questions you would ask this patient which would be helpful in arriving at a diagnosis.**
5.4 **List the physical signs you would elicit.**

Answer 5.1
Central placenta previa

Answer 5.2
The patient will present with sudden onset of painless vaginal bleeding. There may be previous episodes of mild bleeding. In some cases there may be no bleeding till the onset of labour. A morbidly adherent placenta should be suspected in these cases.

Answer 5.3
- Is the bleeding painless?
- Is there a history of recurrent bleeding?
- Was an USS scan performed after 30 weeks and was she informed of a low lying placenta?
- Is she feeling fetal movements?

- Does she have pregnancy induced hypertension?
- Is there a history of abdominal trauma?
- Is she taking addictive drugs?

Answer 5.4

- There may be a high head or a malpresentation.
- The uterus will be soft and non-tender and the fetal parts can be palpated easily.
- The fetal heart rate will be within normal limits.
- Braxton Hicks contractions will be felt.

QUESTION 6

6.1   What is the most appropriate management of a woman who presents with sudden onset of severe continuous painless bleeding and haemodynamic compromise (blood pressure is 90/50 mmHg and the pulse rate is 130) at a POA of 31 weeks? The fetal heart rate is 140 bpm.

6.2   What is the most appropriate management of a woman who presents with sudden onset of painless moderate bleeding which stops after admission, at a POA of 31 weeks? The blood pressure is 100 /60 mm Hg, the pulse rate is 110 beats per minute and the uterus is soft and non-tender. The fetal heart rate is 130 beats per minute.

6.3   What is the most appropriate management of a woman with the condition given in question 5 who presents without bleeding at a POA of 38 weeks?

6.4   What are the complications which could occur in the third stage when a caesarean section is performed for placenta previa? Give your reasons.

6.5   How will you prevent the above complications?

Answer 6.1

Carryout immediate resuscitation and perform an immediate caesarean section.

Answer 6.2

- Perform an USS to confirm the diagnosis of placenta previa
- Carryout expectant management as an in-ward patient at a tertiary care centre.

Answer 6.3

Perform a caesarean section as soon as possible. Perform a MRI scan before performing surgery to exclude a morbidly adherent placenta.

Answer 6.4

Postpartum haemorrhage can occur due to:
- Morbid adhesion of the placenta
- Larger placental area
- Poor contractility of the lower segment

Answer 6.5

The third stage should be managed actively after giving 5 units of oxytocin direct intravenously with the delivery of the baby. An infusion of oxytocin should be commenced. A morbidly adherent placenta should be excluded by MRI scan before performing surgery. If a morbidly adherent placenta has been detected arrangements should be made to perform a hysterectomy or uterine artery embolization.

QUESTION 7

An amniotomy is performed in a woman in labour. This is followed by sudden onset of vaginal bleeding. The fetal heart rate drops to 100 beats per minute. The cervix is thin and dilated to 7 cm. The uterus is not tender. She is getting three uterine contractions per ten minutes. Her pulse rate is 80 beats per minute and the blood pressure is 120/80 mm Hg. There is no previous history of vaginal bleeding.

7.1   What are the conditions you would consider in the differential diagnosis?
7.2   What is the most likely cause? Give reasons for your diagnosis.
7.3   How is the diagnosis confirmed?
7.4   If a CTG is performed what is the expected pattern of the tracing?
7.5   What is the best management option?

Answer 7.1

- Rupture of vasa praevia
- Placenta previa
- Placental abruption
- Traumatic haemorrhage
- Incidental causes

Answer 7.2

Rupture of vasa praevia.

The bleeding occurred suddenly at the time of amniotomy and was associated with sudden fetal bradycardia. The maternal vital parameters are normal. There is no previous history of bleeding.

Placenta previa could cause profuse bleeding, at the onset of labour with commencement of cervical dilatation, but will occur earlier in labour and will not cause fetal bradycardia.

Abruption is unlikely because there is no uterine tenderness or continuous pain.

Traumatic haemorrhage will not cause severe fetal bradycardia. A cervical growth or other surface lesions will be felt at vaginal examination and will not cause fetal bradycardia.

Answer 7.3

Diagnosis is confirmed clinically (*refer* answer to question 7.2)

Presence of fetal blood can be confirmed by performing a Kleihauer test, but is not essential and is time consuming.

Answer 7.4

A sinusoidal pattern or atypical variable decelerations with fetal bradycardia will be present due to fetal hypoxia.

Answer 7.5

A caesarean section should be performed immediately.

QUESTION 8

8.1 List 3 precautions which should be taken before performing a caesarean section for placenta previa.

8.2 What is the best management option for a primiparous woman with a morbidly adherent placenta previa?

8.3 What is the best management option for a third para with a morbidly adherent placenta?

Answer 8.1

- Perform a MRI scan to exclude morbid adhesion of the placenta.
- Crossmatch 5 units of blood.
- The caesarean section should be performed by an experienced senior consultant.
- Perform uterine artery catheterization prior to the caesarean section, if a morbidly adherent placenta is suspected.

Answer 8.2

Perform uterine artery catheterization prior to caesarean section and leave the placenta *in situ*. The caesarean section should be performed without cutting through the placenta. Uterine artery embolization is performed, if bleeding occurs.

Answer 8.3

Perform a caesarean hysterectomy.

References
- *SBA Questions in Obstetrics, Chapter 3.*
- *RCOG Green top Guide line No. 63.*
- *Obstetrics by Ten Teachers, 19th edition, pages 245–247.*

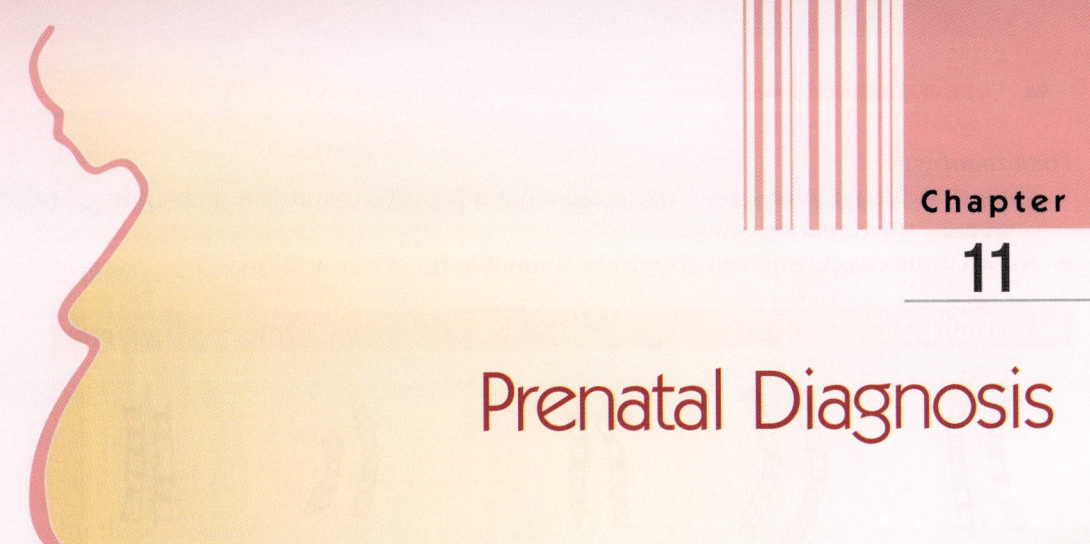

11

Prenatal Diagnosis

QUESTION 1

1.1 Mention 5 prenatal screening tests.
1.2 Mention 4 prenatal diagnostic tests.
1.3 List the advantages and disadvantages of screening tests.

Answer 1.1

- Quadruple test for Down's syndrome (estimation of hCG, AFP, oestriol and inhibin A).
- Measurement of the nuchal translucency by USS for Down's syndrome.
- Measrement of maternal serum alpha fetoprotein levels at 15–19 weeks for neural tube defects.
- Estimation of the fetal sex by analysis of cell free fetal DNA in screening for haemophilia.
- Haemglobin electrophoresis to identify carrier parents of thalassemia.

Answer 1.2

- USS for fetal structural abnormalities at 20 weeks.
- Amniocentesis after 15 weeks to confirm chromosomal and genetic diseases.
- Chorionic villous sampling from 11–13 weeks to confirm chromosomal and genetic diseases.
- Cordocentesis to confirm fetal anaemia after 15 weeks.
- Meternal cell free DNA analysis to determine the fetal blood group.

Answer 1.3

Advantages
- Screening tests are performed on all women in order to identify patients who are at risk of a disorder.
- They are performed for disorders with a high prevalence, for which accurate diagnostic tests are available.
- They are non-invasive tests.
- They do not carry any risk to the pregnancy.

Disadvantages
- Main disadvantage of screening tests is that a positive result is not absolute but can cause unwanted anxiety.
- An accurate diagnostic test should be available for the condition.

QUESTION 2

2.1   The karyotype of a newborn baby with dysmorphic features is given below. Name this condition and give your reasons.
2.2   Mention one characteristic of a mother in whom this condition can occur.
2.3   Mention another genetic type of this condition. Mention one characteristic of parents in whom this condition can occur.
2.4   Mention 3 antenatal screening tests for the above condition.
2.5   Mention 2 confirmatory tests for this condition.

Answer 2.1

Down's syndrome. There are 3 chromosomes at 21—trisomy 21

Answer 2.2

She could be more than 40 years of age.

Answer 2.3

Translocation Down's syndrome where a part or whole of one of the pair of chromosomes 21 become attached to another chromosome.
    One of the parents may carry a balanced translocation.

Answer 2.4

Screening tests include:
- Measurment of the nuchal translucency by USS at 11–13 weeks

- Decreased pregnancy associated plasma protein-A (PAPPA) in the first trimester.
- Quadruple test at 15–18 weeks:
  - Decreased alpha fetoprotein
  - Increased serum beta hCG
  - Increased inhibin A
  - Decreased oestriol

Answer 2.5

Confirmatory tests include:
- Amniocentesis after 15 weeks.
- Chorionic villous sampling from 11th to 13th weeks.
- Analysis of cell free fetal DNA in the maternal serum.

QUESTION 3

3.1 This is the karyotype of a 16-year-old girl. Name this condition.
3.2 Is this condition routinely diagnosed prenatally? Give reasons for your answer.
3.3 Can this condition be diagnosed in the newborn baby? Give reasons for your answer.
3.4 Mention two tests which can be used to diagnose this condition prenatally.

Answer 3.1

Turner's syndrome

Answer 3.2

This condition is not routinely diagnosed prenatally because:
- There are no routine prenatal screening tests for the condition.
- It is usually a chance occurrence.

Answer 3.3

It is not usually diagnosed in the newborn baby as there are no external dysmorphic features at birth. However, this condition should be suspected in a child who is found to have a congenital heart defect.

Answer 3.4

Prenatal diagnosis can be carried out by:
- Chorionic villous sampling from 11 to 13 weeks
- Amniocentesis after 15 weeks

QUESTION 4

4.1 Mention a screening test for haemophilia.
4.2 What is the best method to exclude haemophilia in the fetus if a carrier woman attends the antenatal clinic at 15 weeks?
4.3 Can a father who has haemophilia and a normal mother produce affected sons? Draw a genetic diagram to support your answer.
4.4 Can an unaffected father and a carrier mother produce affected and unaffected sons? Draw a genetic diagram to support your answer.

Answer 4.1

Determination of the fetal sex by analysis of cell free fetal DNA in the maternal blood, from 10 weeks onwards, in carrier women, is helpful because if the fetus is a female the disease can be excluded.

Answer 4.2

Fetal sex should be determined by cell free fetal DNA analysis. Amniocentesis should be performed in a male fetus, to confirm the diagnosis by performing genetic studies on fetal cells.

Answer 4.3

No

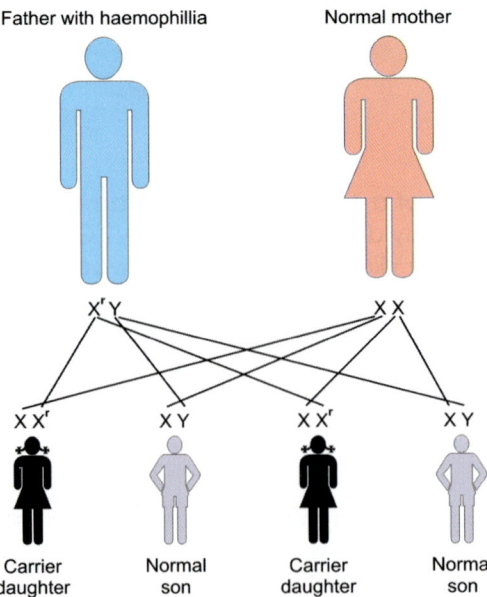

Answer 4.4

Yes

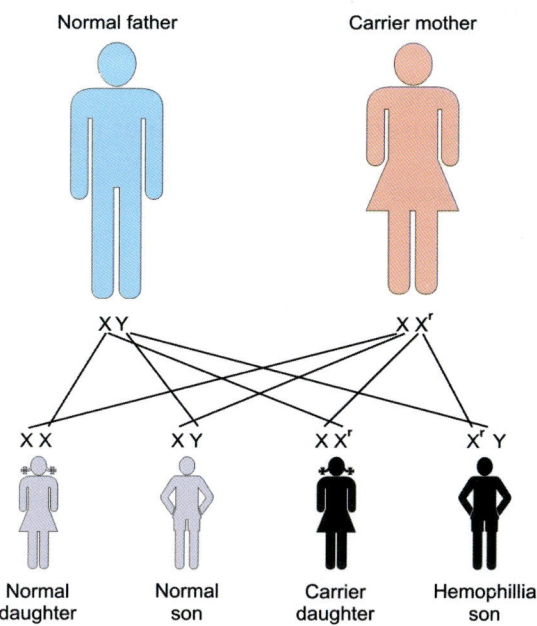

Normal father   Carrier mother

X Y   X X^r

X X   X Y   X X^r X^r Y

Normal daughter   Normal son   Carrier daughter   Hemophillia son

QUESTION 5

5.1   A woman who is a thalassemia trait attends the antenatal clinic at a POA of 10 weeks. What is the next step in the management?

5.2   If the father is also a carrier what are their chances of having a child with thalassemia major? Give reasons for your answer.

5.3   If both parents are carriers what is the first step in the management during each pregnancy?

5.4   What advise will you give the couple regarding future pregnancies?

Answer 5.1

Thalassemia carrier status of the father should be assessed by performing haemoglobin electrophoresis to measure HbA2.

Answer 5.2

Since thalassemia is an autosomal recessive condition there is a 25% chance of having a child with thalassemia major during each pregnancy.

Answer 5.3

Analysis of cell free fetal DNA should be performed at 9 weeks. Chorionic villous sampling may be performed at 12 weeks.

Answer 5.4

Since thalassemia is an autosomal recessive condition there is only a 25% chance of having a child with thalassemia major during each pregnancy. Therefore, they can embark on a pregnancy. An affected child can be identified early by the methods given in 5.3.

QUESTION 6

Mention the prenatal diagnostic tests and POA at which they should be performed for the following conditions.

6.1 Fetal varicella syndrome
6.2 Fetal abnormalities caused by type 1 diabetes mellitus
6.3 Anencephaly
6.4 Congenital heart disease
6.5 Cystic fibrosis

Answer 6.1

USS is performed at 20 weeks or 5 weeks after the infection.

Answer 6.2

USS is performed at 20 weeks.

Answer 6.3

USS is performed after 12 weeks.

Answer 6.4

Fetal echocardiography is performed during the second trimester.

Answer 6.5

DNA analysis is performed on fetal cells obtained by CVS at 11–13 weeks or amniocentesis after 15 weeks.

QUESTION 7

Mention 3 methods available to confirm the antenatal diagnosis of the following fetal abnormalities.

7.1 Down's syndrome
7.2 Thalassemia major
7.3 Mention a method available to detect fetal abnormalities caused by the use of anti-epileptic drugs.
7.4 Name 3 conditions which can be treated if detected in the early neonatal period.

Answer 7.1

- Chorionic villous sampling from 11 to 13 weeks.
- Amniocentesis at 15 weeks.
- Analysis of cell free fetal DNA in the maternal blood from 8 weeks.

Answer 7.2

- Chorionic villous sampling from 11 to 13 weeks.
- Amniocentesis at 15 weeks.
- Analysis of cell free fetal DNA in the maternal blood from 8 weeks.

Answer 7.3

Anti-epileptic drugs cause structural fetal abnormalities which can be diagnosed by ultrasound scanning at 20 weeks.

Answer 7.4

- Congenital hypothyroidism
- Phenyl ketonuria
- Galactosaemia

References
- *SBA Questions in Obstetrics, Chapter 11.*
- *Obstetrics by Ten Teachers, 19th Edition, Chapter 7, page 75–85*

Perinatal Infections

A woman is exposed to chickenpox at a period of amenorrhoea of 10 weeks. She does not give a history of having had the disease previously.

1.1   What is the first step in the management?

1.2   How can you prevent this woman from developing the disease.?

1.3   A woman develops chickenpox at 39 weeks. She has no other pregnancy complications. What is the best method to prevent neonatal infection?

1.4   A woman who has developed chickenpox 2 days ago is admitted in labour. What is the best method to prevent infection in the neonate?

Answer 1.1

Test maternal blood for antibodies against varicella zoster virus.

Answer 1.2

Test her blood for antibodies against varicella zoster virus and administer varicella zoster immunoglobulin as soon as possible after exposure, if the woman does not have IgG antibodies against varicella zoster virus.

Answer 1.3

Continue the pregnancy for at least one week till the acute infection subsides and the mother develops antibodies against the virus.

Answer 1.4

Administer varicella zoster immunoglobulin (VZIG) to the neonate soon after birth.

2.1   What are the fetal risks, if the mother develops chickenpox during the pregnancy?

2.2　A woman develops chickenpox at a POA of 8 weeks. What are the abnormalities which will occur in the fetus and how will you diagnose these abnormalities?

2.3　How will you counsel a woman who develops chickenpox at a POA of 8 weeks?

Answer 2.1

If a pregnant woman develops varicella or shows serological conversion in the first 28 weeks of pregnancy, the fetus has a small risk of developing fetal varicella syndrome (about 0.55% at 8 weeks).

Answer 2.2

The fetus may develop limb deformity, microcephaly, hydrocephalus, soft tissue calcification, scarring of the skin and fetal growth restriction.

She should be referred to a fetal medicine specialist and an USS should be performed at 20 weeks.

Answer 2.3

- She should be informed that the fetus has a small risk of developing fetal varicella syndrome (about 0.55% at 8 weeks). It can be diagnosed by USS at 20 weeks.
- The woman should be advised to avoid contact with others especially other pregnant women and neonates.
- She should get advice from her general practitioner, but should not attend the antenatal clinic.
- She should rest at home, drink plenty of fluid, eat a light diet and take paracetamol to control fever.
- She should get admitted only if she has a persistently high temperature not responding to paracetamol or if she develops respiratory or neurological symptoms.

References for Questions 1 and 2
- *Chickenpox in Pregnancy, RCOG Green-top Guideline No. 13, Published: 21/01/2015.*
- *SBA Questions in Obstetrics, Chapter 10.*

QUESTION 3

A woman complains of discharge and soreness in the vulval region at a period of amenorrhoea of 36 weeks. Examination reveals small discreet, tender ulcers in the labia majora, minora and perineum.

3.1　What is the most likely diagnosis?

3.2　How will you confirm the diagnosis?

3.3　What is the next step in the management?

3.4　What is the best treatment option, if the woman does not have antibodies against the infecting strain?

3.5　What is the best treatment option, if she gives a history of a similar episode before becoming pregnant, and has antibodies against the infecting organism?

3.6　What is the best treatment option, if a woman develops the infection at 20 weeks and does not have antibodies against the infecting strain?

Answer 3.1

Genital herpes

Answer 3.2

The diagnosis is confirmed by identifying the infecting organism and the type by performing a PCR test on swabs taken from the ulcer.

Answer 3.3

Test for type specific IgG antibodies against the infecting organism in the maternal serum.

Answer 3.4

Treat with oral acyclovir (400 mg 3 times a day) and perform an elective caesarean section at 38 weeks.

Answer 3.5

Treat with oral acyclovir and allow vaginal delivery.

Answer 3.6

Allow spontaneous onset of labour and normal vaginal delivery at term as she will develop antibodies against the infecting strain in 6 weeks. Oral acyclovir can be given if the infection is severe, but is best avoided as she is just 20 weeks pregnant. She can be treated with oral aciclovir from 36 weeks onwards to prevent recurrence of ulcers and viral shedding at the time of delivery.

References for Question 3
- *Management of genital herpes in pregnancy RCOG Green-top Guideline No. 30 (September 2007).*
- *SBA Questions in Obstetrics, Chapter 10.*

QUESTION 4

4.1   What is the test you will perform to advise a woman who is 6 weeks pregnant regarding her risk of contacting rubella?

4.2   What is the method you would adopt to diagnose occurrence of the disease in a woman who is exposed to rubella infection at a period of amenorrhoea of 10 weeks? Her immune status is not known.

4.3   What is the risk of the fetus developing congenital rubella, if the mother develops the infection:
a. before 11 weeks of gestation
b. at 11–12 weeks
c. at 15–16 weeks
d. between 16 and 20 weeks
e. after 20 weeks

4.4   A woman whose immune status is unknown is exposed to rubella infection at a period of amenorrhoea of 10 weeks. Serological testing one week after exposure shows rubella specific IgM antibodies. What is the most appropriate management?

4.5   Is there any method of preventing occurrence of the infection in a non-immune woman who is exposed to rubella.

Answer 4.1

Maternal serum should be tested for rubella specific IgG antibodies. If antibodies are present she can be reassured that she is unlikely to develop rubella. If antibodies are absent she should be advised to avoid exposure to rubella and she should be tested for antibodies if she is exposed to rubella.

Answer 4.2

- Since her immune status is not known the first step in the management is, to test maternal serum for rubella specific IgG and IgM antibodies immediately, to determine the immune status and after 3 weeks to detect the occurrence of infection.
- Presence of rubella specific IgG antibodies in the initial serum sample will indicate immunity. Presence of IgM antibodies in the first or second samples will indicate acute infection with a high risk of congenital rubella.
- If IgM is negative and there is a significant increase in IgG in the second sample, infection may have occurred, but there is a reduced risk of congenital rubella.

Answer 4.3

a. Before 11 weeks of gestation—90%
b. At 11–12 weeks—33%
c. At 15–16 weeks—24%
d. Between 16 and 20 weeks—less than 1%
e. After 20 weeks—0%

Answer 4.4

Presence of IgM antibodies indicate acute infection with a high-risk of congenital rubella as her POA is 10 weeks. Therefore, she should be counselled regarding the high-risk of the fetus developing congenital rubella syndrome.

Answer 4.5

There is no known method.

References for Question 4
- *SBA Questions in Obstetrics, Chapter 10*
- *Rubella in pregnancy, SOGC clinical practice guidelines, 203, February 2008.*

QUESTION 5

5.1 A woman who is HIV positive at a period of amenorrhoea of 20 weeks has a viral load of 100, 000 copies per ml of serum. Mention 3 important steps in the management.

5.2 What are the indications for zidovudine monotherapy?

5.3 What are the indications for elective caesarean section?

5.4 When is vaginal delivery allowed?

5.5 What are the precautions which should be taken if vaginal delivery is allowed?

5.6 What precautions will you take to prevent vertical transmission?

Answer 5.1

- Commence combined anti-retroviral therapy.
- Test for other sexually transmitted infections. She should also be tested for antibodies against rubella measles and varicella zoster.
- She should be vaccinated with killed vaccines, against hepatitis B, Pneumococcus and influenza.
- Her sexual contacts should be traced, tested and treated.

Answer 5.2

- The plasma viral load should be less than 10,000 copies per ml.
- The delivery should be by elective caesarean section.

Answer 5.3

LSCS is done between 38 and 39 weeks for women:
- Taking cART, who have a plasma viral load greater than 50 copies/ml.
- Taking ZDV monotherapy.
- With HIV and hepatitis C.

Answer 5.4

Vaginal delivery is allowed for women on cART whose viral load is less than 50 copies/ml.

Answer 5.5

- Insertion of prostaglandins and sweeping of membranes is not contraindicated.
- cART should be given throughout labour.
- Invasive procedures are contraindicated.
- Amniotomy should be delayed till delivery is imminent.
- If instrumental delivery is indicated, low cavity forceps are preferable to vacuum.

Answer 5.6

- Give anti-retroviral therapy for the mother.
- Perform an elective caesarean section.
- Avoid breast feeding.
- Give anti-retroviral therapy for the baby.

References for Question 5
- SBA Questions in Obstetrics, Chapter 10.
- British HIV Association guidelines for the management of HIV infection in pregnant women 2012 (Updated May 2014).

QUESTION 6

6.1   What is the most likely cause for the abnormalities seen in these images?
6.2   List 4 other complications of this condition.
6.3   What are the investigations which should be performed in the baby ?
6.4   What are the investigations you would perform in the mother?
6.5   How will you treat the baby?
6.6   How will you manage the mother?
6.7   At what stage of the disease is vertical transmission more likely?

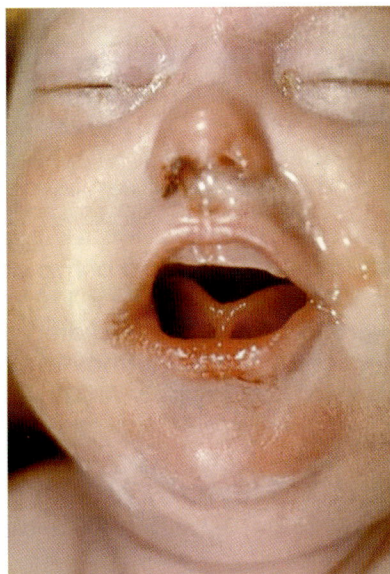 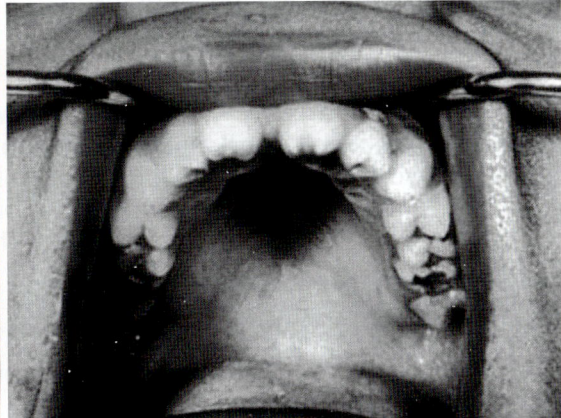

From Wikipedia commons

Answer 6.1

Congenital syphilis

Answer 6.2

- Blindness
- Deafnes
- Bone defects
- Failure to thrive

Answer 6.3

- VDRL test
- Fluorescent treponemal antibody (FTA) test or treponema pallidum haemagglutination (TPHA) test
- Bone X-ray
- Lumbar puncture.

Answer 6.4

- VDRL test
- Confirm the infection with FTA or TPHA
- Perform blood tests for HIV and hepatitis B
- Obtain an endocervical swab for DNA amplification tests to detect Chlamydia and Gonococcus.

Answer 6.5

Give procaine penicillin 50,000 units/kg daily for 7 days.

Answer 6.6

- Give 2.4 mega units of benzathine penicillin as a single dose.

- Trace and test the partners.
- Advise regarding safe sex.

Answer 6.7

It is more likely in the early stages of the disease.

QUESTION 7

A primipara is admitted at a POA of 38 weeks with fever and myalgia of two days duration. She appears flushed. Her temperature is 101°F. Her pulse rate is 110/min, low volume and blood pressure is 100/70 mmHg. She is mildly dehydrated, not icteric and the respiratory system and the abdomen are clinically normal. She has a single live fetus in cephalic presentation. The fetal heart rate is regular and 160 bpm.

The following investigations are available:
- Full blood count-white cell count of 2.5×10^9/L ($4–11 \times 10^9$/L), Hb of 14.5 g/dL (12–16 g/dL) with PCV of 48% and platelet count of 152×10^9/L ($150–400 \times 10^9$/L)
- SGPT–74 U/L (up to 40 U/L)
- SGOT–100U/L(up to 38 U/L)
- UFR–Protein–trace, Pus cells–occasional, red cells–2–4/HPF, organisms not seen
- CTG–160 bpm, non-reactive
7.1   What is the most likely diagnosis? Give your reasons.
7.2   What is your first line management?
7.3   If the diagnosis of dengue is confirmed how will you observe her to detect development of complications early?

Answer 7.1

Viral fever. Dengue should be excluded because she:
- appears flushed with myalgia.
- has a low white cell count with a high PCV.
- has elevated liver enzymes.

Answer 7.2

- Rapid assessment patient's condition. Check for evidence of dengue fever such as flushing, conjunctival petichae and tenderness over the liver.
- Perform an USS and repeat the cardiotocograph to assess fetal well-being.
- Perform an ELISA test for dengue NS 1 antigen.
- Inform the medical team immediately.
- Maintain a fluid balance chart and review 6 hourly. Give 2500 ml of fluid for 24 hours.
- Maintain a temperature chart. Paracetamol can be given to reduce the temperature. NSAIDs and aspirin should not be given.

Answer 7.3

- The patient should be managed in the obstetric high dependency unit.
- A multi-disciplinary approach with active involvement of a physician, anaesthetist, paediatrician/neonatologist, radiologist and haematologist is essential.

- Monitor using dengue monitoring blue chart-monitor BP, pulse rate and respiratory rate continuously, urine output hourly and assess fluid balance 3–6 hourly. Urine output should be maintained at 0.5–1 ml/kg/hour.
- Give 2500 ml of fluid daily. Oral fluids should include fruit juices and king coconut water. Avoid giving plain water. Intravenous fluids should include normal saline or Hartmann's solution and should be given if the patient is unable to tolerate oral fluids
- Perform FBC twice a day, PCV 6 hourly, SGPT/OT and serum electrolytes daily.
- Crossmatch 2 pints of blood.
- Perform ultrasound scanning daily to exclude ascites and pleural effusion.
- Monitor the fetus via CTG and ultrasound scanning. Avoid delivery during the acute phase.
- Explain to the family members about the course of dengue fever and the management.

Diabetes Mellitus Complicating Pregnancy

QUESTION 1

1.1 A 30-year-old multiparous woman with type 2 diabetes mellitus attends the prenatal clinic. List the important steps in the management at the prenatal clinic before allowing her to conceive.

1.2 What are the investigations which should be done to assess the level of control of diabetes in a woman with type 2 diabetes at the booking visit at a POA of 6 weeks? Give your reasons.

1.3 A 25-year-old primipara whose both parents have type 2 diabetes mellitus attends the antenatal clinic at a POA of 12 weeks. What is the best method to detect the occurrence of GDM or diabetes mellitus in this woman?

1.4 What is the range of blood sugar values in the OGTT which would indicate the presence of GDM?

1.5 What are the investigations which should be performed next in a woman with an abnormal OGTT? Give your reasons for performing these investigations.

Answer 1.1

- HbA1c should be 6.5% or lower as this indicates good control. Women whose levels are above 10% should be strongly advised against conception until good glycaemic control is achieved, in view of the higher risk of congenital anomalies.
- Diabetes should be well controlled. Fasting blood sugar should be between 5–7 mmol/L and pre-meal values and blood sugar levels at other times of the day should be between 4 and 7 mmol/L.
- Only metformin and insulin can be used as hypoglycaemic agents.
- Angiotensin-converting enzyme inhibitors and angiotensin-II receptor antagonists and statins should be discontinued before conception, or as soon as pregnancy is confirmed.
- She should be commenced on folic acid 5 mg daily.
- Weight should be reduced if the BMI is above 27 kg/m^2.
- Retinal, renal and cardiac assessment should be done and any abnormalities should be treated.

Answer 1.2

- HbA1c is the first test that should be done at the booking visit in those who are known diabetics, as it indicates the degree of control during the past three months. Good diabetic control during the time of conception and in the first trimester will reduce the fetal and maternal complications including fetal abnormalities.
- A 6 sample blood sugar series (FBS, pre-prandial and postprandial blood sugar after the three main meals) is performed next, to assess the blood sugar levels throughout the day in order to plan the treatment regimen.

Answer 1.3

Perform a 3 point OGTT at the booking visit and if it is normal repeat the test again at 28 weeks.

Answer 1.4

- FBS between 92 and 126 mg/dL (5.1–7 mmol/L)
- 1 hour PPBS >180 mg/dL (10 mmol/L)
- 2 hour PPBS between 140 and 200 mg/dl (7.8–11.1 mmol/L)

The above values are recommended in the NICE guidelines. IADPSG (International Association of Diabetes and Pregnancy Groups) recommend values of FBS 92 mg, 1 hour PPBS 189 mg and 2 hour PPBS 153 mg/dL.

Answer 1.5

- Perform HbA1c to determine whether she has had undetected diabetes previously. If the HbA1c is less than 6.1% pre-existing diabetes can be excluded and a diagnosis of GDM can be confirmed (this is not necessary, if diabetes has been excluded by performing a PPBS earlier during the pregnancy).
- Perform a 6 point blood sugar series to assess the blood sugar levels throughout the day to plan the method of treatment.

QUESTION 2

A multipara with type 2 diabetes mellitus attends the antenatal clinic at 28 weeks. Her fasting blood sugar is 7.5 mmol/L and the post prandial values 2 hours after lunch and dinner are 9 mmol/L and 11 mmol/L respectively. Her BMI is 25 kg/m².
2.1   What are the treatment options? Give your reasons.
2.2   How will you monitor the treatment?
2.3   What are the other tests which should be performed at 28 weeks?

Answer 2.1

- Commence on a diabetic diet and regular exercise which is the first step in the management of all patients with diabetes.
- She should be commenced on insulin immediately as the fasting blood sugar is more than 7 mmol/L. Commence on 3 pre-meal doses of soluble insulin.
- Commence with a small dose of insulin (6 units) and adjust the dose according to the response. Ideally fasting, pre and postprandial blood sugar levels should be done daily before and 1 hour after the main meals. Bedtime blood sugar levels also should be done.
- Add isophane insulin at night, if the post dinner and the fasting sugar levels cannot be controlled with soluble insulin alone.

Answer 2.2

- Diabetics who are on a multiple daily insulin injection regimen should test their fasting, pre-meal, 1-hour post-meal and bedtime blood glucose levels daily during pregnancy.
- However, if the woman is unable to test the blood sugar at home a 6 point BSS is performed one week after commencing treatment. After the effective drug regimen is established blood sugar series should be performed once in 2 weeks.

Answer 2.3

- Renal and retinal assessment should be done.
- USS should be done for fetal growth, macrosomia and liquor volume. USS should be repeated once in 3 weeks.

QUESTION 3

3.1   What are the fetal complications of type 1 and type 2 diabetes mellitus?
3.2   What are the maternal complications of type 1 and type 2 diabetes mellitus?
3.3   How and when will you deliver a woman with type 1 or type 2 diabetes mellitus?
3.4   How will you monitor the blood sugar levels during labour?

Answer 3.1

- Congenital abnormalities occur only in those with pre-existing diabetes especially if the control is poor at the time of conception and in the first trimester. Commonest is cardiovascular, also neural, renal and skeletal defects can occur. Sacral agenesis is rare but specific for diabetes.
- Macrosomia can occur and can cause birth asphyxia and birth trauma.
- Intrauterine growth restriction.
- Sudden intrauterine death.

Answer 3.2

- Pregnancy induced hypertension.
- Aggravation of retinopathy and nephropathy (assessed by serum creatinine and 24 hour protein excretion).
- Infections.
- Polyhydramnios.
- Ketoacidosis.
- Cephalo-pelvic disproportion due to fetal macrosomia.

Answer 3.3

Women with type 1 or type 2 diabetes and no other complications should be delivered by induction of labour, or by elective caesarean section if indicated due to obstetric reasons, between 37 + 0 weeks and 38 + 6 weeks.

Answer 3.4

- Blood glucose should be maintained between 4 and 6 mmol/L.
- Blood glucose is assessed hourly.
- A insulin dextrose drip is needed in resistant cases.

- Intravenous dextrose infusion with potassium chloride 20 mmol/L at the rate of 10 g/hour (100 ml) using a10% solution and human actrapid insulin 6 units in 60 ml of normal saline (1 unit/10 ml) is delivered via an infusion pump.
- Insulin is commenced at the rate of 1 unit/hour if the blood glucose level is between 4 and 6 mmol/L.

  Check the blood glucose hourly, if more than 6 double the insulin dose and if less than 4 halve the dose. Halve the dose soon after delivery.

QUESTION 4

4.1 A woman with type 2 diabetes mellitus attends the antenatal clinic at 20 weeks. Her fasting blood sugar is 5 mmol /liter and the 2 hour post prandial values after lunch and dinner are 6.4 mmol/L and 6.2 mmol/liter respectively. Pre-prandial blood sugar levels before lunch and dinner are 7.4 mmol/L and 7 mmol/L respectively. She is on three pre-meal doses of soluble insulin. What is the best management option? Give your reasons.

4.2 A multipara is found to have GDM at 24 weeks. Her fasting blood sugar is 6 mmol/L and the postprandial values 1 hour after lunch and dinner are 8 mmol/L and 7.9 mmol/L respectively. Her BMI is 30 kg/m^2. What are the treatment options? Give your reasons.

4.3 A multipara with GDM who is on metformin attends the antenatal clinic at 35 weeks. Her fasting blood sugar is 6. 5 mmol/L and the postprandial values 1 hour after lunch and dinner are 9 mmol/L and 8.5 mmol/L respectively. Her BMI is 30 kg/m^2. USS revealed fetal macrosomia and hydramnios. What is the next step in the management? Give your reasons.

4.4 What are the maternal complications of GDM?

4.5 What are the fetal complications of GDM?

4.6 When and how will you deliver a woman with GDM?

Answer 4.1

This woman is most probably taking snacks with a high glycaemic index between meals, resulting in high pre-prandial sugar values. The insulin dose seems to be satisfactory as the fasting and postprandial sugar values are under control.

Advise the woman to avoid taking snacks with a high glycaemic index and perform a 6 point BSS after 3 days.

Answer 4.2

Commence her on a diabetic diet and advise regular exercise.

Perform a blood sugar series after 2 weeks and if the fasting blood sugar is more than 5.1 mmol/L or the 1 hour PPBS values after the main meals is more than 7.8 mmol/L commence on metformin.

Answer 4.3

Continue metformin and add 3 pre-meal doses of soluble insulin.

It is better to add insulin than to increase the dose of metformin because:
- Her blood sugar levels are high.
- She has hydramnios and macrosomia which indicate poor control.
- She is close to term.
- She should be advised to follow the dietary advice.

Answer 4.4

- Pregnancy induced hypertension.
- Infections.
- Polyhydramnios.
- Cephalo-pelvic disproportion due to fetal macrosomia.

Answer 4.5

- Macrosomia can cause birth asphyxia and birth trauma.
- Sudden intrauterine death

Answer 4.6

- Women with gestational diabetes who are well controlled should be delivered by 39–40 weeks by elective induction of labour. Caesarean section is indicated for obstetric reasons.
- Poorly controlled diabetics should be delivered by 37 weeks after a course of corticosteroids.

References

- *Diabetes in pregnancy: Management of diabetes and its complications from preconception to the postnatal period. NICE guidelines [NG3] Published date: February 2015.*
- *Obstetrics by Ten Teachers, 19th Edition page 163–164.*
- *Diabetes and pregnancy—an Endocrine Society Clinical Practice Guideline (optional reading)*
- *SBA Questions in Obstetrics, Chapter 6.*

Pregnancy Induced Hypertension

A 30-year-old primipara is admitted with generalized fits at a POA of 32 weeks.

1.1 What is the first step in the management?
1.2 Mention 5 questions you would ask the accompanying person.
1.3 What are the initial examinations you would perform?
1.4 How will you diagnose eclampsia in this woman?
1.5 Mention your immediate management if this woman is having eclamptic fits.
1.6 What precautions should be taken when a woman is given magnesium sulphate? How will you determine magnesium toxicity?
1.7 How will you manage magnesium toxicity?
1.8 What is the definitive management of this woman?
1.9 What are the complications of eclampsia?
   (This type of long questions are asked at postgraduate examinations but can be divided into several questions for undergraduates.)

Answer 1.1

Maintain a patent airway and breathing by:
• Turning to the lateral side.
• Sucking out secretions.
• Inserting an oropharyngeal airway.
• Oxygen inhalation with a face mask.

Answer 1.2

• Did she have high blood pressure during the antenatal period?
• Is she known to have epileptic fits?
• Did she have fever or a fall with a head injury?
• Has she had headaches recently?
• What is the LRMP and are her antenatal records available?

Answer 1.3

• Check the blood pressure.

- Assess the level of consciousness.
- Examine the lung bases for crepitations as she may have aspirated.
- Perform an obstetric abdominal and vaginal examination.
- Perform a complete nurological examination.

Answer 1.4

Eclampsia is diagnosed in a pregnant woman who is having fits, by the presence of elevated blood pressure and significant proteinuria (++) in the urine ward test.

Answer 1.5

- Maintain a patent airway. Insert 2 intravenous canuulae.
- Control fits by giving a bolus dose of 4 g of magnesium sulphate by slow intravenous injection and commence an infusion at the rate of 1 g hourly.
- Control the blood pressure by giving labetalol 20 mg by slow intravenous injection. The dose can be repeated at 15 minute intervals up to a maximum of 80 mg.
- Obtain blood for coagulation profle, liver function tests, renal function tests, full blood count and random blood sugar. Crossmatch 1 pint of blood.
- Insert an indwelling catheter and maintain an intake output chart.
- Perform an USS to determine the gestational age and the viability of the fetus.
- Admit to the ICU.
- Prepare for caesarean section.
- Monitor:
  - The pulse and respiratory rates, blood pressure, oxygen saturation and fetal heart rate continuously.
  - Patellar reflex hourly and observe for fits
  - Urine output hourly.

Answer 1.6

Treatment should be monitored by hourly assessment of the patellar reflex and continuous monitoring of oxygen saturation and respiratory rates. Monitoring of serum levels are needed only if the patient has oliguria. Urine output is measured hourly. Nifedipine should not be used with magnesium sulphate as both block calcium channels.

Respiratory depression is the first sign of magnesium toxicity. The drug should be stopped if

- The respiratory rate reaches 16/minute.
- There is loss of deep tendon reflexes. This occurs when the serum levels exceed 5 mmol/L
- The urine output is less than 30 ml/hour

Answer 1.7

- The first step in treating magnesium toxicity is to stop the drug.
- The next step is to give 10 mg of 10% calcium gluconate intravenously.

Answer 1.8

- Delivery should be carried out as soon as possible if the fetus is alive.
- The best method of delivery is by caesarean section under general anaesthesia as the POA is 32 weeks. General anaesthesia is used for brain protection as she has

fits. Spinal anaesthesia is not used because the intracranial pressure may be elevated and a coagulopathy may be present.
- If the fetus is dead delivery can be postponed till the mother is stable.
- The mother should be monitored in the ICU for 48 hours as fits can occur and she can develop complications such as liver, coagulation and renal impairment.

Answer 1.9

- Cerebrovascular accidents
- Respiratory failure due to aspiration
- Liver failure
- Renal failure
- Disseminated intravascular coagulation
- HELLP syndrome
- Placental abruption
- Heart failure
- Fetal distress
- Fetal death

QUESTION 2

A primipara has a blood pressure of 160/105 mmHg at 38 weeks. The fetus is in cephalic presentation. The head is engaged. There is no proteinuria.
2.1 What are the investigations you would perform?
2.2 When should the fetus be delivered?
2.3 How will you decide the mode of delivery?
2.4 What is the best management option if the Bishop score is 3?

Answer 2.1

- Urine albumin ward test
- Full blood count and coagulation profile
- Renal function tests—serum electrolytes and creatinine
- Liver function tests—SGPT, serum bilirubin
- Ultrasound scan and Doppler studies
- Cardiotocograph

Answer 2.2

It is better to deliver the fetus at 38 weeks as she has moderately severe pregnancy induced hypertension.

Answer 2.3

Vaginal delivery is possible as she has no other obstetric problems. A vaginal examination should be performed to assess the Bishop score and the pelvis.

Answer 2.4

Insert 3 mg of dinoprostone to the vagina to ripen the cervix and to induce labour. Repeat the dose in 6 hours. Amniotomy can be done once labour is well established and the cervical dilatation is about 5–6 cm. Oxytocin should not be commenced till 6 hours after inserting prostaglandin.

QUESTION 3

A 25-year-old primipara attends the antenatal clinic at a period of amenorrhoea of 32 weeks. Her blood pressure is 150/95 mmHg. Urine examination revealed a moderate amount of albumin (++). She has a single fetus in the cephalic presentation.

3.1   What is the first step in the management?
3.2   What are the investigations you would perform?
3.3   How will you treat the hypertension?
3.4   How will you monitor the fetus?
3.5   How and when will you plan to deliver this woman?

Answer 3.1

Admit to hospital.

Answer 3.2

1. 24 hours urine protein estimation/urine ward test for protein should be done daily.
2. Full blood count and coagulation profile
3. Renal function tests—serum electrolytes and creatinine
4. Liver function tests—SGPT, serum bilirubin
5. Ultrasound scan and Doppler studies
6. Cardiotocograph
   - 2–4   should be done twice weekly
   - 5   should be done weekly
   - 6   should be done if the fetal movements are not satisfactory.

Answer 3.3

If the blood pressure remains above 149/99, 24 hours after admission to hospital commence anti-hypertensive drugs. Methyldopa (1–2 gm daily in 3 divided doses), nifedipine (40 mg per day in 2 divided doses up to a maximum of 120 mg per day) or labetalol (300 mg per day in 3 divided doses) are the recommended drugs. Labetalol is the drug of choice.

Answer 3.4

- Advise the woman to maintain a fetal movement chart.
- Perform a cardiotocograph if the movements are reduced.
- Perform USS for amniotic fluid volume and Doppler studies once a week.
- Perform USS for fetal growth once in three weeks.

Answer 3.5

- A course of corticosteroids should be given.
- Delivery is best carried out by 36 weeks by caesarean section.
- Earlier delivery is indicated if:
  - Blood pressure rises rapidly.
  - There are signs of impending eclampsia.
  - There are signs of other organ involvement.
  - There is reduced or absent diastolic flow.
  - The CTG is abnormal.

QUESTION 4

4.1 What are the indications to use anti-hypertensive drugs in pregnancy induced hypertension?

4.2 What are the recommended drugs and the doses?

4.3 What are the contraindicated drugs?

4.4 What are the indications for rapid reduction of blood pressure and what are the recommended drugs?

4.5 What are the drugs which can be used during breast feeding?

Answer 4.1

Antihypertensives should be commenced if the blood pressure remains elevated beyond 150/90 mmHg for 24 hours.

Answer 4.2

Labetalol is the first line drug. The other recommended drugs are methyl dopa and nifedepine (*refer* answer to question 3.3).

Answer 4.3

- Angiotensin receptor blockers—losartan
- Angiotensin converting enzyme inhibitors—enalapril and captopril
- Diuretics
  All these drugs can cause congenital abnormalities.

Answer 4.4

Rapid reduction of blood pressure is indicated if the diastolic blood pressure is greater than 110 mmHg.

The drugs used for rapid reduction of blood pressure include:
- Intravenous labetalol
- Intravenous hydrallazine
- Sublingual nifedepine if the woman is not having fits

Answer 4.5

- Labetalol
- Enalapril
- Captopril
- Atenolol
- Metoprolol

References
- *Hypertension in pregnancy: The management of hypertensive disorders during pregnancy. NICE guidelines (CG107). Published date: August 2010.*
- *SBA Questions in Obstetrics, Chapter 6.*

Fetal Surveillance

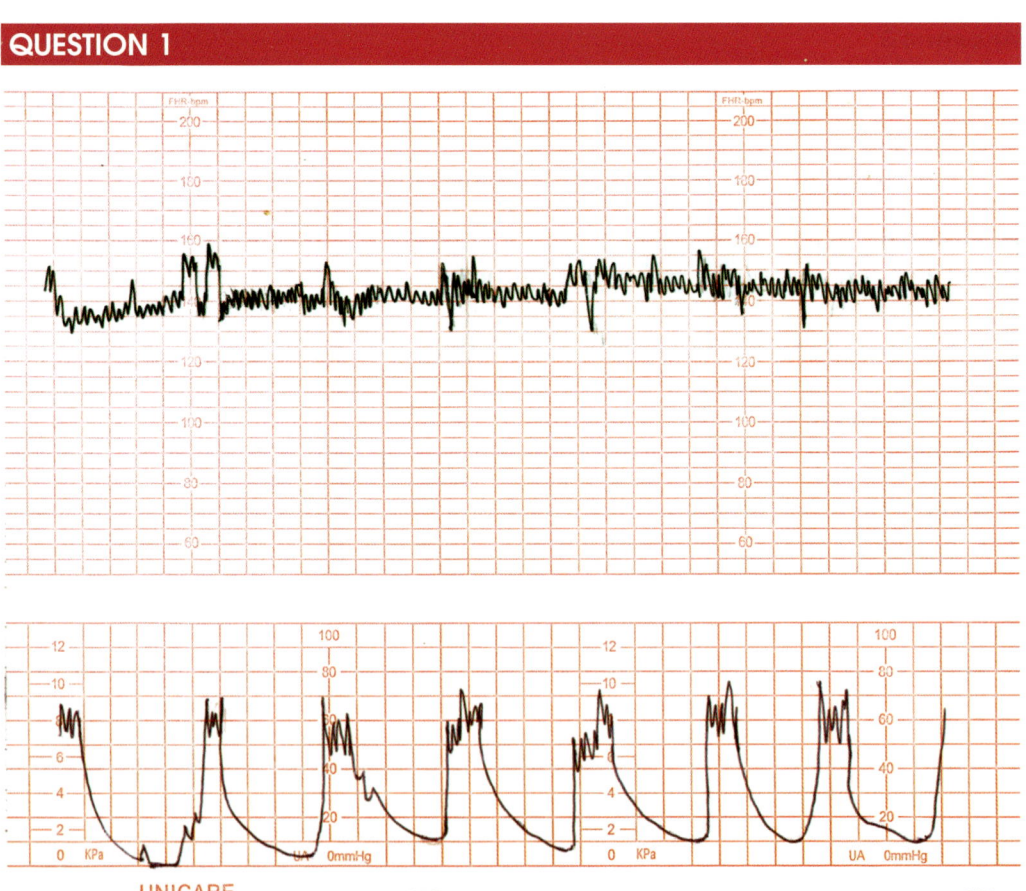

UNICARE

1.1 Write your observations regarding this CTG which was obtained during the first stage of labour.

1.2 How will you manage this patient? Give your reasons.

Answer 1.1

The CTG is normal because:
- The fetal heart rate is between 130 and 140 beats per minute.
- The beat to beat variability is more than 10 beats per minute.
- There are 2 accelerations.
- There are no decelerations.
- There are regular uterine contractions at a frequency of about 3–4 per 10 minutes.

Answer 1.2

Allow labour to progress anticipating normal vaginal delivery because:
- The fetal heart tracing is normal.
- There are regular frequent uterine contractions suitable for a patient in the active phase of the first stage.

QUESTION 2

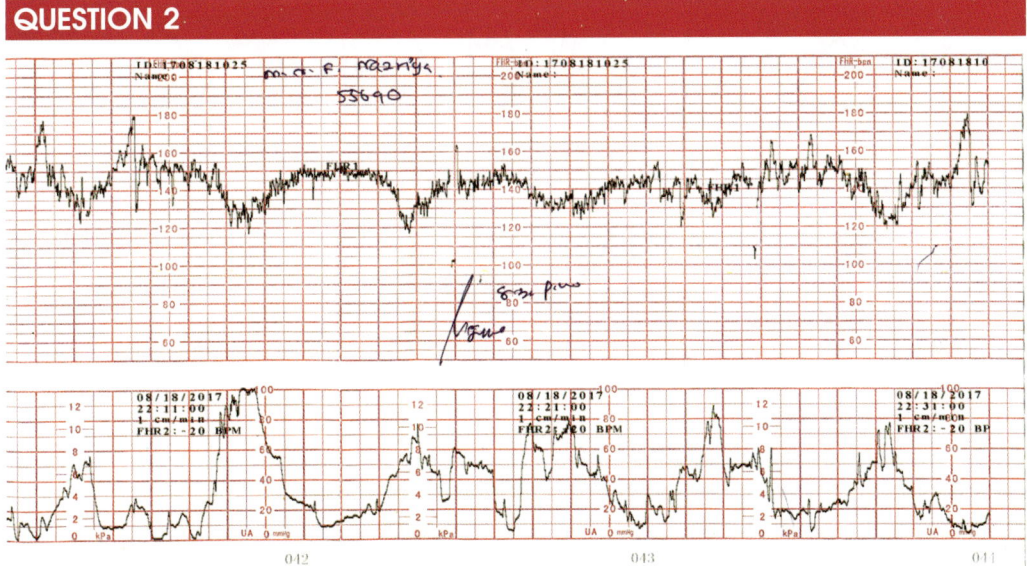

This is the cardiotocograph of a woman in the first stage of labour.
2.1   What are the abnormalities seen in this cardiotocograph?
2.2   What is the first-line management?
2.3   How will you manage this woman if the first-line treatment fails?

Answer 2.1

There are recurrent typical variable decelerations in the fetal heart rate and in-coordinate, frequent uterine contractions.

Answer 2.2

- If an oxytocin drip is running it should be discontinued.
- Turn the patient to the left lateral side to improve the placental blood flow and to relieve any cord compression
- Give oral gliceryl trinitrate or intravenous ritodrine or subcutaneous terbutaline to reduce the contractions. Commence an infusion of Hartmann's soulution.

- Perform fetal scalp blood sampling.
- Commence continuous fetal heart rate monitoring.

Answer 2.3

Perform a caesarean section if the abnormality persists or the fetal scalp blood pH is less than 7.2.

QUESTION 3

3.1 Write your observations regarding this cardiotocograph.
3.2 What is the first-line management?
3.3 How will you manage this woman if the first-line treatment fails?

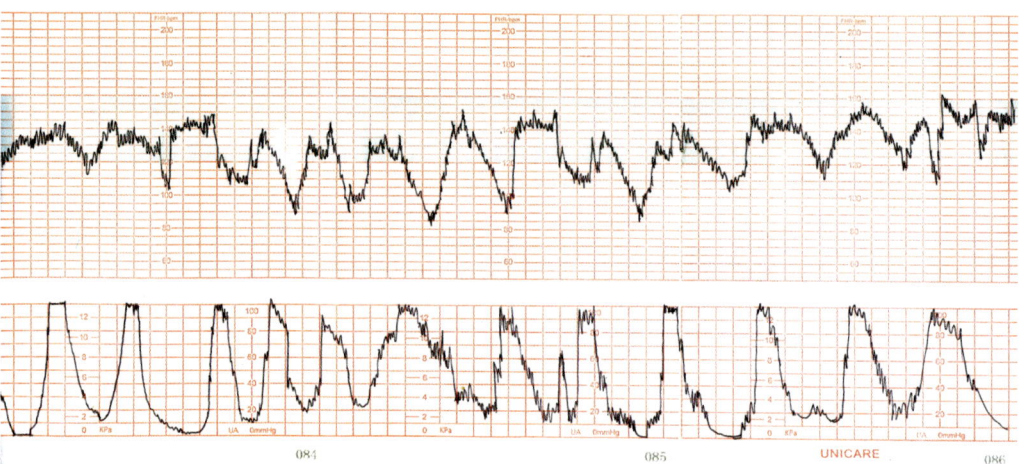

Answer 3.1

There are deep and frequent variable decelerations. The decelerations are atypical because they are U-shaped and there is slow return to the baseline.

There are strong and frequent uterine contractions with a frequency of more than 5 per 10 minutes.

Answer 3.2

- If an oxytocin drip is running it should be discontinued to reduce the frequency of uterine contractions.
- Give oral glyceryl trinitrate or intravenous ritodrine or subcutaneous terbutaline to reduce the contractions.
- Turn the patient to the left lateral side to improve the placental blood flow and to relieve any cord compression.
- Improve hydration with intravenous crystalloids.

Answer 3.3

Immediate delivery should be carried out. Fetal scalp blood sampling is not essential as the CTG pattern indicates acute fetal compromise. Perform a vaginal examination.

- Apply Simpson's forceps, if the patient is in the second stage and all the criteria for foceps delivery are satisfied.

- Perform a caesarean section if the patient is in the first stage or if the criteria for forceps delivery are not satisfied.

QUESTION 4

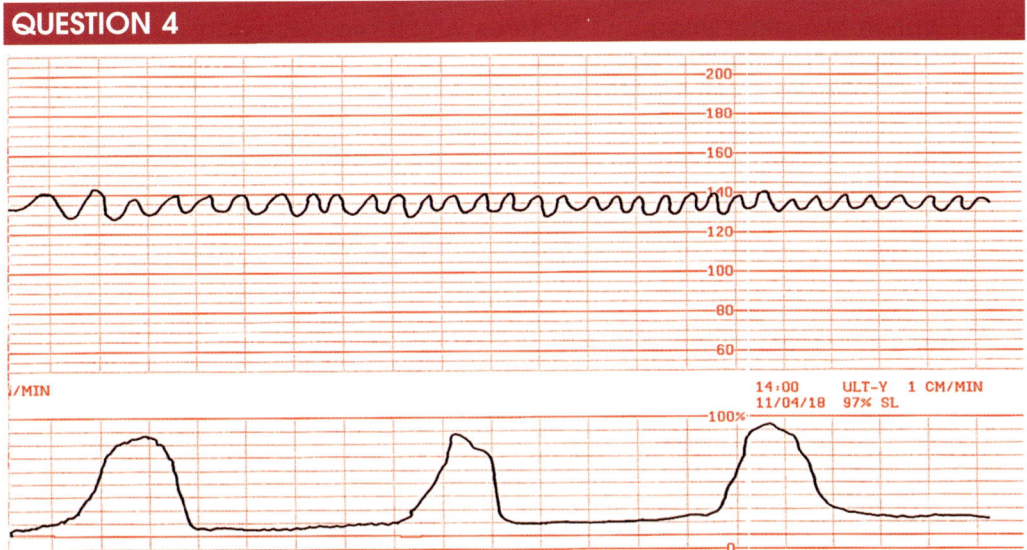

4.1 What is this abnormality?
4.2 What are the diagnostic criteria of this abnormality?
4.3 What are the causes of this abnormality?
4.4 What is your management?

Answer 4.1
Sinusoidal pattern of the fetal heart rate tracing

Answer 4.2
- The baseline fetal heart rate should be within the normal range of 120–160 bpm.
- The amplitude of the waves is rarely greater than 5–15 bpm.
- The frequency of the waves is between 2 and 5 cycles per minute.
- The short-term variability is fixed or flat.
- There are no areas of normal FHR variability or reactivity.
- Oscillation of the waves should be above and below a baseline.

Answer 4.3
- Severe fetal anaemia due to rupture of vasa praevia.
- Severe fetomaternal haemorrhage causing hydrops fetalis.
- Severe fetal hypoxia due to cord prolapse.
- Use of narcotic drugs.
- Fetal cardiac anomalies.
- Severe fetal infection.

Answer 4.4
Immediate delivery should be carried out by caesarean section or forceps delivery if the patient is in the second stage.

QUESTION 5

5.1   Mention one clinical situation in which a baseline bradycardia of 100–110 can be regarded as normal.

5.2   Mention two other important features which are necessary to regard this fetal heart rate pattern as normal.

5.3   What is the significance of (a) presence of accelerations, (b) absence of accelerations in a CTG?

5.4   What is meant by (a) reduced variability, (b) increased variability and (c) decelerations.

Answer 5.1

- Post-maturity
- Maternal hypothermia
- Administration of beta blockers

Answer 5.2

- There should be no decelerations.
- The baseline variability should be between 5 and 25 bpm

Answer 5.3

a. Presence of accelerations indicate a neurologically responsive fetus without hypoxia or acidosis.

b. Absence of accelerations is of uncertain significance.

Answer 5.4

a. Reduced variability is a band width <5 bpm for >50 min in baseline segments, or for >3 min during decelerations.

b. Increased variability (saltatory pattern) is a band width >25 bpm for >30 min.

c. A deceleration is a fall in the fetal heart rate of >15 bpm for >15 seconds.

QUESTION 6

6.1   How do you identify type 1 decelerations?

6.2   How do you identify type 2 decelerations?

6.3   How do you identify variable decelerations?

6.4   List 5 disadvantages of internal fetal heart rate monitoring.

6.5   List an advantage of internal fetal heart rate monitoring.

6.6   What is the recommended method of fetal heart rate monitoring?

Answer 6.1

Type 1 (early) decelerations are shallow, short-lasting, have normal variability, rapid recovery to the baseline and are coincident with uterine contractions. They begin early in the contraction and return to the baseline at the end of the contraction.

Answer 6.2

Type 2 (late) decelerations are U-shaped with reduced variability, start towards the middle or end of the uterine contraction with a gradual onset, have a nadir 20s after the acme of the contraction, and return to the baseline gradually after the end of the contraction with >30s from nadir to baseline.

Answer 6.3

Typical variable decelerations have a rapid drop to nadir within 30s after onset, good variability, rapid return to the baseline, are V-shaped but vary in shape, size and relation to uterine contractions.

Atypical variable decelerations: When variable decelerations develop features which increase the likelihood of fetal hypoxia/acidosis, they are described as atypical or complicated variable decelerations. These complicating features are:
- Baseline tachycardia.
- Persistent large amplitude (>60 bpm in depth) or long duration (>60 seconds) decelerations
- U-shaped decelerations
- Reduced variability within the deceleration
- Slow return to the baseline after the contraction has finished
- Disappearance of "shoulders" where it was initially present
- Smooth post-deceleration shoulders ("overshoots")

Answer 6.4

- It is more expensive because it requires a disposable electrode.
- The fetal electrode should be applied after clear identification of the presenting part and delicate fetal structures such as the sutures and fontanelles should be avoided.
- The membranes should be ruptured for application of the electrode and cannot be used in cases where amniotomy is contraindicated as in the presence of a high head.
- Since there is an increased risk of vertical transmission of infections, it should not be used in patients with active genital herpes infection and in those who are seropositive for hepatitis B, C, D, E, or to human immunodeficiency virus.
- It is best avoided in suspected fetal blood disorders and in prematurity.

Answer 6.5

It provides a more accurate interpretation of the fetal rate pattern.

Answer 6.6

External fetal heart rate monitoring is recommended.

QUESTION 7

List the indications for continuous fetal heart rate monitoring.

Answer

Indications for continuous fetal heart rate monitoring are:
- Maternal pulse over 120 beats/minute on 2 occasions 30 minutes apart.
- Temperature of 38°C or above on a single reading, or 37.5°C or above on 2 consecutive occasions 1 hour apart.
- Suspected chorioamnionitis or sepsis.
- Pain reported by the woman that differs from the pain normally associated with contractions.

- The presence of significant meconium.
- Fresh vaginal bleeding that develops in labour.
- Hypertension/pre-eclampsia
- Confirmed delay in the first or second stage of labour.
- Contractions that last longer than 60 seconds (hypertonus), or more than 5 contractions in 10 minutes (tachysystole).
- Oxytocin use.
  Continuous EFM should be commenced in women previously monitored with intermittent auscultation:
- If there is baseline bradycardia (less than 110 bpm) or tachycardia (greater than 160 bpm).
- If decelerations are detected on auscultation.
- If any intrapartum risk factors develop.
  (from NICE guidelines on CTG monitoring)

QUESTION 8

8.1   List the characteristics which are used in the interpretation of a CTG
8.2   List the characteristics of a non-reassuring CTG.
8.3   List the characteristics of a pathological CTG.

Answer 8.1

- Heart rate
- Baseline variability
- Presence/absence of decelerations
- Presence/absence of accelerations

Answer 8.2

- Fetal heart rate between 100–109 or 161–180 beats per minute
- Baseline variability less than 5 beats per minute for more than 40 minutes but less than 90 minutes.
- Presence of early decelerations, variable decelerations or a single prolonged deceleration up to 3 minutes.

Answer 8.3

- Fetal heart rate less than 100 or more than 180 beats per minute
- Baseline variability less than 5 beats per minute for more than 90 minutes.
- Presence of late decelerations, atypical variable decelerations or a single prolonged deceleration for more than 3 minutes.

QUESTION 9

How will you manage a woman with a:
9.1   Non-reassuring CTG
9.2   Pathological CTG

Answer 9.1

- Stop the oxytocin drip.
- If there is uterine hyper-contractility commence tocolytic drugs.

- Exclude maternal pyrexia, hypotension and dehydration.
- Commence intravenous crystalloids.
- Turn to the left lateral position.
- If the CTG does not improve carry out fetal blood sampling.

Answer 9.2

- Delivery should be performed.
- Perform fetal scalp blood sampling and deliver if the pH is less than 7.2.

References

- *FIGO guidelines on intrapartum fetal monitoring.*
- *NICE guidelines on fetal monitoring during labour.*

Caesarean Section

Describe how you would advise a registrar on the precautions which should be carried out when performing a second stage caesarean section (*surgical skills and teaching module for postgraduates but undergraduates should know the basic procedure.*)

Answer

- Inquire whether he has performed or seen a second stage caesarean section before.
- The operation should preferably be performed by a senior registrar/consultant.
- Check whether an urinary catheter has been inserted.
- It is better to try to disimpact the head by pushing it up before commencing the surgery.
- Stand on a step or lower the table. The table may be tilted into the Trendelenburg position.
- Commence the surgery in the usual manner. A transverse skin incision can be used.
- Care should be taken when opening into the peritoneal cavity as the bladder could be high.
- The peritoneum of the lower uterine segment should be opened into taking care not to damage the bladder. The bladder is pushed down and a lower segment incision is performed at a higher level.
- The head should be delivered in between uterine contractions. Intravenous glyceryl trinitrate may be given to relax the uterus.
- Delivery of the head can be done using one of the three methods described below.
  - Get an assistant to cup the head in the palm of the hand vaginally and push it up towards the surgeon's hand which is inserted between the anterior flap of the uterine incision and the fetal head, or
  - Perform internal podalic version and breech extraction.
    - o The surgeon inserts a hand into the fundus of the uterus grabs one foot and gently brings it out of the uterine incision. Traction on this leg will deliver

the other leg. Deliver the fetal trunk and the head in the manner in which a breech is delivered at caesarean section.

– Perform Patwardhan's technique

  o This is especially helpful if the anterior shoulder comes out of the uterine incision as happens in most cases. With gentle traction on this shoulder, the posterior shoulder is also delivered out. Next, the surgeon hooks the fingers through both the axillae and with gentle traction, aided by fundal pressure applied by the assistant, the body of the fetus is brought out of the uterus.

Now the baby's head which is the only part of the fetus which is still inside the uterus, is gently lifted out of the pelvis.

- A T extension may be performed in difficult cases .
- Inspect for tears after the delivery is completed. The uterus should be delivered out of the incision to obtain a good view to suture any deep tears.
- Close the uterus in the usual manner.
- If a T extension has been performed or if tears occur the patient should be informed regarding the implications for a future pregnancy.

QUESTION 2

Describe how you would teach a registrar the precautions which should be taken when performing a caesarean section for a transverse lie (*surgical skills and teaching module for postgraduates but undergraduates should know the basic procedure.*)

Answer

- Inquire whether he has performed or seen a caesarean section for transverse lie.
- The operation should preferably be performed by a senior registrar/consultant.
- Commence the surgery in the usual manner. A transverse skin incision can be used.
- The lower segment may be poorly developed due to the high presenting part. Therefore once the abdomen is opened check the development and the capacity of the lower segment.
- In most cases, it may be possible to deliver the fetus through a lower segment incision.
- Try to turn the fetus into a longitudinal lie. If this fails internal podalic version and breech extraction can be done as described in Question 1. This could be aided if necessary with intravenous glyceryl trinitrate.
- A T extension may be performed in difficult cases.
- If the lower segment is poorly formed a vertical incision will have to be made. It should be commenced low down and extended into the upper segment.
- Examine for tears after the delivery is completed.
- If an upper segment incision or a T extension has been performed the patient should be informed regarding the implications for a future pregnancy.

QUESTION 3

A second para who has previously had a caesarean section is found to have a central placenta previa at 36 weeks. There is no history of vaginal bleeding.

3.1   **What is the POA at which a caesarean section should be performed?**

3.2   **List the precautions which should be taken before performing a caesarean section for placenta previa.**

3.3   **List the specific risks of caesarean section for placenta previa which should be included in the consent form.**

3.4   **When is vaginal delivery possible in a woman with placenta previa?**

Answer 3.1

If a morbidly adherent placenta is suspected LSCS should be performed between 36–37 weeks. In others LSCS should be performed at 38 weeks.

Answer 3.2

- The patient should be informed regarding all the additional risks.(*see* answer 3.3)
- The operation should be performed by a consultant obstetrician. A consultant anaesthetist should be present.
- The preoperative haemoglobin level should be more than 12 gm/dL.
- A morbidly adherent placenta should be excluded by performing a MRI scan.
- A catheter should be inserted into the uterine artery if profuse bleeding is anticipated or if a morbidly adherent placenta is suspected.
- Five units of blood should be cross matched.
- An ICU bed should be available.

Answer 3.3

The woman should be informed regarding the risk of:
- Profuse bleeding during and after the delivery.
- The need to transfuse large volumes of blood.
- The possibility of a morbidly adherent placenta with the associated risks such as:
  - Profuse haemorrhage
  - The need to perform a hysterectomy.
  - The need to leave the placenta *in situ* especially in primiparous women with the risk of bleeding and infection.
  - Bladder injury in cases of placenta percreta invading into the bladder.
- The need to perform an upper segment caesarean section in some cases and the problems it could cause in subsequent pregnancies.
- Of death due to uncontrolled haemorrhage.

Answer 3.4

Normal vaginal delivery may be possible if the placental edge is more than 4 cm away from the internal os and the placenta is thin.

QUESTION 4

Describe how you would advise a registrar on the precautions which should be carried out when performing a caesarean section for a major degree placenta previa (*surgical skills and teaching module for postgraduates but undergraduates should know the basic procedure.*)

Answer

- The operation should be performed by a consultant obstetrician.
- Check whether:
  - The patient has been informed of all the risk factors when consent was taken.
  - Blood is available
  - A morbidly adherent placenta has been excluded. It is better if the placental site is accurately mapped ultrasonically before commencing the operation.
  - Uterine artery catheterization has been performed.
  - An ICU bed is available.
- A transverse skin incision is usually performed. A vertical incision may be performed in a woman with several previous surgeries or if a transverse lie is present.
- Once the abdomen is opened check the lie of the fetus and whether the lower segment is well formed.
- Attempt version if the lie is transverse.
- A bladder flap should not be made due to the increased vascularity of the lower segment and the high presenting part.
- A high lower segment incision is made. Try to avoid large blood vessels.
- If an anterior or a central placenta is present it will be encountered when the uterus is opened.
- Do not cut through the placenta.
- Displace the placenta laterally or upwards with the right hand to reach the fetus.
- Maintain a longitudinal lie of the fetus. Use the right hand to maintain a fetal pole in the lower segment of the uterus while applying fundal pressure with the left hand.
- Rupture the membranes.
- Deliver the fetus by extracting either the breech or the head.
- Perform an internal podalic version and a breech extraction if the lie is still transverse.
- The assistant should apply fundal pressure at the appropriate time.
- Give a bolus of 10 units of oxytocin intravenously and commence an oxytocin infusion.
- Apply Green-Armytage clamps on bleeding sinuses.
- Apply angle sutures as soon as possible.
- Suture the uterus quickly in the normal manner.
- Apply figure of eight sutures to any bleeding points.
- Check whether the uterus is well contracted. Misoprostol 800 µg can be inserted into the rectum if the uterus is not well contracted.
- If oozing is present from the uterine incision the uterine arteries should be ligated followed by bilateral internal iliac artery ligation.
- If the uterus remains relaxed carry out the management for atonic postpartum haemorrhage (*refer* to Chapter 2, Questions 2 to 5)
- The patient should be carefully observed in the ICU/HDU during the postoperative period.

QUESTION 5

5.1 How will you prepare a woman on the day prior to an elective caesarean section?
5.2 What is your check list immediately before sending the patient to the theatre?
5.3 What are the drugs which are used for premedication in an emergency caesarean section?

Answer 5.1

- Informed consent should be taken.
- Only a full blood count is carried out in the absence of complications.
- Blood should be sent for cross matching before 9 am on the previous day and 1 pint is reserved.
- The operation list should be sent.
- Premedication is given in the night and in the morning
  - Oral domperidone or metoclopramide 10 mg and famotidine or omeprazole 20 mg is given in the night and in the morning. 15 ml of sodium citrate is given in the theater.
- The patient is kept fasting for 6 hours. High energy drinks may be taken till 2 hours before surgery.
- Shave the area of the incision.
- Dress in clean clothes—be ready before the time for surgery.

Answer 5.2

Check whether:
- It is the correct patient.
- The patient is fasting.
- The patient has given consent.
- Blood is available.
- All the investigation reports are available.
- Dentures and jewellery have been removed.
- The area is properly shaved.
- The baby's clothes are sent to the theatre.

Answer 5.3

Ranitidine 50 mg and metoclopramide 10 mg are given intravenously. 15 ml of sodium citrate is given in the theatre.

QUESTION 6

6.1 What is the commonest cause of bleeding after caesarean section?
6.2 What are the complications which can occur during the first 24 hours after caesarean section?
6.3 What are the complications which can occur between 24 and 72 hours?
6.4 What are the complications which can occur between days 4 and 7?

Answer 6.1

- Postpartum haemorrhage due to uterine atony is the commonest cause.

- Retained placental tissue is a rare complication because the placenta is removed under direct vision.
- Bleeding from the uterine incision is rare.

Answer 6.2

Anaesthetic complications	incomplete recovery
	respiratory difficulties
	hypotension
Bleeding	postpartum haemorrhage
	bleeding from the uterine incision (rare)
Pain	
Renal complications	retention
	oliguria
	true incontinence due to a direct cut in the bladder

Answer 6.3

- Paralytic ileus
- Urinary tract infection
- Respiratory tract infection
- Peritonitis

Answer 6.4

- Breast engorgement
- Cracked nipples
- Wound infection
- Urinary tract infection
- Respiratory tract infection
- Deep vein thrombosis and pulmonary embolism
- Pelvic abscess formation

Primary Amenorrhoea

1.1   A 16-year-old girl has not attained menarche. Mention the important points in the history.

1.2   Mention physical signs which would be helpful in arriving at a diagnosis.

1.3   List the first-line investigations you would perform in each case and give your reasons. (*This type of long question is commonly asked at the MD and MRCOG examinations.*)

Answer 1.1

Inquire regarding:

- Development of breasts and axillary and pubic hair.
- Occurrence of a growth spurt.
- Presence of hirsutism or virilism.
- Occurrence of monthly abdominal pain.
- Occurrence of headaches and visual disturbances.
- Weight gain or weight loss.
- Psychological stress.
- Excessive exercise.
- Illnesses during childhood such as meningitis, encephalitis, epilepsy, and malnutrition. History suggestive of heart disease.
- Use of drugs such as hormones, corticosteroids, anti-psychotic drugs or cytotoxic drugs.
- Use of performance enhancing or addictive drugs.
- Head injuries.
- Intelligence and success at school.
- Family history of amenorrhoea in other siblings.
- Results of investigations which have been performed.

Answer 1.2

Physical signs which are helpful to arrive at a diagnosis include:

- Height and weight.
- Presence or absence of breast development. Mention the Tanner stage.
- Occurrence of scanty body hair.
- Presence of hirsutism or virilism.
- Webbing of the neck, increased carrying angle, wide spaced nipples.
- Presence of an abdominal mass.
- Palpation of a haematocolpos on rectal examination/presence of a bluish bulging membrane at the introitus/absence of the vagina.
- Presence of ambiguous external genitalia.

Answer 1.3

Investigations depend on the clinical picture and the tentative diagnosis.

- If the secondary sexual characteristics are present an obstructive lesion of the genital tract or androgen insensitivity should be suspected.
  - An USS scan of the genital tract should be done to detect the site of the obstruction.
  - If the uterus and the vagina are absent, Meyer-Rokitansky syndrome or complete androgen insensitivity should be considered in the differential diagnosis. Karyotyping is performed to confirm the diagnosis in these patients. The karyotype will be XX in Meyer-Rokitansky syndrome and XY in complete androgen insensitivity syndome. Body hair will be absent or scanty in the latter.
  - In all patients with structural abnormalities of the genital tract an USS of the renal tract should be performed to exclude co-existing abnormalities.
- If secondary sexual characteristics have developed up to about Tanner stage 3, delayed menarche should be considered.
  - If the USS does not show a structural abnormality, hormone profile should be done.
  - If the results are in the low normal range she should be observed for 6 months for menstruation to occur.
- If secondary sexual characteristics are absent the first investigation is to perform FSH, LH and prolactin levels, to determine whether the lesion is in the hypothalamus/pituitary or in the ovary.
  - If the FSH and LH levels are low or the prolactin levels are high, the lesion is in the hypothalamus or the pituitary. GnRH levels and other pituitary hormones should be estimated, to determine the exact site and extent of the lesion. CT/ MRI scans should be done, to exclude tumours or other intracranial lesions.
  - If the FSH and LH levels are high the lesion is in the ovary. A karyotype should be done to exclude Turner syndrome (XO) or XY gonadal agenesis. If the karyotype is XX premature ovarian failure, resistant ovary syndrome or XX gonadal agenesis could be the cause.
- If virilising features are present, the individual can be a male or a female.
  - The first step is to perform a karyotype.
  - If the karyotype is XY the individual is male with impaired testicular functions.
  - If the karyotype is XX the individual is a female.
  - If the patient is a female the next step is to perform serum 17 hydroxy-progesterone levels.
  - If 17 hydroxyprogesterone is elevated, diagnosis of congenital adrenal hyperplasia is confirmed. Serum electrolytes should be done to exclude salt loss.
  - If CAH is excluded an USS should be performed to exclude adrenal tumours or androgen secreting ovarian tumours.

QUESTION 2

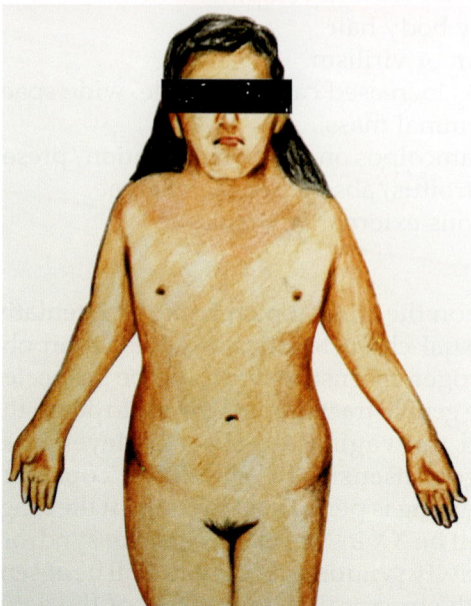

This 16-year-old girl complains of failure to attain menarche. Her height is 4 feet.

2.1 What is the first investigation you would carry out? Give your reasons.
2.2 What are the expected results and what is the most likely diagnosis?
2.3 Give 3 other reasons for arriving at this diagnosis.
2.4 State 2 conditions which should be considered in the differential diagnosis.
2.5 How will you confirm the diagnosis?
2.6 What are the other pathological conditions which can occur in this girl?
2.7 State three steps in the treatment of this condition.
2.8 State a function which cannot be directly restored by treatment.
2.9 State 3 functions which can be restored by treatment.
2.10 How do you counsel this child and her parents? (*This type of long questions are commonly asked at the MD and MRCOG examinations. However, a shortened version is commonly asked at undergraduate examinations.*)

Answer 2.1

Secondary sexual characteristics are absent indicating the absence of circulating estrogens. Hence the lesion is either due to failure of the pituitary to provide gonadotropins to stimulate the ovaries (hypogonadotropic amenorrhoea) or due to failure of the ovary to respond to pituitary gonadotropins (hypergonadotropic amenorrhoea). Therefore, a hormone profile, (FSH, LH, prolactin, TSH and estrogen levels) should be performed first to decide the site of the lesion.

Answer 2.2

The FSH and LH levels will be high, estrogen level will be low and the prolactin level will be normal. The TSH level will be normal.
• Turner's syndrome.

Answer 2.3

Presence of:
- Short stature
- Wide spaced nipples
- Increased carrying angle
- Webbed neck

Answer 2.4

- Gonadal agenesis
- Premature ovarian failure

Answer 2.5

Perform a karyotype. It will be XO.

Answer 2.6

- Cardiac structural defects–coarctation of the aorta, bicuspid aortic valve, dissection of the aorta
- Hypertension
- Type 1 diabetes
- Structural renal malformations, including horseshoe kidney and duplication of the collecting system
- Hearing defects and ear infections
- Cataracts and nystagmus

Answer 2.7

- Reassurance and explanation is the first step in the management.
- Growth hormone levels should be assessed. Even if the levels are normal the height could be improved by treating with recombinant growth hormone before commencing estrogen.
- Commence 0.25–0.5 mg of ethinyl estrodiol and continue till breasts develop up to tanner stage 2–3 or till break through bleeding occurs.
- Commence long term treatment with sequential combined HRT to maintain bone mineral density and monthly menstruation.
- Regular exercise and calcium supplements are helpful to maintain bone mineral density.
- Other defects should be treated appropriately.

Answer 2.8

Fertility

Answer 2.9

- Menstruation
- Slight breast development
- Slight increase in height

Answer 2.10

The girl and her parents should be told that:
- She is a female with a genetic abnormality causing disordered sexual development.

- It is a chance occurrence and is not an inherited condition.
- The illness is due to ovarian failure and that the uterus and the vagina are intact.
- A complete cure is not possible though some functions can be restored.

They should be informed:
- Of the need to take life-long HRT.
- That it is possible to have some degree of breast development and increase in height with treatment.
- That it is possible to have monthly menstruation by taking combined HRT or combined oral contraceptive pills cyclically.
- That it is possible to get married and have normal sexual intercourse, but fertility is possible only at a high cost in centers which carry out IVF with ovum donation.
- That the husband should be counseled regarding her condition before marriage.

QUESTION 3

3.1   Mention 4 conditions which could cause primary amenorrhoea in a 16-year-old girl who has good secondary sexual characteristics.
3.2   What is the first investigation you would perform?
3.3   Physical examination and investigations reveal an abdominal mass with absence of the vagina. What is the best treatment option?
3.4   This is the appearance of the external genitalia of a 14-year-old girl who presented with primary amenorrhoea. Name this condition.

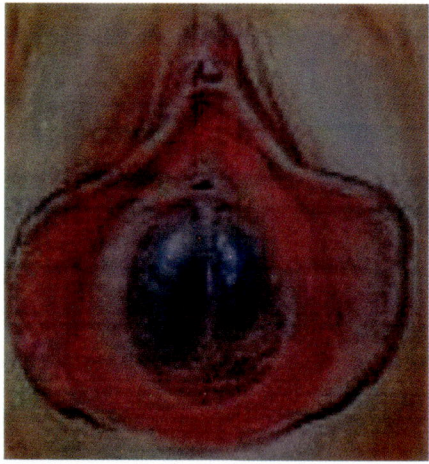

3.5   Mention 3 symptoms.
3.6   How will you confirm the diagnosis?
3.7   What is your management?
3.8   What are the functions which can be restored by treatment?

Answer 3.1

- Complete androgen insensitivity syndrome
- Meyer-Rokitansky syndrome
- Imperforate hymen
- Occurrence of a vaginal septum
- Absence of the vagina with a functioning uterus.

Answer 3.2

Perform an ultrasound scan to exclude structural abnormalities of the genital tract and cryptomenorrhoea.

Answer 3.3

It is most probably due to a haematometron. Confirm the diagnosis by performing an USS. Carry out reconstruction of a vagina which communicates with the uterus.

Answer 3.4

Imperforate hymen

Answer 3.5

- Failure to attain menarche in spite of developing normal secondary sexual characteristics.
- Occurrence of monthly abdominal pain.
- Difficulty in passing urine/retention.

Answer 3.6

Perform an USS to demonstrate the haematocolpos with normal uterus, vagina and ovaries.

Answer 3.7

Perform a cruciate incision of the hymenal membrane. A drain should not be inserted. The blood should be allowed to drain gradually.

Answer 3.8

- Menstruation
- Sexual activity
- Fertility

QUESTION 4

4.1   State 2 conditions you would consider in the differential diagnosis in an 18-year-old girl with primary amenorrhoea and good breast development, if the uterus and the vagina are not seen on the ultrasound scan.

4.2   What is the next step in the investigation?

4.3   The karyotype of a 16-year-old girl with good breast development who presented with primary amenorrhoea is shown below. What is the most likely diagnosis?

4.4   Mention two other physical signs you could elicit to support your diagnosis.

4.5   Mention another investigation you would perform to confirm your diagnosis.

4.6   Mention functions which cannot be restored by treatment.

4.7   What is the best treatment option?

4.8   Is it possible to have sexual intercourse?

4.9   What is your advice if the woman requests fertility?

4.10 Will this woman become virilised? Give reasons for your answer.

4.11 Can this condition cause a threat to her life?

4.12 How will you counsel this woman? (*This type of long questions are commonly asked at the MD and MRCOG examinations. However, a shortened version is commonly asked at undergraduate examinations*).

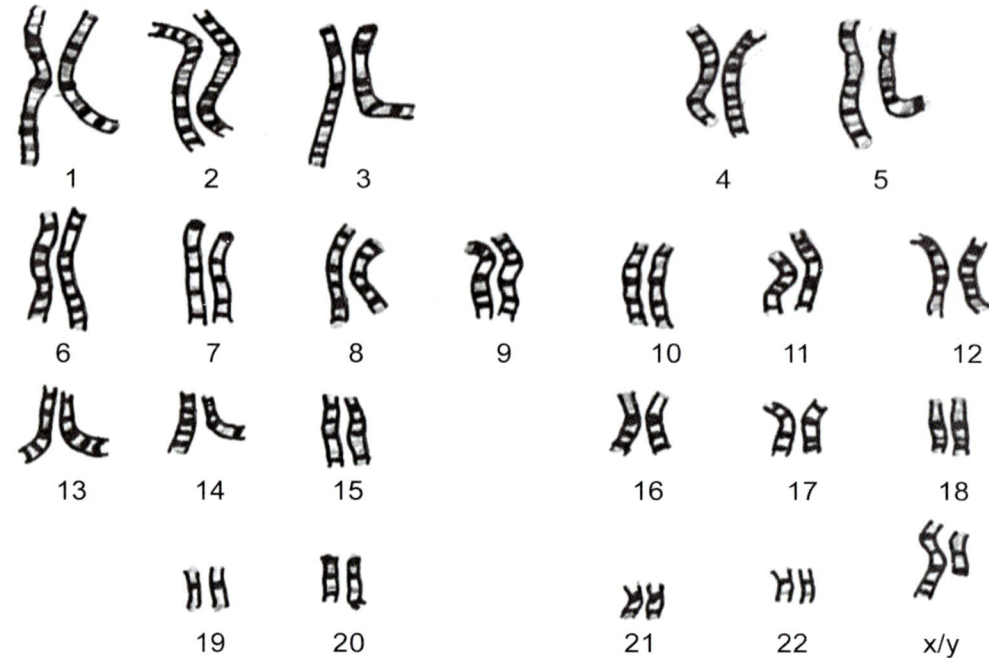

Answer 4.1

Complete androgen insensitivity syndrome
Meyer-Rokitansky syndrome

Answer 4.2

Perform a karyotype.

Answer 4.3

XY disorder of sexual development—complete androgen insensitivity syndrome

Answer 4.4

- Normal height.
- Absence of pubic and axillary hair, scanty body hair and absence of virilisation.
- Absence of the uterus can be demonstrated by performing a rectal examination.

Answer 4.5

Perform serum testosterone levels which will be high.

Answer 4.6

Fertility and menstruation

Answer 4.7

Reassurance, explanation and removal of abnormal gonads.

Answer 4.8

These women have a short blind cloacal vagina which may be adequate for sexual intercourse. If difficulties are encountered vaginal dilatation or reconstruction of an artificial vagina should be considered.

Answer 4.9

Adoption or surrogacy are the only options. IVF with ovum donation is not possible as she does not have an uterus.

Answer 4.10

She will not develop virilism as the functions of testosterone are prevented due to a genetic abnormality.

Answer 4.11

She can develop a dysgerminoma in the abnormal testis, if the gonads are not removed soon after breast development is complete.

Answer 4.12

The girl and her parents should be told that:
- She is a male with a congenital condition of disordered sexual development.
- It is a chance occurrence and the parents are not responsible for this condition.
- She has testes and the uterus and the vagina are absent.
- The disorder is because testosterone produced by the testis is not functioning normally due to a defect in her genes.
- She has female features due to estrogen produced by the testes and the other organs such as the adrenals, which is unopposed by testosterone as in normal males.
- A complete cure is not possible though some functions can be restored.
- She should continue as a female as she has female external features and she cannot perform male sexual functions.

She should be informed that:
- Fertility is not possible because she has no uterus and adoption or surrogacy are the only options.
- Gonads should be removed after puberty because of the risk of developing a malignant tumour.
- She has a short vagina which may be adequate for sexual intercourse. If difficulties are encountered vaginal dilatation can be carried out.
- She will not develop masculine features because testosterone is not functioning.
- Her husband should be counselled regarding her condition before marriage.

QUESTION 5

5.1   State 3 reasons for this appearance of the external genitalia in a newborn child.

5.2   What is the next step in the management?

5.3   If the karyotype is XX what is the next step in the management and what is the most likely condition?

5.4 How do you treat the condition you have mentioned?

5.5 If the karyotype is XY what is the management?

5.6 How will you counsel the parents if the karyotype is XY? (*This type of question is asked at the MD and MRCOG examinations. However, a shortened version can be asked at undergraduate examinations.*)

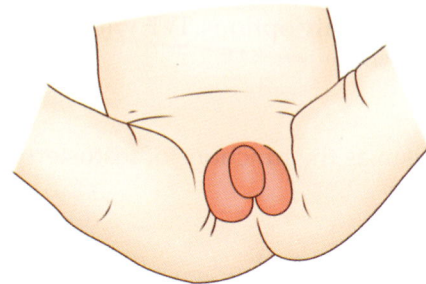

Answers 5.1

- Congenital adrenal hyperplasia
- XY disorder of sexual development.
- True hermaphroditism
- Exposure of a female fetus to exogenous androgens *in utero*

Answer 5.2

Perform a karyotype.

Answer 5.3

Perform blood 17α-hydroxyprogesterone levels to exclude/confirm congenital adrenal hyperplasia. If the blood alpha-hydroxyprogesterone levels are high diagnosis of congenital adrenal hyperplasia can be confirmed.

Answer 5.4

- Commence a high dose of corticosteroids.
- Exclude/treat salt loss. Commence normal saline infusion.
- Perform surgical correction of the external genitalia during infancy. Counsel the parents regarding her condition.

Answer 5.5

- This case should be managed in collaboration with a paediatric endocrinologist
- Perform FSH, LH and testosterone levels. Perform an USS to exclude the presence of the uterus and the vagina. If true hermaphroditism is suspected laparoscopy and gonadal biopsy may be necessary.
- If it is a treatable condition like hypogonadotropic hypogonadism with low FSH and LH levels, the child can be reared as a male. Treatment with gonadotropins can be commenced at the age of 11–16 years and fertility can be restored by the same method later.
- If the FSH and LH levels are high and the testosterone levels are low primary testicular failure can be diagnosed. It is best to rear this child as a female because it is difficult to restore male sexual functions.

- If FSH and LH levels and the testosterone levels are within normal limits partial androgen insensitivity should be suspected. The sex of rearing depends on the severity of the condition and the ability of the penis to perform male sexual functions. Testosterone can be supplemented at the pubertal age.
- If the child is reared as a male infertility can occur.

If the child is reared as a female:
- The gonads should be removed during childhood to prevent further virilisation and malignant transformation.
- Estrogen should be given at about 11 years of age to develop the breasts.
- If the uterus and vagina are present menstruation can be induced with lifelong treatment with OCP or sequential combined HRT.
- If the uterus and vagina are absent she will need HRT with estrogen alone to maintain bone mineral density.
- The cloacal vagina may be adequate for sexual intercourse or the vagina can be dilated or an artificial vagina can be reconstructed.
- Fertility is not possible. If the uterus is present IVF with ovum donation may be considered.

Answer 5.6

Parents should be informed that:
- This child is a genetic male with a congenital condition of disordered sexual development.
- Only a few conditions are treatable. If such a condition is found the child can be reared as a male and treatment can be commenced at the pubertal age.
- If there is testicular failure it is not treatable. It would be difficult for this child to perform sexual functions as a male as the testicular functions are defective.
- Female sexual role may be easier as a cloacal vagina may be present. The short vagina can be dilated or an artificial vagina can be reconstructed.
- Fertility is not possible as a male or a female. If an uterus is present there is a remote possibility of fertility at a high cost in centres which carry out IVF with ovum donation.
- Female secondary sexual characteristics can be developed to some extent by treatment with estrogens at the appropriate age. If a uterus and a vagina is present menstruation can be induced at the appropriate age.
- The testes will have to be removed at an early age if the child is reared as a female as virilisation can occur.

QUESTION 6

The karyotype of an 18-year-old girl who presented with primary amenorrhoea is given below. Development of her breasts are at Tanner stage 5. She has no other complaints.
6.1   What is the most likely diagnosis? Give reasons for your diagnosis.
6.2   What are the tests you would perform to confirm your diagnosis and what are the expected results?
6.3   What are the treatment options?

1   2   3   4   5

6   7   8   9   10   11   12

13   14   15   16   17   18

19   20   21   22   X   Y

Answer 6.1

Meyer-Rokitansky syndrome.

If there is primary amenorrhoea with good breast development and no other complaints such as monthly abdominal pain the diagnosis is most probably Meyer-Rokitansky syndrome or complete androgen insensitivity syndrome. If the woman has normal body hair, the former condition is more likely. Since the karyotype is XX a diagnosis of Meyer-Rokitansky syndrome can be made.

Answer 6.2

- Ultrasound scanning should be done in all cases. The uterus and vagina will be absent with the presence of normal ovaries. Structural abnormalities of the renal tract and other abdominal organs should be excluded.
- Examination under anaesthesia and laparoscopic examination may be performed as a supplementary investigation. Examination under anaesthesia will reveal absence of the vagina and uterus. Laparoscopy will reveal absent or streaky uterus, absent vagina and normal ovaries.

Answer 6.3

There is no definitive treatment.

The woman should be counseled that:

- She is a genetic female and would not have any hormonal changes till the age of menopause as she has normal functioning ovaries.
- The uterus is absent but she has a short vagina. Menstruation cannot be restored.

- Sexual intercourse may be possible with the short vagina or vaginal dilatation or construction of an artificial vagina can be carried out.
- Fertility is not possible because she has no uterus and adoption or surrogacy are the only options.
- The partner should be informed of her disabilities before legal marriage.

Reference
- *Dewhurst's Textbook of Obstetrics and Cynaecology, 8th edition, chapter 37. SBA Questions in Gynaecology, Chapter 2.*

Vaginal and Pelvic Infections

A 40-year-old multiparous woman presents with vaginal discharge.
1.1　State the important questions you would ask her.
1.2　How will you examine her to determine the cause?
1.3　How will you investigate this woman?
　　　(*This type of questions will be asked at the MD and MRCOG examinations*).

Answer 1.1

Question her regarding:
- The duration and amount of the discharge and past history of similar episodes.
- Relationship to the menstrual cycle.
- The appearance of the discharge. Is it purulent, blood stained, white and mucoid or white and curdy? Is it offensive or non-offensive?
- The presence of pruritus/burning sensation.
- A history of insertion of foreign bodies such as IUCD or pessary.
- Use of contraceptives.
- A history of diabetes, sexually transmitted diseases and sexual promiscuity.
- A history suggestive of pelvic inflammatory disease such as pregnancy terminations, miscarriages, pelvic surgeries, abdominal pain and fever.
- Results of previous investigations and response to previous treatment.
- The last cervical smear report.

Answer 1.2

- Presence of fever and/or abdominal tenderness would indicate the possibility of pelvic inflammatory disease.
- Speculum examination could reveal:
  - A local lesion such as an ectropion, polyp or a carcinoma.
  - Cervicitis in infections with gonococcus or chlamydia.
  - Greenish frothy offensive discharge of trichomoniasis.
  - Yellow/greyish discharge of bacterial vaginosis.

– Offensive discharge of surface growths/trichomonas/bacterial vaginosis.
– White curdy discharge of candidiasis.
– White mucoid discharge of chlamydial infection or leucorrhoea.
– Foreign bodies such as IUCD threads or pessaries.
• Bimanual vaginal examination may reveal bilateral adnexal tenderness or masses, if PID is present.

Answer 1.3

• Perform a speculum examination. If there is no local lesion, perform a high vaginal and an endocervical swab. Perform a cervical smear if not performed within the previous 3 years. Perform a TVS to exclude an endometrial lesion.
• A PCR test is performed on the endocervical swab to exclude *Chlamydia trachomatis* and *Neisseria gonorrhoeae*.
• A direct wet smear is performed immediately from the high vaginal swab to exclude *Trichomonas vaginalis*, clue cells of bacterial vaginosis or fungal hyphae in candidiasis
• A Gram stained smear is examined from the high vaginal and endocervical swabs. Gram-positive yeasts will be seen in infection with *Candida albicans*. Clue cells with attached bacteria will be seen in bacterial vaginosis. Gram-negative intracellular diplococci will be seen in the endocervical swab in gonococcal infections.
• A culture and an ABST should be performed on blood and high vaginal and endocervical swabs if the patient is ill with acute pelvic infection.
• WBCDC and C reactive protein levels should be done if acute/chronic pelvic inflammatory disease is suspected.

QUESTION 2

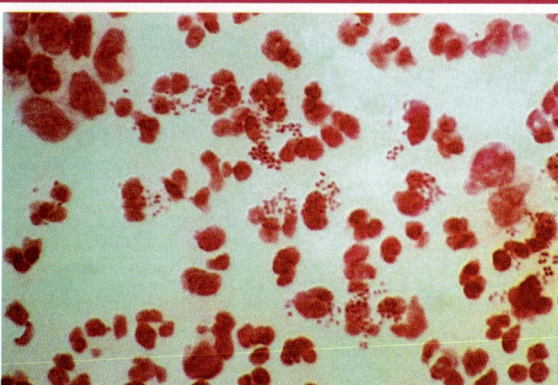

A 30-year-old multiparous woman complains of lower abdominal pain and a purulent vaginal discharge of two weeks duration.
2.1　What is the first investigation you would perform to determine the infecting organism?
2.2　The above smear is obtained from this patient. What is your diagnosis? Give your reasons.
2.3　State two other tests which can be performed to confirm the diagnosis.
2.4　Can you use material obtained from a high vaginal swab to confirm the diagnosis?
2.5　What are the physical signs you would expect?

2.6 **Which other infection could also be present?**
2.7 **State two effective drug regimes.**
2.8 **State two sequelae of this infection.**

Answer 2.1

Obtain an endocervical swab for PCR test and Gram staining and microscopy. Perform culture and ABST.

Answer 2.2

This is a Gram stained smear showing Gram-negative intracellular diplococci. Therefore, she is infected with *Neisseria gonorrohoea*.

Answer 2.3

- Perform nuclear acid amplification test on material obtained from an endocervical swab.
- Culture the organism in blood agar in an atmosphere of CO_2.

Answer 2.4

It can be done by performing a DNA detection based test.

Answer 2.5

- Abdominal examination may reveal bilateral tenderness if ascending infection has resulted in acute pelvic infection.
- Speculum examination will show a red inflamed cervix and purulent discharge.
- Vaginal examination will reveal bilateral adnexal tenderness if PID has occurred.

Answer 2.6

Chlamydial infection could be present. She should be tested for other sexually transmitted infections.

Answer 2.7

- Ceftriaxone 500 mg IM as a single dose *plus* azithromycin 1 g orally as a single dose
- Oral cefixime 400 mg as a single dose *plus* azithromycin 1 g orally as a single dose.

Answer 2.8

- Acute pelvic infection due to ascending infection.
- Infertility due to tubal damage.

QUESTION 3

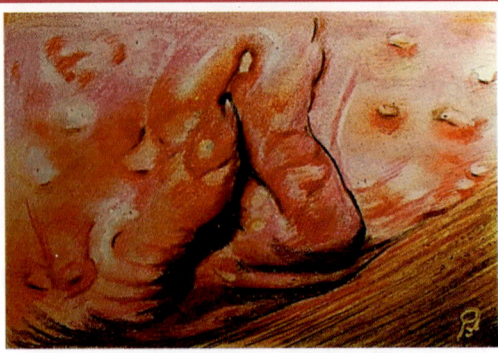

3.1   What is this infection?
3.2   Mention 3 symptoms of this condition.
3.3   How is the infection confirmed?
3.4   What is best treatment option?
3.5   Mention two other important aspects of management of this patient.
3.6   How will you manage if this woman is 36 weeks pregnant?

Answer 3.1

Genital herpes

Answer 3.2

- Painful ulcers
- Mild fever
- Discharge
- Dysuria

Answer 3.3

The infection is confirmed by performing electron microscopic examination or a PCR test on material scraped from the ulcers. Culture can be performed to type the organism.

Answer 3.4

Acyclovir 800 mg 5 times a day for five days is the treatment of choice. Analgesics and antibiotics may be necessary if pain or infection is present.

Answer 3.5

Test for HIV, syphilis and hepatitis B infections. Trace and treat sexual contacts. Advise regarding safe sex.

Answer 3.6

- Identify the organism by performing electron microscopic examination or PCR on material scraped from the ulcers. Perform a culture to identify the type of the organism. Test the maternal serum for type specific antibodies.
- If the maternal serum contains antibodies the infection is a secondary one and vaginal delivery can be allowed.
- If antibodies are absent deliver by caesarean section at 38–39 weeks (before membranes rupture) to prevent neonatal infection.
- If the infection is severe the woman can be treated with acyclovir.

QUESTION 4

This is an microscopic image of a Gram stained smear of vaginal discharge obtained from a 30-year-old multiparous woman.
4.1   Name the cells seen in the image.
4.2   What is the diagnosis?
4.3   Mention the other diagnostic criteria of this condition.
4.4   What are the organisms, which are involved?
4.5   What is the best treatment option?
4.6   What are the complications of this condition?

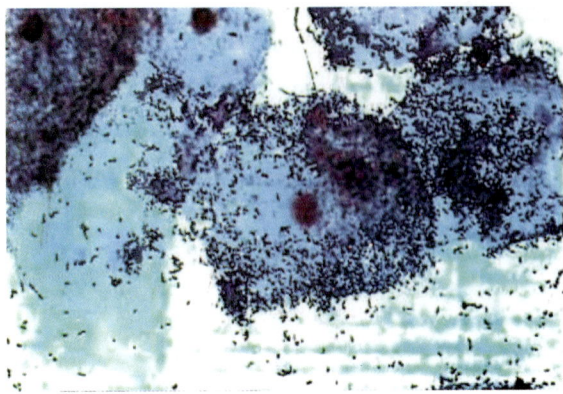

Answer 4.1

Clue cells.

Answer 4.2

Bacterial vaginosis

Answer 4.3

- Presence of a yellowish grey discharge with a fishy odour, without pruritus.
- pH of vaginal fluid >4.5.
- Release of a fishy odour on adding 10% potassium hydroxide (KOH).

Answer 4.4

- *Gardnerella vaginalis* (most abundant)
- Bacteroides
- *Mobiluncus* spp.
- *Mycoplasma hominis*

Answer 4.5

Metronidazole 400 mg twice daily for 7 days

Answer 4.6

- Pregnancy complications:
  - Preterm labour
  - Second trimester miscarriages
  - Chorioamnionitis
  - Pre-labour rupture of membranes
- Increased risk of acquiring other sexually transmitted infections because of the change in normal vaginal flora.
- Increased tendency to develop PID.
- Reduced success rate at IVF and increased risk of miscarriage.

QUESTION 5

A 25-year-old parous woman presents with white vaginal discharge without pruritus.
5.1   State 2 conditions you would consider in the differential diagnosis.

5.2   Name the organism seen in the image.
5.3   What is the main presenting complaint?
5.4   State 3 predisposing factors for this condition.
5.5   What is the best treatment option?

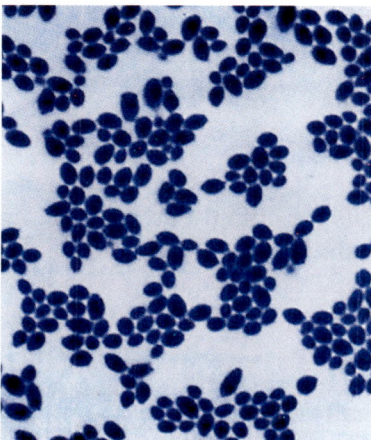

Answer 5.1

- Chlamydial infection
- Leucorrhoea

Answer 5.2

Candida albicans.

Answer 5.3

Occurrence of a white curdy vaginal discharge with pruritus.

Answer 5.4

- Immunosuppression-HIV, immunosuppressive therapy, e.g. steroids.
- Diabetes mellitus.
- Broad-spectrum antibiotic therapy
- Increase in oestrogen due to pregnancy or use of high dose combined oral contraceptive pills.

Answer 5.5

- A single dose of treatment with clotrimazole 500 mg vaginal tablet is adequate.
- If oral treatment is required at the time of menstruation or in an unmarried woman, a single 150 mg tablet of fluconazole is effective.

QUESTION 6

A woman who has had a miscarriage one month ago is admitted with a history of purulent vaginal discharge, lower abdominal pain and fever.
6.1   What is the most likely cause?
6.2   What are the initial tests you would perform to investigate this woman?
6.3   What is the best treatment option?

6.4   What is the most likely diagnosis if this woman develops high swinging fever and diarrhoea?

6.5   How will you confirm the diagnosis?

6.6   Mention in the correct order the steps you would carry-out to manage this woman.

Answer 6.1

Acute pelvic inflammatory disease.

Answer 6.2

Perform:
- DNA detection based tests for chlamydia and gonorrhoea on material obtained from an endocervical swab.
- Perform a culture and ABST on blood and an endocervical swab.
- Perform C-reactive protein levels, serum lactate levels and a full blood count.

Answer 6.3

A single intramuscular injection of ceftriaxone 500 mg together with oral doxycycline 100 mg twice daily and metronidazole 400 mg twice daily for 14 days. This is the treatment of choice as it covers gonococcus, chlamydia and anaerobes. However, culture and ABST should be performed on blood and an endocervical swab before antibiotics are commenced.

Answer 6.4

A pelvic abscess

Answer 6.5

The diagnosis is confirmed by performing an USS.

Answer 6.6

- Perform a culture and ABST on blood and an endocervical swab.
- Commence intravenous broad spectrum antibiotics.
- Aspirate the abscess under ultrasound guidance.
- Perform a repeat USS once daily to exclude refilling.
- Continue intravenous antibiotics for one week and oral antibiotics for another 2 weeks.
- Open drainage is required only if
  - The pus is too thick for aspiration.
  - The abscess is inaccessible.
  - There is free pus in the peritoneal cavity.

References
- *UK National Guideline for the Management of Pelvic Inflammatory Disease 2011 (updated June 2017).*
- *SBA Questions in Gynaecology, Chapter 9.*

Abnormal Uterine Bleeding

A 44-year-old multiparous woman complains of irregular frequent vaginal bleeding for 4 months.

1.1 What are the important points in the history?
1.2 What are the important aspects in the examination?
1.3 What are the initial investigations you would perform?
   (*This type of question will be asked at the MD and MRCOG examinations*)

Answer 1.1

- Commence from the last normal period and describe the progress of the illness.
- Is she maintaining a menstrual diary?
- Is the bleeding heavy or mild?
- Inquire regarding:
  - Dysmenorrhoea and dyspareunia (to exclude endometriosis).
  - Vaginal discharge or postcoital bleeding to exclude a surface lesion.
  - Bleeding from other sites, personal or family history of bleeding disorders or use of aspirin, clopidogrel and other anticoagulant drugs.
  - Iotrogenic causes such as use of hormones for contraception (OCP/DMPA/ Implant) or for treatment at initial stages of the disease.
  - Presence of a copper IUCD.
  - Cervical smear tests.
  - Known aetiological factors for cervical carcinoma.
  - Symptoms suggestive of anaemia.
  - Disturbance of day to day activities.
  - Details of previous investigations and results.
  - Details of previous treatment and the response.

Answer 1.2

- *General examination:*
  - Pallor of the mucous membranes.
  - Signs of bleeding disorders such as purpura and enlarged lymph nodes.

- Abdominal examination
  - Masses
    - o Fibroids, endometrioma
- Pelvic examination
  - Speculum examination
    - o Cervical polyp
    - o Cervical carcinoma
    - o Perform a cervical smear if there is no visible lesion or bleeding
  - Bimanual vaginal examination
    - o Uterine enlargement due to fibroids
    - o Adnexal masses due to endometriosis or hormone secreting ovarian tumours.

Answer 1.3

- Full blood count and coagulation profile
- Transabdominal and transvaginal USS.

QUESTION 2

A 40-year-old multiparous woman complains of irregular frequent vaginal bleeding for 5 months. Abdominal and vaginal examinations are normal
2.1   List 5 causes for this condition.
2.2   What are the first-line investigations?
2.3   What information can you obtain from a TVS in this patient?
2.4   What is the first-line, best management option if the image given below is seen on the transvaginal scan?

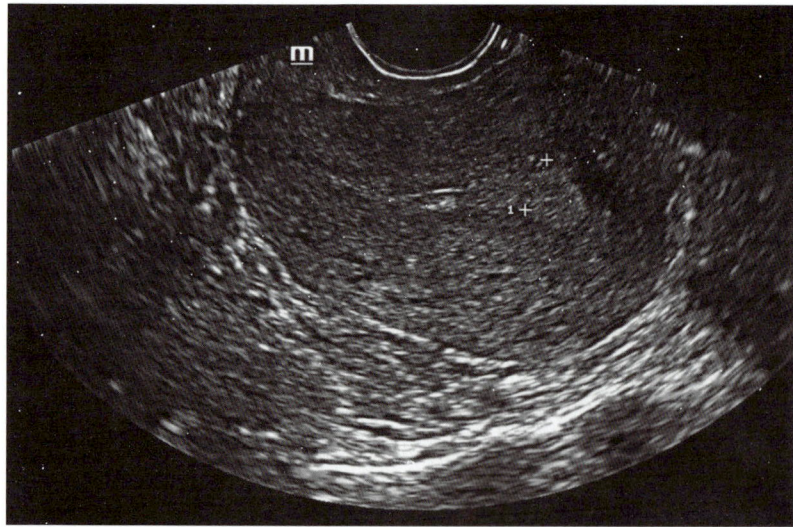

2.5   Mention two other management options.
2.6   What is your management if she does not respond to your initial treatment options?

Answer 2.1

- Endometrial polyp/small submucous fibroid
- Stage 1A endometrial carcinoma

- Use of hormonal contraceptives
- Ovulatory disorders
- Use of anticoagulant drugs/coagulopathy

Answer 2.2

Perform a:
- Full blood count
- Coagulation profile
- Transvaginal and transabdominal ultrasound scan.

Answer 2.3

- Size of the uterus
- Submucus fibroids/fibroid polyps
- Endometrial polyps
- Endometrial thickness/endometrial hyperplasia
- Endometrial carcinoma
- Hormone secreting ovarian tumours.

Answer 2.4

Insert a levonorgestrel releasing intrauterine system as there are no structural lesions in the uterus and the endometrial thickness appears to be normal.

Answer 2.5

- Treat with norethisterone 5 mg twice daily for 3 cycles of 21 days.
- Treat with oral contraceptive pills for 3 cycles.

Answer 2.6

- Perform Pipelle aspiration/hysteroscopy to exclude endometrial hyperplasia or carcinoma.
- Perform a hysterectomy with conservation of the ovaries.
- Endometrial ablation is an option in the absence of atypical endometrial hyperplasia or any other uterine pathology.

QUESTION 3

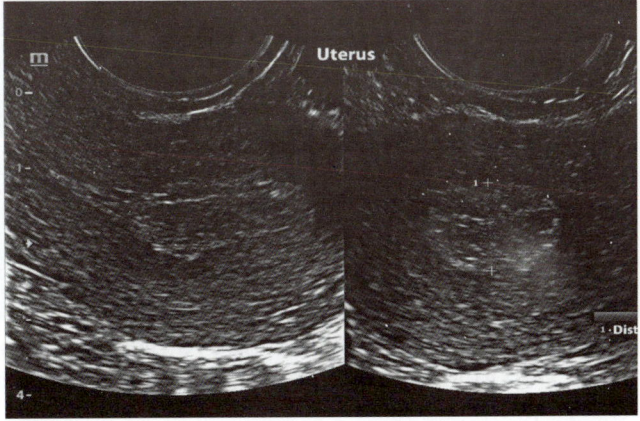

3.1 Describe the abnormality seen in this ultrasound image obtained from a 48 year old woman.
3.2 Mention two clinical conditions which could cause this abnormality.
3.3 Describe another ultrasound feature which will be helpful in the diagnosis
3.4 What is the next step in the management?

Answer 3.1

There is well defined focal thickening of the endometrium.

Answer 3.2

- Endometrial polyp
- An early endometrial carcinoma.

Answer 3.3

Blood flow studies will show a single blood vessel in the case of a polyp while there will be increased vascularity over the entire mass in an endometrial carcinoma.

Answer 3.4

- Perform hysteroscopy and polypectomy if an endometrial polyp is seen.
- Perform hysteroscopy and biopsy if an endometrial carcinoma is suspected.

QUESTION 4

A 40-year-old woman complains of heavy regular menstrual bleeding for 4 months.
4.1 Mention 5 causes for this condition
4.2 If the abdominal and vaginal examinations are normal what is the next step in the management?

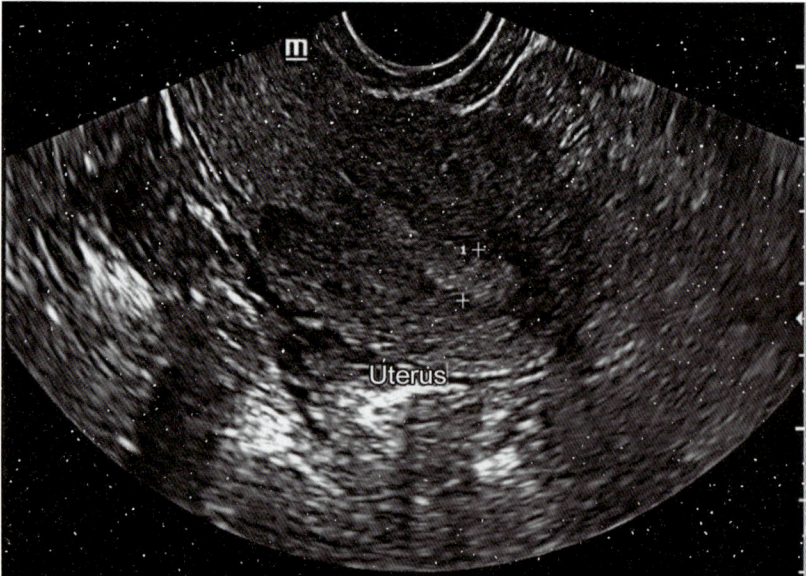

4.3 What is the first-line management if the above picture is seen on the TVUS?
4.4 What is the next step in the management, if the first-line management fails to relieve her symptoms?

Answer 4.1

- Uterine fibroids
- Adenomyosis
- Coagulopathy
- Ovulatory disorders
- Local disorders in the endometrium.

Answer 4.2

- Perform a transvaginal ultrasound scan.
- Perform a full blood count to exclude anaemia.
- Perform a coagulation profile.

Answer 4.3

- As there are no structural lesions in the uterus and the endometrial thickness appears to be normal, treat with mefenamic and/or tranexamic acid 500 mg 8 hourly during menstruation for 3–6 months.
- Give oral iron if the haemoglobin is less than 12 gm%.

Answer 4.4

Insert a levonorgestrel releasing intrauterine system.

QUESTION 5

A 17-year-old girl complains of heavy regular menstrual bleeding for 4 months.

5.1   Mention 2 causes for this condition.
5.2   List the preliminary investigations you would perform.
5.3   Mention the first-line treatment option.
5.4   What are the likely causes if this girl is complaining of frequent, irregular bleeding?
5.5   What is the best treatment option if this girl is complaining of frequent, irregular bleeding?

Answer 5.1

- Ovulatory disorders
- Coagulopathy

Answer 5.2

Perform a:
- Full blood count
- Coagulation profile
- Transabdominal USS

Answer 5.3

Treat with mefenamic and/or tranexamic acid 500 mg 8 hourly during menstruation for 3–6 cycles.

Answer 5.4

- Ovulatory disorders
- Coagulopathy

Answer 5.5

Treat with oral contraceptive pills for 3–6 cycles (cyclical or continuous).

QUESTION 6

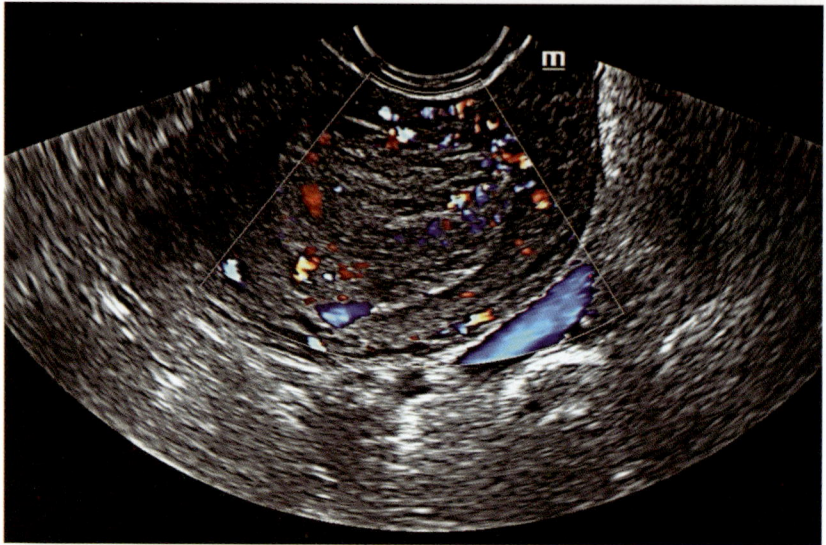

6.1 Describe the abnormality seen on this transvaginal image?

6.2 Mention 2 clinical conditions which could cause this abnormality. Give reasons for your diagnosis.

6.3 What is the next step in the management?

6.4 What is the best treatment option if an endometrial carcinoma is found in this patient?

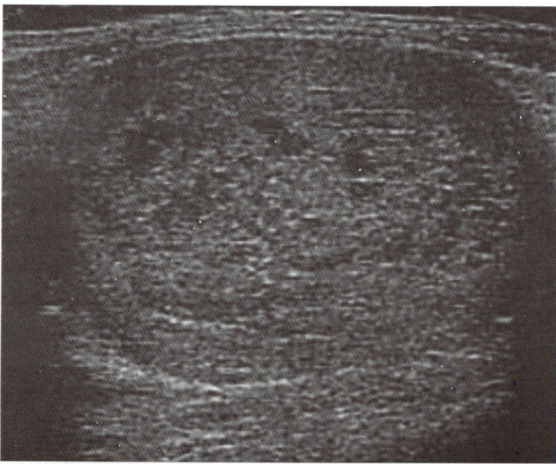

Reproduced with permission from ultrasound cases.info

6.5 What is the most likely diagnosis if the above image is seen on the transvaginal scan performed on a 55-year-old woman who presents with postmenopausal bleeding?

6.6 What is the most appropriate option to treat this woman?

Answer 6.1

There is a well-defined mass with a significant blood flow filling the endometrial cavity.

Answer 6.2

- Endometrial carcinoma. The mass is vascular and is filling the entire endometrial cavity even though it appears well-defined.
- Endometrial polyp. The mass is within the endometrial cavity and though large, it is well defined and there is no appearance of necrosis or infiltration. However, a polyp would be less vascular and will have a single blood vessel.

Answer 6.3

Perform hysteroscopy and biopsy if an endometrial carcinoma is suspected or hysteroscopy and polypectomy if a polyp is seen.

Answer 6.4

If an endometrial carcinoma is found the treatment depends on the histology type, grade and the stage of the tumour. A MRI scan should be performed to stage the tumour before surgery is planned.

Total abdominal hysterectomy and bilateral salpingo-oophorectomy is performed if the tumour is stage 1A, G1 or G2 and endometrioid type. The pelvic and para-aortic lymph nodes should be palpated and sampled if required. Peritoneal washings are taken for cytology. Radical hysterectomy is indicated if it is a G3 tumour or is clear cell in type.

Answer 6.5

Advanced endometrial carcinoma stage 1B or beyond.

Answer 6.6

- The diagnosis should be confirmed by hysteroscopy and biopsy.
- A MRI scan should be performed to determine the spread of the tumour.
- Radical hysterectomy, BSO, pelvic and para-aortic lymphadenectomy, combined with adjuvant radiotherapy is the treatment for stages 2 and 3 tumours.
- Total abdominal hysterectomy, BSO, pelvic and para-aortic lymphadenectomy and peritoneal washings for cytology, is the standard treatment for women with stage 1B tumours. Postoperative brachytherapy may be needed.

References
- *Up to date–August 2014—Approach to abnormal uterine bleeding in nonpregnant reproductive-age women—Author Andrew M Kaunitz, MD.*
- *The Journal of the American Board of Family Medicine. Abnormal Uterine Bleeding: A Management Algorithm—John W. Ely, MD.*
- *SBA Questions in Gynaecology, Chapter 1.*

Postmenopausal Bleeding and Endometrial Carcinoma

A 56-year-old woman complains of a single episode of postmenopausal bleeding.

1.1 What are the possible causes?

1.2 State the questions you would ask in the history to reach a diagnosis.

1.3 What are the abnormalities which can be detected on physical examination?

1.4 If the abdominal and vaginal examinations are normal what is the first step in investigating this woman? What are the abnormalities which can be detected?

(*This type of question will be asked at the MD and MRCOG examinations*)

Answer 1.1

- Surface lesions of the genital tract
  - Carcinoma of the vagina
  - Cervical polyps
  - Cervical carcinoma
  - Endometrial polyps
  - Endometrial carcinoma
  - Senile vaginitis and senile endometritis
  - Decubitus ulcer
- Irregular use of HRT
- Retained foreign bodies such as a copper IUCD or a pessary
- Granulosa cell tumour of the ovary
- Bleeding disorders or use of anticoagulants
- Genital tract trauma

Answer 1.2

- Was the menopause gradual or did she have perimenopausal bleeding? Did she previously have symptoms suggestive of PCOS?
- Is she on hormone replacement therapy?
- Does she have an offensive/blood stained discharge?

- Has she got postcoital bleeding?
- Does she have a retained IUCD/pessary?
- Does she feel a lump at the vulva?
- Is she on anticoagulant drugs? Is there bleeding from other sites?

Question regarding:
- Risk factors for endometrial and cervical carcinoma
- Cervical screening
- Family history of cancers.
- Investigations which have been performed and the results.

Answer 1.3

- Look for evidence of bleeding disorders such as petichae/enlarged lymph nodes.
- Abdominal examination:
  - In most cases the abdominal examination is normal.
  - However, the uterus may be felt if she has previously had uterine fibroids.
  - The uterus will be palpable abdominally only in later stages of endometrial carcinoma.
  - Hormone secreting ovarian tumours are small and may not be palpable during early stages.
- Speculum examination:
  - Look for surface growths of the genital tract such as carcinoma of the vagina, cervical polyps and cervical carcinoma.
  - Look for the appearance of petichae in senile vaginitis.
  - Look for IUCD threads.
- Vaginal examination:
  - Feel for surface lesions of the genital tract. Exclude uterovaginal prolapse with a decubitus ulcer or a retained pessary.
  - The uterus may be bulky in endometrial carcinoma.
  - An adnexal mass may be palpable if a hormone secreting ovarian tumour is present.

Answer 1.4

Perform a TVUS to detect:
- Endometrial polyps
- Endometrial thickness/endometrial hyperplasia
- Endometrial carcinoma
- Fibroids
- Hormone secreting ovarian tumours

A cervical smear should be performed if there is no active bleeding or visible lesion on the cervix and if a smear has not been performed within 3 years.

QUESTION 2

What is the most appropriate next step in the management, if the following images are seen on the TVS during investigation of a woman with postmenopausal bleeding? Give your reasons.

2.1

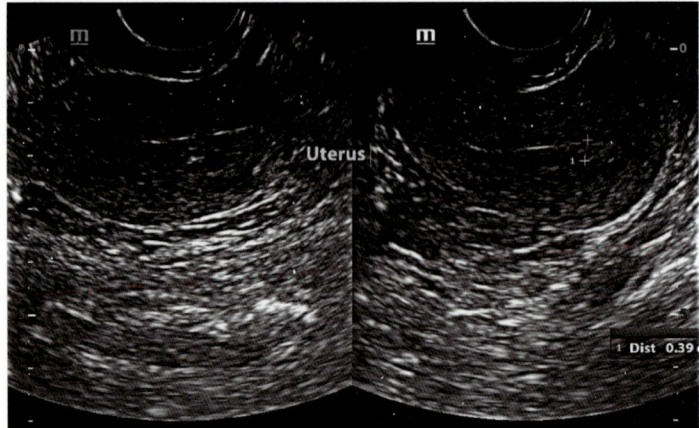

2.2

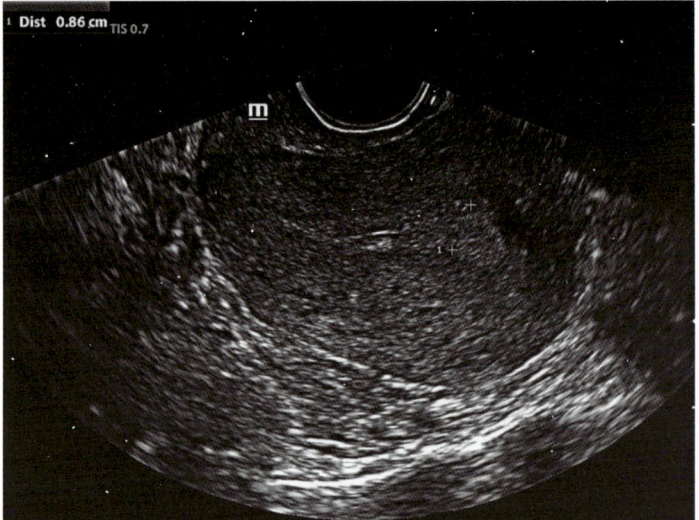

The following image is seen on the TVS during investigation of a woman with postmenopausal vaginal discharge.

2.3 Describe this appearance

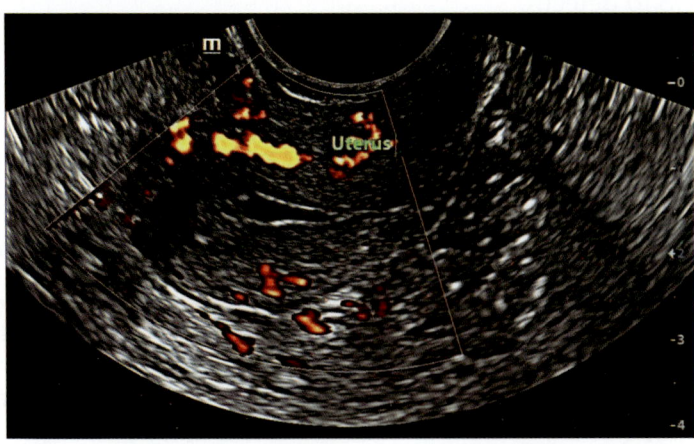

2.4 What are the most likely causes?
2.5 What is the next step in the management?

Answer 2.1

The endometrial thickness is .39 cm. Therefore, if the bleeding stops the patient can be reviewed in 3 months with a TVS. However, if the woman has high risk factors for endometrial carcinoma hysteroscopy and biopsy should be done.

Answer 2.2

Perform a hysteroscopy and biopsy as the endometrial thickness is 0.86 cm (more than 4 mm).

Answer 2.3

There is a collection of fluid in the endometrial cavity. There is increased vascularity.

Answer 2.4.

It could be due to cervical stenosis caused by:
- Cervical surgeries such as biopsy or amputation
- Endocervical carcinoma
- Endometrial carcinoma
- Previous obstetric injuries
- Menopausal atrophy

Answer 2.5

Perform hysteroscopy, endometrial and endocervical biopsy and drain the collected fluid.

QUESTION 3

Hysteroscopy and biopsy reveals an endometrial carcinoma during investigation of a woman with postmenopausal bleeding.
3.1 What is the next step in the management?
3.2 Biopsy reveals a G2 endometrioid carcinoma confined to the fundus. After MRI scanning the tumour is found to be confined to the endometrial cavity. What is the most appropriate management?
3.3 What modifications should be made in the surgical procedure if more than 50% myometrial invasion is found in a preoperative MRI scan?
3.4 State 3 indications for pelvic and para-aortic lymph node dissection.
3.5 State 3 indications for adjuvant radiotherapy.
3.6 How will you treat a woman with stage 3 endometrial carcinoma?

Answer 3.1

Perform a MRI scan to assess the spread.

Answer 3.2

Perform TAH and BSO. The pelvic and para-aortic lymph nodes should be palpated and sampled, if required. Peritoneal washings are taken for cytology.

Answer 3.3

TAH and BSO should be combined with pelvic and para-aortic lymph node dissection.

Answer 3.4

- Stage 1A G3 tumours
- Stage 1A serous, papillary or clear cell tumours.
- Stage 1B tumours

Answer 3.5

- G3 tumours.
- Stage of the tumour stage 2 or above.
- Serous papillary or clear cell tumours.

Answer 3.6

Perform surgery to debulk as much as possible of the tumour and send for adjuvant chemoradiotherapy.

QUESTION 4

A 55-year-old woman who is on continuous combined hormone replacement therapy complains of spotting on and off for 2 months.
4.1   What is the most likely cause?
4.2   Why is it necessary to investigate this woman?
4.3   How will you investigate this woman?
4.4   What are your treatment options?

Answer 4.1

Irregular use of HRT and missing tablets on and off, can cause irregular spotting due to occurrence of withdrawal bleeding. However, there could be a co-existent surface lesion of the genital tract which should be carefully excluded.

Answer 4.2

This woman should be investigated as there could be a co-existent structural lesion of the genital tract. Genital tract malignancies are common at this age.

Answer 4.3

- A careful history should be taken to find out whether this woman has been missing pills on and off.
- A careful history should be taken to exclude causes of postmenopausal bleeding. (*refer* to Question 1)
- An abdominal, speculum and a bimanual vaginal examination should be performed (*refer* to Question 1)
- A transvaginal scan and a coagulation profile should be performed.
- A cervical smear should be performed if there is no visible lesion on the cervix and if a smear has not been performed within 3 years.

Answer 4.4

Once a structural lesion has been excluded advise the woman to take the pills regularly at the same time every day. If the pills are marked according to the days of the week she should take the appropriate pill as it would help to realize if she misses a pill. A pill with a higher dose may be indicated to prevent break through bleeding. If a structural lesion is found it should be treated appropriately.

References
- *Staging classifications and clinical practice guidelines of gynaecologic cancers- FIGO Committee on Gynaecologic Oncology JL Benedet, H Bender, H Jones III, HYS Ngan, S Pecorelli.*
- *Endometrial Hyperplasia, Management of (Green-top Guideline No. 67).*
- *SBA Questions in Gynaecology, Chapter 16.*

Uterine Fibroids

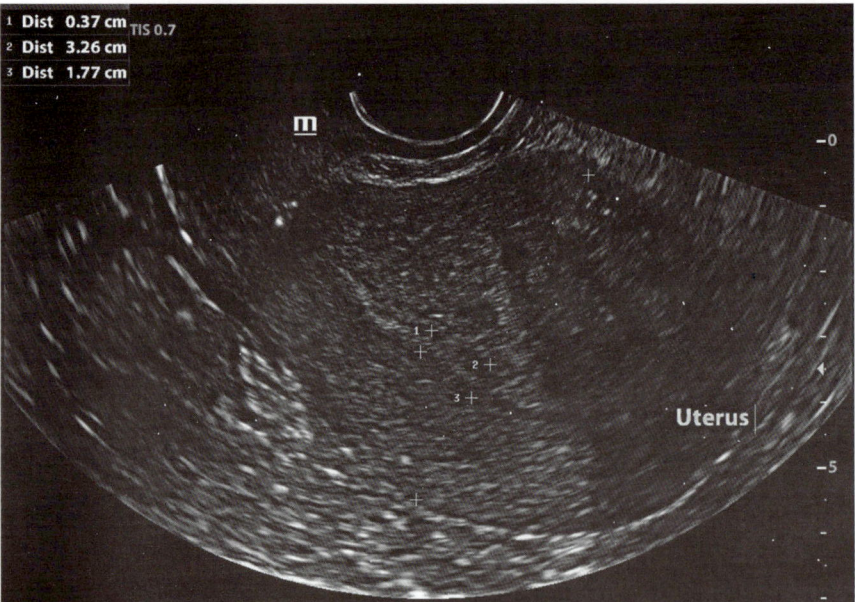

1.1 What is the abnormality seen in the ultrasound image?
1.2 List the complaints this woman may have.
1.3 What are the treatment options if this woman is 35 years of age with one child?
1.4 Is it possible to resect this lesion through the hysteroscope? Give reasons for your answer.

Answer 1.1

The uterus is enlarged due to an interstitial fibroid which is pressing into the endometrial cavity.

Answer 1.2

- Heavy menstrual bleeding
- Presence of an abdominal mass
- Pressure symptoms on the bladder
- Recurrent miscarriages

Answer 1.3

- Myomectomy by laparotomy or laparoscopy.
- Uterine artery embolization.

Answer 1.4

The fibroid cannot be resected through the hysteroscope because it is mainly interstitial.

QUESTION 2

2.1   What is the abnormality seen in the ultrasound image?

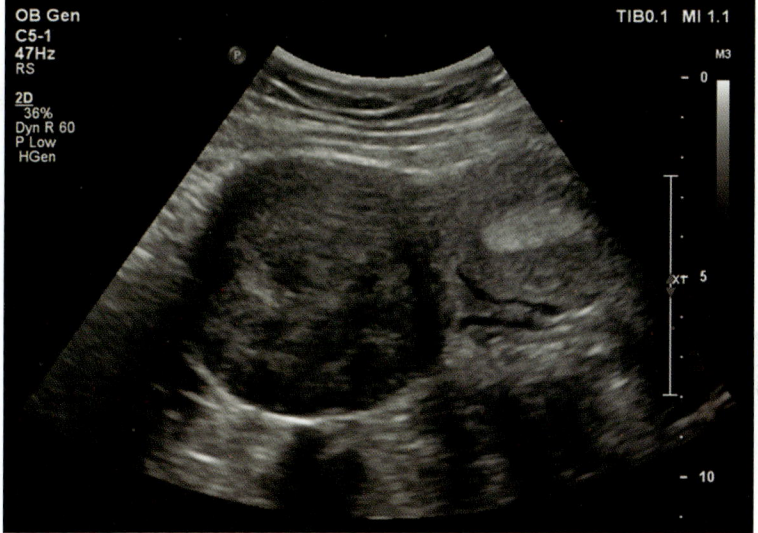

2.2   What would be the presenting complaints?
2.3   What are the treatment options if this woman is 28 years of age, has no symptoms and is infertile for 1 year?
2.4   What is the treatment option if this woman is 51 years of age and has reached menopause 6 months ago? She has not had abnormal uterine bleeding.
2.5   Mention 2 methods to reduce bleeding at myomectomy.

Answer 2.1

The uterus is enlarged due to a fundal fibroid.

Answer 2.2

- Pressure symptoms on the bowel and the bladder.
- She may feel a mass or may be asymptomatic and the fibroid may be detected at a routine clinical examination.

Answer 2.3

- The available options should be discussed with the woman
- Though she is asymptomatic the fibroid is moderate in size. It may interfere with fertility and red degeneration can occur during a pregnancy
- Myomectomy can be performed by laparotomy or laparoscopy.
- Myomectomy can result in adhesions and interfere with fertility.

Answer 2.4

If she does not have any pressure symptoms, she may be reviewed with an ultrasound scan in 1 year as the fibroid may shrink after menopause.

Answer 2.5

- The vascularity of fibroids can be reduced by pre-treatment with GnRH analogues for 3 months.
- Intraoperative bleeding can be reduced by application of a tourniquet round the uterine arteries.
- A catheter can be placed in the uterine arteries so that embolization can be carried out if bleeding occurs.

QUESTION 3

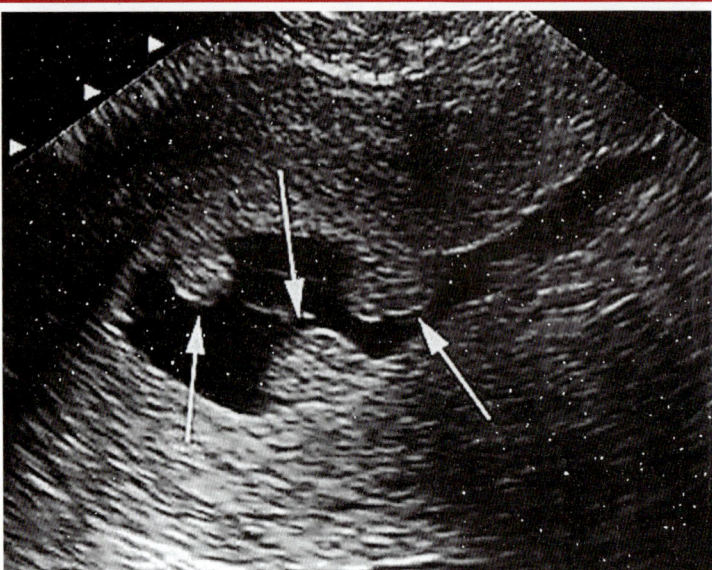

3.1   Describe this image.
3.2   What would be the main presenting complaint?
3.3   Mention 2 other complaints she may have.
3.4   What would be the best treatment option if this woman is 45 years of age?
3.5   What would be the best treatment option if this woman is 32 years of age?

Answer 3.1

This is an image of a hysterosonogram showing 3 small submucous fibroids or endometrial polyps.

Answer 3.2

Heavy menstrual bleeding

Answer 3.3

- Frequent, heavy, irregular menstrual bleeding, vaginal discharge
- Infertility
- Recurrent miscarriages
- Abdominal pain

Answer 3.4

Hysteroscopic resection of the tumours is the best treatment option since they are submucosal and small.

Answer 3.5

Hysteroscopic resection of the tumours is the best treatment option since they are submucosal and small.

QUESTION 4

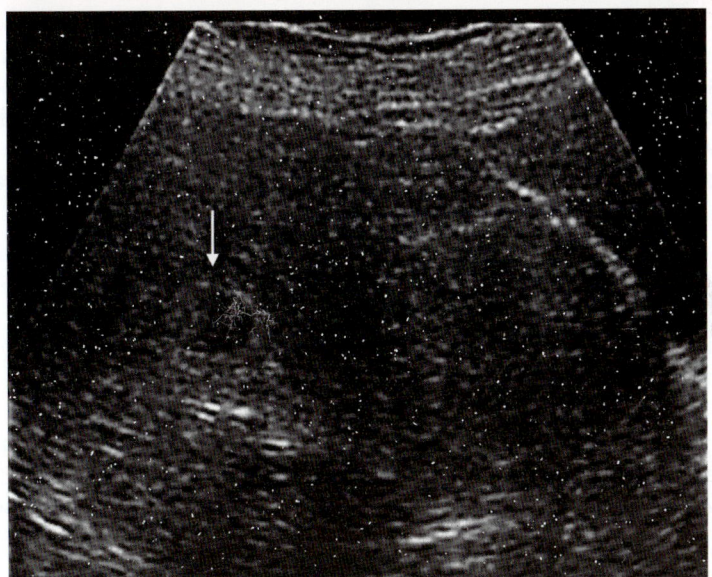

Reproduced with permission from: http://www.ultrasoundcases.info

This image was obtained from a 40-year-old primipara who had a POA of 6 weeks.

4.1   What is the abnormality seen in the ultrasound image?

4.2   Mention 3 changes which can occur in this lesion as the pregnancy proceeds.

4.3   Name the pathological condition which occurs as a result of these changes.

4.4   Mention 3 symptoms of the above condition.

4.5   State your management of this condition.

Answer 4.1

There is an intrauterine pregnancy in an uterus containing a fibroid.

Answer 4.2

- Enlargement in size
- Increase in the vascularity
- Necrosis of the centre of the fibroid due to inadequate blood supply.

Answer 4.3

Red degeneration

Answer 4.4

Recurrent episodes of:
- Abdominal pain
- Mild fever
- Vomiting.

Answer 4.5

- Reassurance and explanation is essential.
- Conservative management is carried out with analgesics and intravenous fluids.

QUESTION 5

5.1 What is the most suitable method of delivery for a woman with a fundal fibroid?
5.2 What is the best method of management if a large lower segment fibroid is found at caesarean section? State the reason/s for your decision.
5.3 When will you perform a myomectomy in this woman?
5.4 What are the postpartum problems of fibroids complicating pregnancy?

Answer 5.1

Vaginal delivery can be allowed in the absence of an obstetric problem, as the fibroid is in the fundal region.

Caesarean section should be performed if there is an obstetric problem or prolonged subfertility.

Answer 5.2

Try to place a lower segment incision avoiding the fibroid. Perform an upper segment caesarean section if the fibroid cannot be avoided when performing a lower segment incision.

Fibroids become very vascular during pregnancy. Therefore, entering into the uterine cavity by cutting through the fibroid or close to the fibroid can result in profuse bleeding. Myomectomy cannot be performed at caesarean section for the same reason.

Answer 5.3

Myomectomy is performed 6 months after delivery by which time the fibroid will be less vascular and smaller.

Answer 5.4

Complications occur mainly with submucous fibroids as they protrude into the uterine cavity. Postpartum haemorrhage and infection can occur.

QUESTION 6

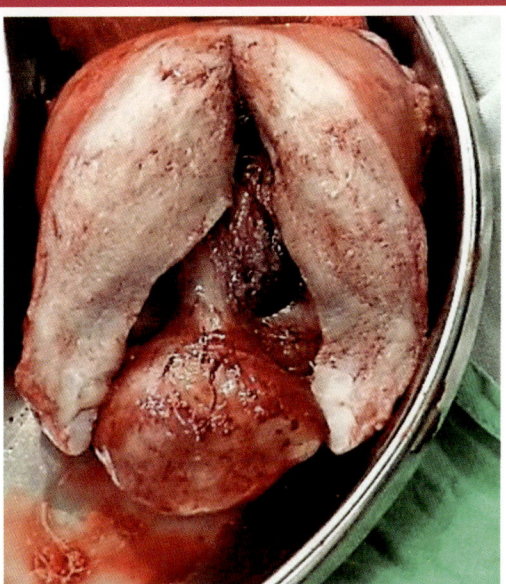

6.1   Describe this image.
6.2   What are the presenting symptoms of this condition?
6.3   What is the best management option?

Answer 6.1

This image shows an uterus with a submucous fibroid polyp. The endometrium appears to be normal. There is hypertrophy of the myometrium but there are no other fibroids.

Answer 6.2

- Irregular frequent or continuous vaginal bleeding.
- Abdominal pain
- Dysmenorrhoea
- Recurrent miscarriages

Answer 6.3

Perform polypectomy through the hysteroscope.

Reference
- *SBA Questions in Gynaecology, Chapter 1.*

Contraception

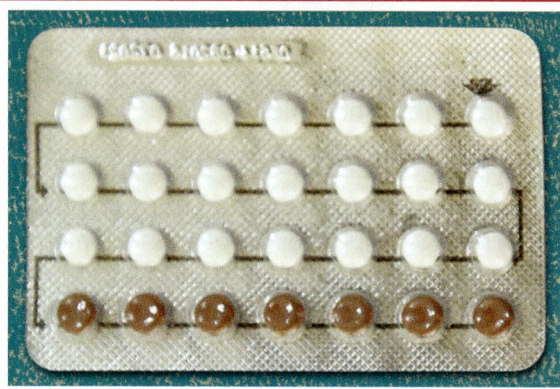

1.1 What is the composition of the above pills and the placebo pills?
1.2 List absolute contraindications for use of the pill.
1.3 List important aspects of counselling before commencing a woman on OCP.
1.4 List 3 non-contraceptive uses of OCP.
1.5 List the non-contraceptive benefits of using the pill.
1.6 How will you advise a woman to commence and continue OCP?
1.7 What are the causes of spotting/irregular bleeding while taking OCP in a previously healthy woman?
1.8 How will you treat such a woman?

Answer 1.1

Ethinyl estradiol 30 µg and levonorgestrel 0.15 mg

The placebo pill contains iron as iron supplements are required during menstruation.

Answer 1.2

• Current history of stroke.

- Current history of ischaemic heart disease.
- Current or past history of deep vein thrombosis.
- Breast cancer.
- Diabetes with nephropathy, retinopathy, neuropathy or vascular disease.
- Systemic lupus erythematosus/antiphospholipid syndrome.
- Migraine with aura.
- Acute viral hepatitis/cirrhosis/malignant liver tumours.
- Breast feeding less than 6 weeks postpartum.
- Severe hypertension (systolic more than 160 or diastolic more than 100).

Answer 1.3

- Exclude absolute contraindications. Reconsider the decision if there are relative contraindications.
- Advise her:
  - To commence the first pill on the first day of menstruation.
  - To take a pill daily at the same time.
  - Regarding minor and major side effects.
  - That the contraceptive efficacy may be reduced by certain drugs, notably anti-epileptic drugs and certain antibiotics. Therefore, she should inform the doctor before taking other drugs.
  - Regarding the procedure which should be followed if she misses a pill.
    o The correct procedure to follow when a woman misses one or two pills is to take the most recent missed pill immediately, use condoms for 7 days and continue the packet. If 7 or more pills are remaining in the packet, finish the remaining tablets and start the next packet after a 7 day gap. If there are fewer than 7 pills remaining in the packet, finish the remaining tablets and start the next packet the next day without taking the placebo tablets.
  - That fertility usually returns soon after stopping the pill.
  - That the pregnancy rate is 1/1000 if properly used without missing any pills.
  - That there are many non-contraceptive benefits.

Answer 1.4

- Treatment of abnormal menstrual bleeding in the absence of a structural lesion. The pill is given for 3–6 cycles.
- The pill is administered cyclically for the treatment of primary dysmenorrhea.
- The pill is given continuously for 6 months without placebo tablets in the treatment of endometriosis.
- It can be used to cause cyclical menstruation in women with hypergonadotropic amenorrhoea.
- It can be used to treat premenstrual syndrome.

Answer 1.5

- The menstruation will occur regularly and primary dysmenorrhea will improve.
- It will protect against endometrial, ovarian and colorectal cancer.
- It will improve acne and hirsutism.
- It will improve bone mineral density in older women.

Answer 1.6

- She should commence the first pill on the first day of menstruation.
- A pill should be taken daily at the same time.
- If the pills are marked according to the days of the week, she should take the pill appropriate to the day, as this will help her to realize that she has missed a pill.
- If the packet has 28 tablets a pill should be taken daily and she will get menstruation when she is taking the placebo pills (containing vitamins and iron) which will be of a different colour. If the packet contains 21 tablets she should leave a gap of 7 days before commencing the next packet. Menstruation should occur during this period.
- She should follow the correct procedure if she misses a pill (*refer* answer to question 1.3)
- She should consult a doctor if she gets side effects.
- She should inform the doctor before taking any other drugs, as most drugs can interfere with the contraceptive effects of the pill.

Answer 1.7

Break through bleeding can occur due to:
- Missing pills or taking them at different times of the day.
- The low estrogen content of the pill.
- Using drugs which interact with the pill to reduce its efficacy.

Answer 1.8

She should commence a new packet.

She should be advised to take a pill daily at the same time. If the pills are marked according to the days of the week she should take the pill appropriate to the day as this will help her to realize that she has missed a pill.

If the bleeding continues with the regular use of the pills advise the woman to change over to a pill with a higher estrogen content after excluding any structural lesions by performing an ultrasound scan.

QUESTION 2

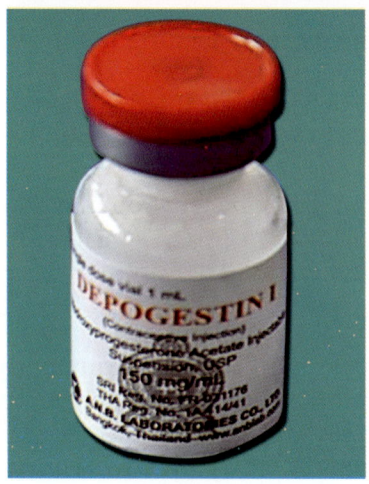

2.1 What is the composition of this contraceptive preparation, the dose and the frequency of administration?

2.2 List 5 advantages of using injectable preparations.

2.3 List 2 non-contraceptive uses.

2.4 List 3 common adverse effects.

2.5 List 5 contraindications.

2.6 How do you commence and continue this preparation?

2.7 How will you treat irregular bleeding caused by DMPA?

Answer 2.1

Depot medroxyprogesterone acetate 150 mg.
    It is given by deep intramuscular injection once in 3 months.

Answer 2.2

- It can be commenced six weeks after partus in breast feeding women.
- The duration of action is 3 months and it is not necessary to remember to take a pill daily.
- It reduces the menstrual blood loss in women with heavy or frequent menstrual bleeding.
- Its effect is not impaired by anti-epileptic or anti-retroviral drugs or antibiotics and hence can be used by patients who are on these drugs.
- It can be used in women with many disease conditions such as hypertension, diabetes, depression, valvular heart disease, endometrial hyperplasia and fibroids.

Answer 2.3

It is used in the treatment of endometrial hyperplasia and endometriosis.

Answer 2.4

- Irregular spotting
- Amenorrhoea
- Weight gain
- Increased risk of breast cancer
- Loss of bone mineral density

Answer 2.5

- Stroke
- Breast cancer
- Liver tumours/cirrhosis
- Current history of ischaemic heart disease or stroke
- Unexplained vaginal bleeding
- Multiple risk factors for arterial cardiovascular disease
- Vascular disease
- Antiphospholipid syndrome
- Diabetes with nephropathy, neuropathy, retinopathy or other vascular disease

Answer 2.6

DMPA should be commenced after excluding pregnancy and other contraindications and re-administered once in 85–90 days. A protective back-up contraceptive method is not necessary for a delay up to 14 days. If it is more than 2 weeks late a urine hCG test should be performed before the injection is administered. Additional contraceptive protection should be used for the next 7 days.

Answer 2.7

Give OCP for 3 cycles after excluding a co-existent structural lesion. OCP can be continued for contraception if there are no contraindications and the woman can be relied to take pills regularly.

QUESTION 3

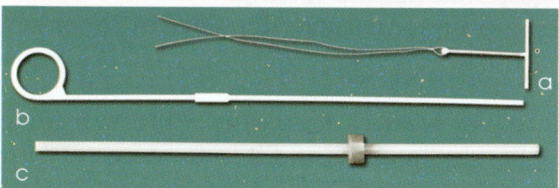

3.1   List the important aspects of counselling before inserting a copper IUCD.
3.2   Name the parts of the IUCD.
3.3   List in the appropriate order the steps required to load a IUCD.

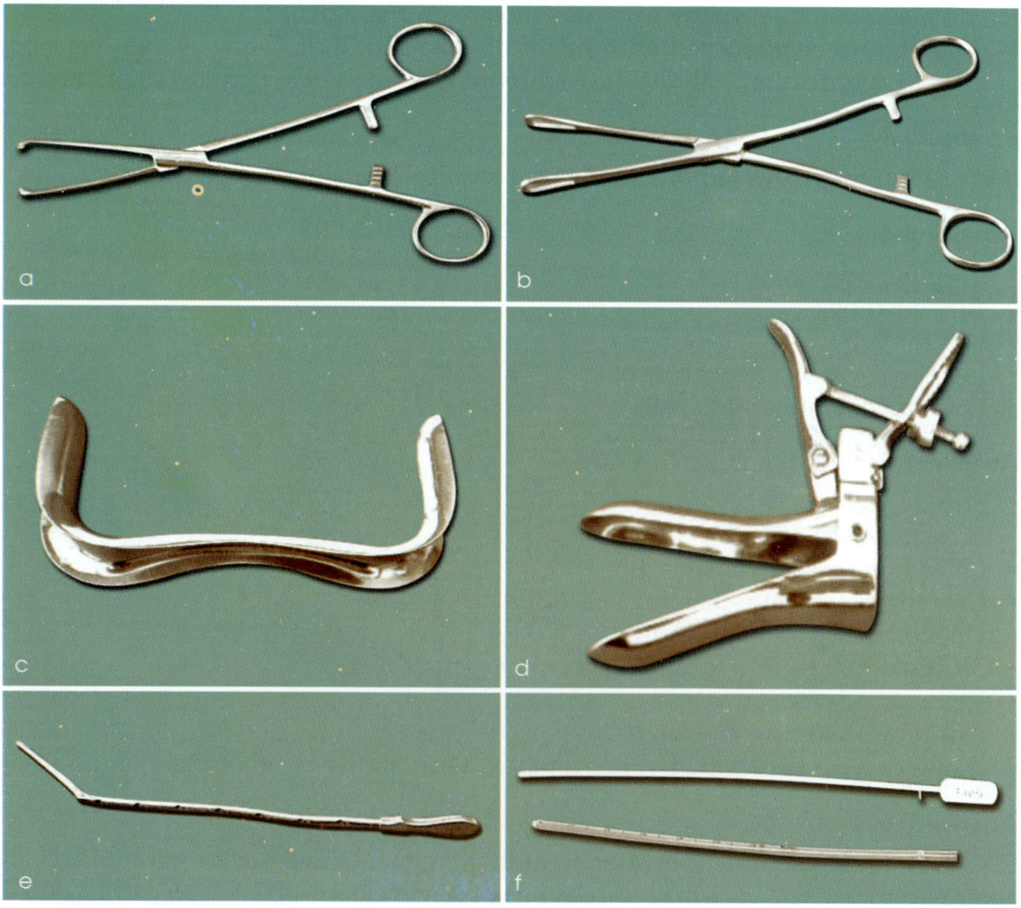

3.4 Select and name the instruments required to introduce a copper IUCD. Arrange them in the order of use during insertion.

3.5 List the steps which should be followed during insertion of a copper IUCD after the preliminaries are completed, the IUCD is loaded and the speculum is inserted.

3.6 What is the first line treatment of a woman who develops heavy menstrual bleeding 3 months after insertion of an IUCD?

Answer 3.1

The woman should be informed that:
- There will be some discomfort during the procedure.
- There may be mild pain and mild bleeding soon after insertion. Pain will subside in 24–48 hours and bleeding will subside in 3–7 days. Paracetamol can be taken for the pain. She should consult a doctor if these symptoms become severe or last for a longer duration.
- She should consult a doctor if she develops fever, abdominal pain and vaginal discharge as there is a possibility of pelvic inflammatory disease.
- There will be some increase in leucorrhoea.
- The IUCD should be checked by a doctor after the first menstrual period .
- Heavy or frequent menstrual bleeding can occur in the first 3 months, but will subside thereafter.
- She should frequently feel for the thread in the vagina especially after a menstrual period. She should consult a doctor if she cannot feel the thread.
- It can be retained for 10 years.

Answer 3.2

a IUCD
b Solid rod
c Introducer

Answer 3.3

- Insert the threads and the vertical arm of the IUCD into the introducer tube.
- Bend and insert the horizontal arms into the introducer tube.
- Insert the solid rod (plunger) into the introducer tube and place it in contact with the IUCD.

Answer 3.4

a. Vulsellum forceps
d. Cusco's bivalve speculum
e. Uterine sound
d, a, e

Answer 3.5

- Hold the cervix with a vulsellum forceps
- Insert the uterine sound to assess the direction and length of the uterus.
- Adjust the marker on the introducer according to the length of the uterus measured by the sound.

- Insert the introducer containing the loaded IUCD into the uterus.
- Hold the rod (plunger) steadily and withdraw the introducer a little.
- Next withdraw the rod followed by the introducer tube.
- Cut the threads to the appropriate length with a pair of sterile scissors.
- Finally close the blades and remove the speculum.

Answer 3.6

Give tranexamic and/or mefenamic acid during menstruation.

QUESTION 4

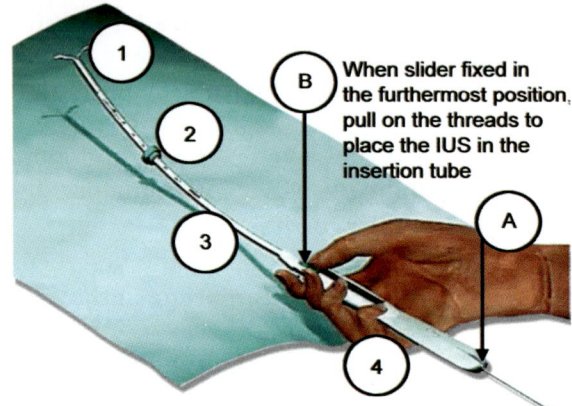

4.1 Name the components of the Mirena set.
4.2 What is the composition of mirena and how much of hormone is released daily?
4.3 List the steps required to load the Mirena.
4.4 List the steps required to insert Mirena after it is loaded and a speculum is inserted exposing the cervix.
4.5 What is the mode of action?
4.6 List 3 situations in which Mirena is regarded as the ideal method of contraception.
4.7 For how long can it be retained in the body?

Answer 4.1

1 The Mirena IUCD
2 Flange
3 Introducer
4 Handle
B Slider
A Thread cleft with thread

Answer 4.2

It contains 52 mg of levonorgestrel and releases 20 µg daily.

Answer 4.3

- Open the packet.

- Wear sterile gloves.
- Release the threads from the thread cleft.
- Hold the slider at the furthermost position.
- Pull the threads to insert the arms into the introducer tube.
- The knobs on the Mirena should close the introducer tube when properly loaded.
- Maintain the slider at the furthermost position till the Mirena is inserted into the uterus.

Answer 4.4

- Hold the cervix with a tenaculum.
- Insert the uterine sound to measure the length and the direction of the uterus.
- Adjust the flange at the appropriate place according to the length of the uterine cavity.
- Insert the introducer up to a distance about 1.5 cm from the cervix.
- Pull the slider to the mark to release the Mirena.
- Hold in the same place for 15 seconds to complete the release of the Mirena.
- Push the introducer gently until a resistance is felt at the fundus.
- Pull the slider to the bottom.
- Remove the introducer.
- Cut the threads about 3 cm from the cervix.
- Remove the tenaculum and the speculum.

Answer 4.5

- It has little effects on the ovarian activity.
- It causes endometrial atrophy and prevents implantation.
- It increases the thickness of the cervical mucus and prevents sperm transport.

Answer 4.6

- Women who need long-term reversible contraception after the age of 40 years.
- Women with abnormal uterine bleeding in the absence of structural lesions in the genital tract, who need long-term reversible contraception.
- Women at high risk of thromboembolism.

Answer 4.7

5 years

QUESTION 5

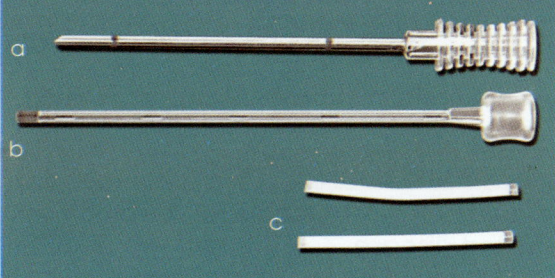

5.1 Name the parts of this contraceptive device.

5.2 For how long can it be retained in the body?
5.3 What is the dose of hormones which enter the body daily?
5.4 Mention the steps of inserting this device after the area is cleaned and anaesthetized.
5.5 What are the side effects?
5.6 How will you treat the side effects caused by this device ?

Answer 5.1

a. Trocar with a sharp end
b. Introducer
c. Contraceptive rods each containing 75 mg of levonorgestrel

Answer 5.2

5 years

Answer 5.3

The initial dose during the first month is about 100 μg/day. This is followed by a decline to about 40 μg/day at 1 year and to about 30 μg/day from 2 years of insertion.

Answer 5.4

- The skin is punctured with the trocar.
- The trocar is inserted under the skin in the shape of a V till the second mark is reached.
- The introducer is removed.
- A contraceptive rod is loaded into the trocar.
- The introducer is re-inserted and the rod is pushed in till a resistance is felt.
- The introducer is removed.
- Palpate to make sure that the rod is just under the skin.
- The trocar is withdrawn up to the first mark.
- Reinsert the trocar under the skin in a direction to complete the V.
- Introduce the second rod in the same manner.
- Withdraw the introducer and then the trocar and place a small plaster at the site.

Answer 5.5

Irregular spotting and amenorrhoea

Answer 5.6

Irregular bleeding is treated with OCP for 3 cycles after excluding a co-existent structural lesion.
    Amenorrhoea does not need any treatment and the woman should be reassured.

QUESTION 6

List 2 contraceptive methods most suitable for a woman with:
6.1 Sexually transmitted disease.
6.2 Severe mitral stenosis who has delivered her first child 6 weeks ago.
6.3 Severe diabetes.

6.4 Breast cancer.
6.5 Frequent irregular bleeding without a structural lesion at the age of 20 years.
6.6 Frequent irregular bleeding without a structural lesion, 6 months after the third pregnancy at the age of 35 years.
6.7 Venous thromboembolism.
6.8 Prolonged immobilization.

Answer 6.1

Use of condoms by the male partner would be the best option as it will protect her from contacting STD in the future.

However, another contraceptive method should always be used to ensure protection as the male partner may not use condoms regularly. A progesterone implant (Jadelle) is a good option as it will provide long term reversible contraception.

Answer 6.2

• Progesterone implant
• DMPA

Answer 6.3

• Copper IUCD
• LNGIUS

Answer 6.4

• Copper IUCD
• Condom

Answer 6.5

• Oral contraceptive pills
• Progesterone implant

Answer 6.6

• Oral contraceptive pills
• LNGIUS

Answer 6.7

• Copper IUCD
• LNG IUS

Answer 6.8

• Copper IUCD
• LNG IUS

QUESTION 7

List non-contraceptive uses of:
7.1 Copper IUCD
7.2 LNG IUS

Answer 7.1

Copper IUCD can be used to:
- Prevent formation of endometrial adhesions after hysteroscopic resection of submucous fibroids
- Prevent re-formation of endometrial adhesions after hysteroscopic resection of adhesions in Asherman's syndrome.
- Prevent formation of endometrial adhesions after postpartum curettage.

Answer 7.2

LNG IUS can be used to:
- Treat abnormal uterine bleeding in the absence of structural lesions.
- Cause regression of simple endometrial hyperplasia.
- Protect the endometrium during hormone replacement therapy with estrogen.

QUESTION 8

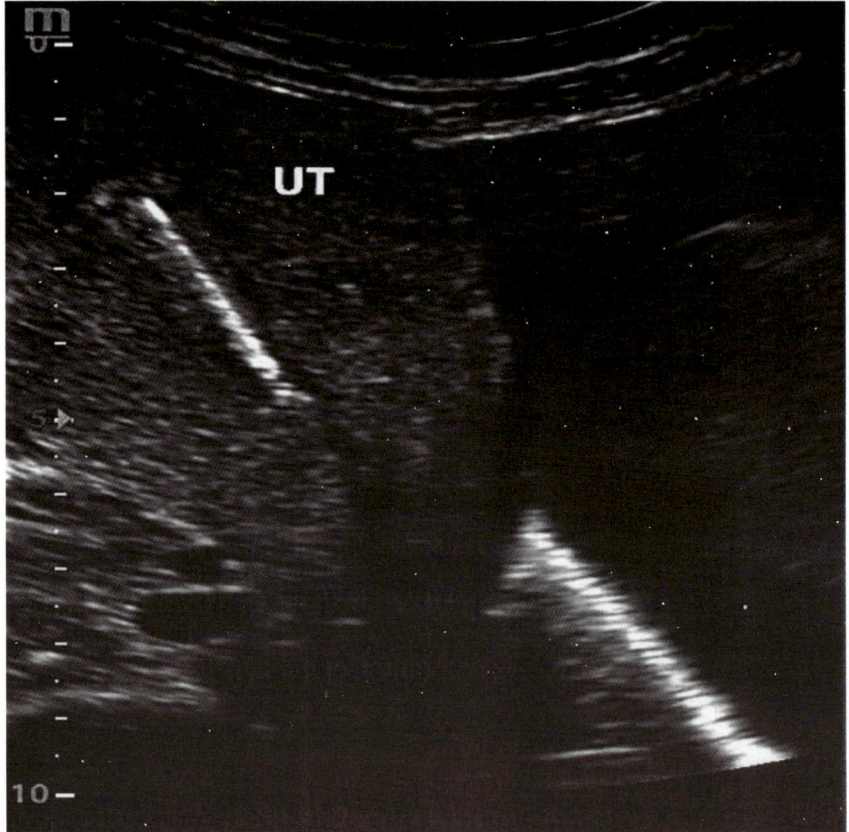

This is the ultrasound scan of a woman who wishes to conceive soon.
8.1   Describe this image.
8.2   List the methods you would adopt to treat this woman.

Answer 8.1

This is an USS image showing an IUCD within the endometrial cavity.

Answer 8.2

- The IUCD has to be removed as she wishes to conceive.
- Insert a Cusco's speculum and try to visualize the thread. If the thread is visible grasp it with a long artery forceps and pull to remove the IUCD.
- If the thread is not visible perform a vaginal examination and try to feel for the IUCD in the lower part of the cervical canal. If it is felt low down in the cervical canal, it can be removed by using a long artery forceps to grasp it and pull it out.
- If the IUCD cannot be felt try to remove by inserting a thread retriever into the cervical canal. If the threads are coiled within the cervical canal the IUCD can be removed in this manner.
- If the above method fails insert 400 µg of misoprostol into the vagina. The IUCD can be removed by inserting a long artery forceps into the uterus once the cervix dilates.
- If this too fails the IUCD should be removed after dilating the cervix under general anaesthesia.

QUESTION 9

9.1 List 4 methods of contraception which can be commenced before a woman is discharged from the postnatal ward.

9.2 List 3 advantages of using a copper IUCD as a method of postpartum contraception.

9.3 List 2 hormonal contraceptives which do not interfere with lactation.

9.4 What is the best method of postpartum contraception? Give your reasons.

9.5 When can a breast feeding woman be commenced on OCP?

9.6 When can an IUCD be inserted if not inserted within the first 48 hours? Give your reasons.

Answer 9.1

- Copper IUCD
- LNG IUS
- Progesterone implant

Answer 9.2

- It can be inserted soon after delivery of the placenta in a normal delivery or a LSCS. It can also be inserted in the postnatal ward up to 48 hours after delivery.
- It does not interfere with breast feeding.
- It does not increase the risk of thromboembolism.
- It provides long term reversible contraception without any commitment by the patient.
- Fertility returns soon after the IUCD is removed.

Answer 9.3

- DMPA
- Progesterone implant
- LNG IUS

Answer 9.4

Copper IUCD is the best method of postpartum contraception because:
- It can be inserted at the time of delivery or within 48 hours after delivery.
- It can be kept for 10 years without any commitment by the patient.
- Fertility returns soon after the IUCD is removed.
- It has no hormones and, therefore, does not interfere with breast feeding or increase the risk of thromboembolism.

Answer 9.5

After 6 months.

Answer 9.6

It should be inserted after 4 weeks because the risk of perforation of the uterus is high, if insertion is carried out between 48 hours and 4 weeks after partus.

QUESTION 10

10.1 What are the available methods of emergency contraception?
10.2 What are the complications of postinor?
10.3 What are the contraindications for the use of postinor?
10.4 How will you counsel a woman before prescribing postinor?

Answer 10.1

- Postinor 1
- Postinor 2
- Combined oral contraceptive pills 2 doses of 2 tablets taken 12 hours apart
- Ulipristol 30 mg
- Insertion of an IUCD

Answer 10.2

Nausea, vomiting, dizziness and menstrual irregularities in the same cycle.

Answer 10.3

- Duration after intercourse more than 72 hours.
- Pregnancy
- Acute liver disease
- Ischaemic heart disease
- Stroke
- Breast cancer
- Diabetes mellitus with nephropathy
- Malabsorption syndrome

Answer 10.4

She should be advised that:
- It should be taken as soon as possible after intercourse. It is not effective if taken after 72 hours.
- It should not be taken if the above contraindications are present.

- It may not be effective if she is taking other drugs such as anti-epileptic drugs, anti-TB drugs or anti-retroviral drugs.
- It will not harm a pregnancy
- It does not cause abortion
- If vomiting occurs within 3 hours another tablet should be taken.
- Condoms should be used for the remainder of the month.
- It can cause nausea breast tenderness and vomiting
- It can cause menstrual irregularity.
- The doctor should be consulted if the period does not occur within 3 weeks.
- It should be taken only for emergency contraception. Frequency of administration should be only about once a month.
- She should commence a reliable method of contraception.

References
- *UK Medical Eligibility Criteria for Contraceptive Use. Faculty of Sexual and Reproductive Healthcare, Royal College of Obstetricians and Gynaecologists.*
- *Medical eligibility criteria for contraceptive use Fifth edition 2015. World Health Organisation.*
- *US. Selected Practice Recommendations for Contraceptive Use, 2013. Adapted from the World Health Organization Selected Practice Recommendations for Contraceptive Use, 2nd Edition.*
- *SBA Questions in Gynaecology, Chapter 5.*

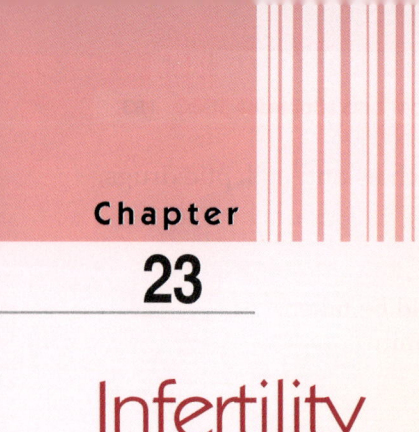

Chapter

23

Infertility

A woman complains of inability to conceive after 2 years of marriage.
1.1 List the important points in the history you would take from this woman.
1.2 What are the important points in the examination?
1.3 State the initial investigations in the order you would perform.
   (This type of question will be asked at the MD and MRCOG examinations.)

Answer 1.1

Inquire regarding:
- Previous marriages/partners
- Previous miscarriages/terminations.
- The duration of unprotected regular intercourse with the intention of conceiving.
- Use of contraceptives.
- The frequency of intercourse, occurrence of dyspareunia or any other coital problems.
- The occurrence of regular 28 day cycles, oligomenorrhoea or amenorrhoea.
- Smoking and intake of alcohol.
- A history suggestive of previous pelvic inflammatory disease, sexually transmitted disease, diabetes mellitus, renal disease, psychiatric disorders, thyroid disorders, tuberculosis or any other chronic illnesses.
- Previous surgeries.
- Weight gain, weight loss, hirsutism.
- Use of drugs, especially, unprescribed drugs, addicting drugs, hormones and antipsychotic drugs.
- Exposure to toxins and radiation.
- Details of previous investigations and results. Ex: Seminal fluid analysis, tests for ovulation and tubal patency tests.
- Details of previous treatment.

History regarding the male partner should include:
- Previous history of fathering a child.
- Use of prescribed and unprescribed drugs.
- Problems associated with intercourse.
- History of mumps, orchitis, chronic illnesses and surgeries.
- Exposure to heat, radiation and toxins.
- Smoking and intake of alcohol.
- Previous investigations and previous treatment.

Answer 1.2
- General examination
  - BMI, hirsutism, thyroid enlargement
- Abdominal examination
  - Abdomino-pelvic masses—fibroids, endometrioma
- Pelvic examination
  - Vaginal discharge—pelvic inflammatory disease
  - Uterine enlargement—fibroids
  - Adnexal masses—endometrioma, inflammatory masses
  - Nodules in the pouch of douglas—endometriosis
  - Cervical excitation pain—endometriosis, pelvic inflammatory disease

Answer 1.3
- Seminal fluid analysis in the male partner.
- Tests for Chlamydia, HIV and hepatitis B.
- Day 21 progesterone levels.
- Hysterosalpingogram in women with no evidence of pelvic pathology or laparoscopy if pelvic pathology is suspected.

QUESTION 2

2.1 Mention two reliable tests to detect ovulation and the time of the cycle during which they should be performed.

2.2 Mention the hormones which should be tested if the woman has irregular cycles.

2.3 List 3 categories of ovulatory disorders.

Answer 2.1
- Serum progesterone levels are usually performed on the 21st day. This could be performed on the 28th day or later if the woman has longer cycles.
- TVS is performed for follicular tracking. This is performed between day 12 and 15. It can be repeated at a later day if the woman has longer cycles.

Answer 2.2
FSH, LH, prolactin, testosterone and thyroxine levels.

Answer 2.3
The World Health Organization classifies ovulation disorders into 3 groups.

- *Group I:* Hypothalamic pituitary failure (hypothalamic amenorrhoea or hypogonadotropic hypogonadism).
- *Group II:* Hypothalamic-pituitary-ovarian dysfunction (predominately polycystic ovary syndrome).
- *Group III:* Ovarian failure.

QUESTION 3

3.1 What are the causes of group 1 anovulatory disorders?
3.2 State the first line management of group 1 ovulatory disorders.
3.3 Describe the first line method of inducing ovulation in these patients.
3.4 Describe the other methods of inducing ovulation if the first line method fails.

Answer 3.1

- Psychological stress
- Eating disorders
- Use of anti-psychotic and performance enhancing drugs
- Excessive exercise
- Intracranial tumours
- Head injuries, irradiation

Answer 3.2

- Increase the body weight if the BMI is less than 19.
- Moderate the exercise levels in women who undertake high levels of exercise.
- Treat psychological stress.
- Omit or reduce drugs.
- Perform CT/MRI scan if an intracranial lesion is suspected.

Answer 3.3

Treat with clomiphene citrate 100 mg daily for 5 days from the second day of the menstrual cycle. Perform TVS for follicular tracking and give 5000 IU of human chorionic gonadotropin when the dominant follicle reaches 1.8–2 cm.

Answer 3.4

- Administer FSH 75 IU intramuscularly daily from the third day of the period. Transvaginal scanning is performed daily to determine the growth of the dominant follicle and to exclude ovarian hyperstimulation. If the dominant follicle does not reach 0.8 cm by the 7th day, the dose is stepped up gradually to a maximum of 150 IU. Give hCG 5000 IU intramuscularly when the follicle reaches 1.8 cm.
- Administer GnRH in a pulsatile fashion by means of a computerized infusion pump intravenously. 1.25–20 µg (2.5–5 µg) administered every 60–90 minutes for 5–6 days, can induce ovulation in anovulatory conditions, such as hypothalamic amenorrhea and polycystic ovarian disease. It has the advantage of not causing ovarian hyperstimulation.

QUESTION 4

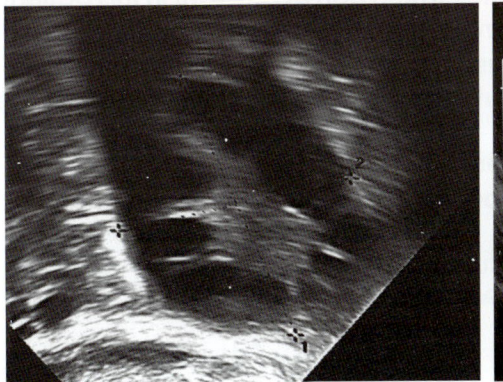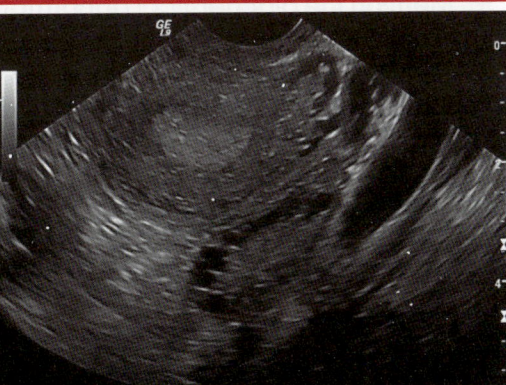

From: Wikipedia commons

These are images obtained by performing an ultrasound scan on a 30-year-old woman.

4.1   What is the clinical condition?
4.2   Give reasons for your diagnosis.
4.3   What are the other criteria required to confirm the diagnosis?
4.4   State the presenting complaints she may have.

Answer 4.1

Polycystic ovarian syndrome.

Answer 4.2

The ovary is enlarged with multiple subcapsular follicles.

Answer 4.3

- Presence of clinical evidence of oligo or anovulation.
  - A history of oligomenorrhoea or amenorrhoea
  - Anovulation is confirmed by performing day 21 progesterone levels.
- Clinical or biochemical evidence of hyperandrogenism.
  - Presence of hirsutism
  - Increase in the levels of free testosterone

Answer 4.4

- Oligo or amenorrhoea
- Obesity
- Infertility
- Hirsutism

QUESTION 5

5.1   A 26-year-old woman whose BMI is 35 kg/m² is complaining of infertility and infrequent periods for 2 years. What is the most likely cause?
5.2   Give reasons for your diagnosis using the above information
5.3   How will you confirm the diagnosis?

5.4   What are the Rotterdam criteria?

5.5   Mention the biochemical abnormalities which can be present in this patient.

5.6   What is the first step in the management?

5.7   Mention 3 first-line drugs which are used to induce ovulation in this woman.

5.8   Mention 4 steps which are carried out during induction of ovulation with the above drugs.

5.9   What is the maximum duration of treatment?

5.10 What are the other drugs which can be used to induce ovulation if treatment with the first-line drugs fail?

5.11 What are the options if ovulation induction fails.
      (This type of long questions will be asked at the MD and MRCOG examinations.)

Answer 5.1

Polycystic ovarian syndrome.

Answer 5.2

Presence of infertility oligomenorrhoea and obesity

Answer 5.3

Diagnosis is confirmed by demonstrating ultrasound evidence of polycystic ovaries:
• Presence of 10 or more sub-capsular follicles less than 10 mm in diameter.
• Increase in the ovarian stroma.

Answer 5.4

Rotterdam criteria include:
• Ultrasound evidence of 10 or more sub-capsular follicles less than 10 mm in diameter with increase in the ovarian stroma.
• Presence of clinical evidence of oligo or anovulation.
   – A history of oligomenorrhoea or amenorrhoea
   – Anovulation is confirmed by performing day 21 progesterone levels.
• Clinical or biochemical evidence of hyperandrogenism
   – Presence of hirsutism
   – Increase in free testosterone levels
   Two of the three criteria should be present to confirm the diagnosis of PCOS.

Answer 5.5

The following hormones are elevated:
• Free testosterone
• LH
• LH: FSH ratio
• Fasting insulin
• Prolactin
• Estradiol and oestrone

Answer 5.6

Lifestyle modification and weight reduction is the first step in the management. Metformin should be given for several months.

Answer 5.7

- Clomiphene citrate
- Letrozole
- Human chorionic gonadotropin injections are given at midcycle when the pre-ovulatory follicle reaches 1.8–2 cm.

Answer 5.8

- Commence clomiphene citrate 50–100 mg daily or letrozole 5 mg daily for 5 days from the second day of the menstrual cycle.
- Commence transvaginal scanning for follicular tracking from the 12th day.
- Give 5000 IU of hCG by intramuscular injection when the follicle reaches 1.8–2 cm in size.
- Perform intrauterine insemination or advise to have sexual intercourse 36 hours after the hCG injection.

Answer 5.9

6 cycles

Answer 5.10

- Administer FSH 75 IU intramuscularly daily from the third day of the period. Transvaginal scanning is performed daily to determine the growth of the dominant follicle and to exclude ovarian hyperstimulation. If the dominant follicle does not reach 0.8 cm by the 7th day, the dose is gradually stepped up to a maximum of 150 IU. Give hCG 5000 IU intramuscularly when the follicle reaches 1.8 cm.
- Administer GnRH in a pulsatile fashion by means of a computerized infusion pump intravenously. 1.25–20 µg (2.5–5 µg) administered every 60–90 minutes for 5–6 days can induce ovulation in anovulatory conditions, such as polycystic ovarian disease. It has the advantage of not causing ovarian hyperstimulation.

Answer 5.11

- Perform diathermy cauterization of polycystic ovaries.
- Perform IVF

QUESTION 6

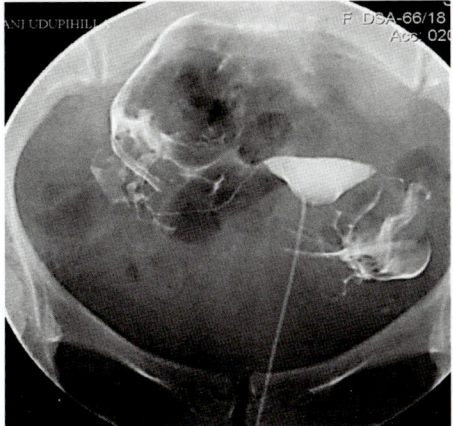

6.1   Comment on this hysterosalpingogram

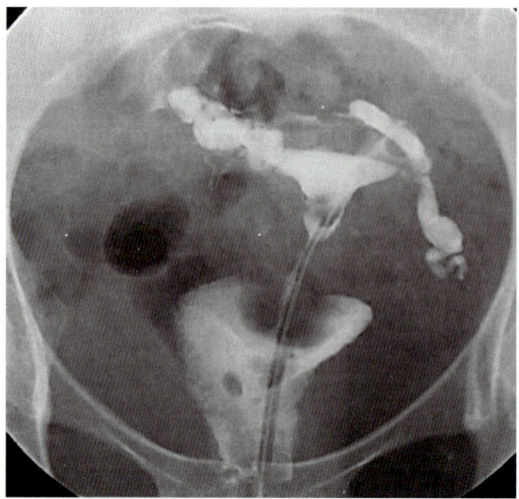

6.2   Comment on this hysterosalpingogram.
6.3   What is the best treatment option if this woman is 38 years of age and has been infertile for 5 years?
6.4   Give 3 reasons for your answer.
6.5   What is the best treatment option if this woman is 25 years of age and has had a termination of pregnancy 5 years ago?

Answer 6.1

- The uterine contour is normal
- The tubes are normal in length and patent with free spill of the dye on both sides.

Answer 6.2

- The uterine contour is normal
- Both tubes are blocked and dilated with hydroslpinges.

Answer 6.3

In vitro fertilization after performing bilateral clip occlusion of the tubes or bilateral salpingectomy.

Answer 6.4

IVF is the preferred option because of:
- Advanced age of the patient.
- Bilateral gross tubal damage.
- Danger of occurrence of an ectopic pregnancy if reconstruction is performed.

Answer 6.5

Tubal reconstruction can be tried. However, there will be damage to the mucosa of the tube because the tubal damage is the result of pelvic infection following the termination. Therefore, she may not conceive even after reconstruction. An ectopic pregnancy should be excluded if conception occurs.

IVF can be performed as the first-line procedure or if surgical correction fails.

QUESTION 7

7.1   List 5 conditions which can be diagnosed by the performing a HSG.

7.2   List 5 conditions which cannot be diagnosed by the performing a HSG.

7.3   What is the period of the menstrual cycle during which a HSG should be performed?

7.4   Give 2 reasons for your answer.

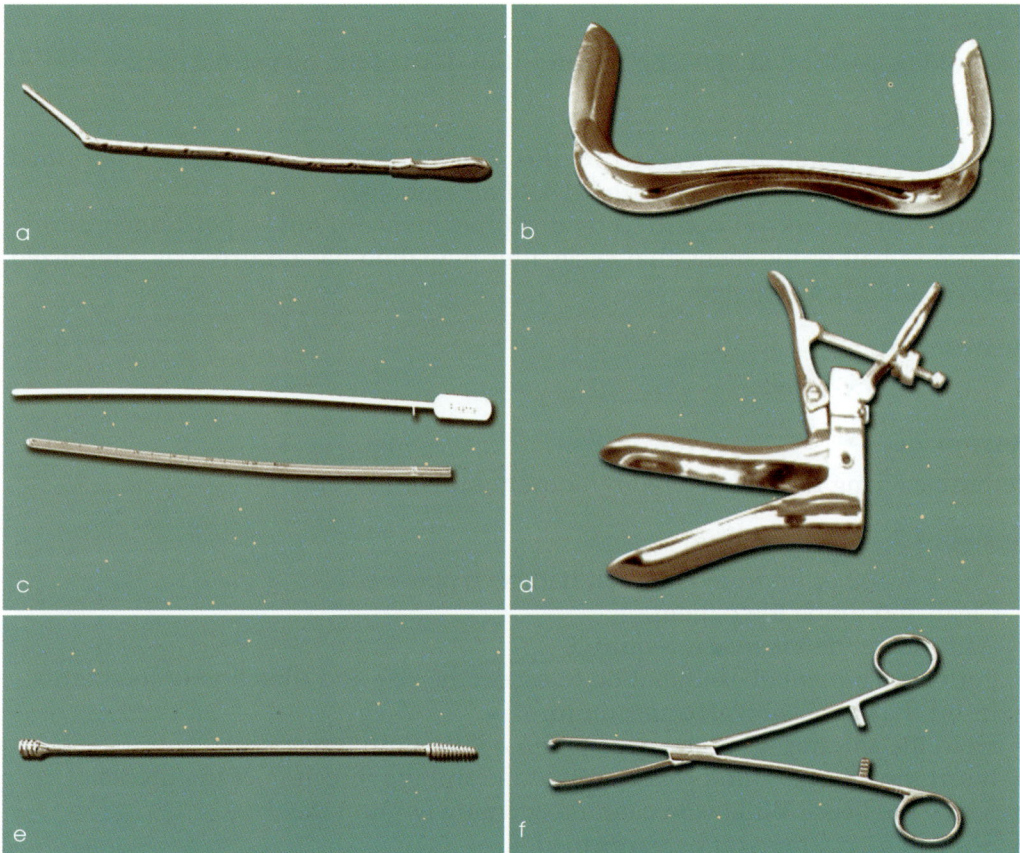

a

b

c

d

e

f

7.5   Pick the instruments required to perform a HSG and place them in the correct order of use.

7.6   What is the anaesthetic agent which is used?

7.7   Mention the steps of performing an HSG after the patient is anaesthetized and placed in the lithotomy position.

Answer 7.1

- Tubal patency
- Tubal length
- Tubal dilatation
- Kinking of the tubes
- Uterine abnormalities
- Uterine septa
- Submucous fibroids

Answer 7.2

- Peritubal adhesions
- Ovarian cysts/polycystic ovaries
- Endometriotic deposits
- Pelvic inflammatory disease
- Sub-serous and interstitial fibroid.

Answer 7.3

It should be performed between 7th and 10th days of the menstrual cycle.

Answer 7.4

Menstruation would have ceased by this time. A HSG should not be performed during menstruation because of the risk of air embolism.

Ovulation has not yet occurred by this time. It should not be performed during the second half of the menstrual cycle after ovulation has occurred as a fertilized embryo could be irradiated.

Answer 7.5

d, f, a, e

Answer 7.6

Pethidine 75 mg is administered by intramuscular injection.

Answer 7.7

- Check whether informed consent had been obtained.
- Clean and drape the patient.
- Catheterise the bladder if required.
- Perform a bimanual examination to assess the size and direction of the uterus.
- Insert the Cusco's bivalve speculum.
- Hold the anterior lip of the cervix with a vulsellum forceps.
- Insert the uterine sound to assess the size and the direction of the uterus.
- Screw the Leech Wilkinson cannula and slowly inject the dye.
- Screening or X-ray will be performed.

QUESTION 8

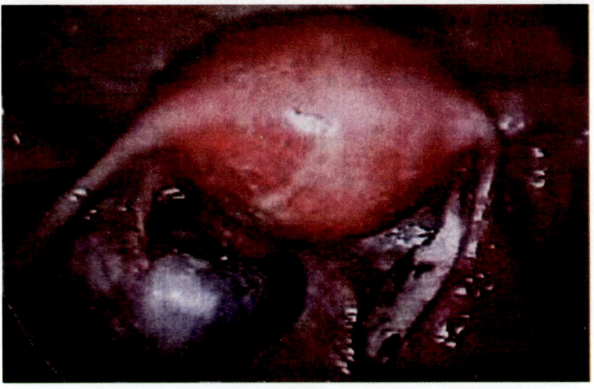

8.1   What is the best test for tubal patency in an infertile woman who has no other symptoms?

8.2   What is the best test for tubal patency in an infertile woman who has secondary dysmenorrhea and deep dyspareunia? Give your reasons.

8.3   What is the condition seen in this laparoscopic image?

8.4   What is the best treatment option if this woman is infertile?

8.5   What are the dyes which are injected during:
       a. HSG
       b. Laparoscopy

Answer 8.1

HSG

Answer 8.2

Laparoscopy and dye test is the best test as this will allow visualisation of the pelvis. Disease conditions such as endometriosis, pelvic inflammatory disease and polycystic ovaries can be diagnosed and certain conditons such as endometriosis can be treated.

Answer 8.3

There is a left sided ovarian endometriotic cyst and endometriotic deposits on the right ovary.

Answer 8.4

Ovarian cystectomy and cauterization of endometriotic deposits should be performed through the laparoscope.

Answer 8.5

a. An iodine containing radio-opaque dye.
b. Methylene blue

QUESTION 9

A couple complains of inability to conceive after 2 years of marriage.

9.1   What is the first investigation you would perform? Give your reasons.

9.2   How will you advise the male partner to collect a sample of seminal fluid?

9.3   Give the normal value for the following:
       a. Sperm count
       b. Progressive sperm motility
       c. Sperm vitality
       d. Normal forms
       e. Pus cells

Answer 9.1

Perform seminal fluid analysis.

   It is an easy non-invasive investigation and male factor is a common cause of infertility.

Answer 9.2

- The test should be performed after 4 days of abstinence from sexual intercourse.
- The sample should be collected into a sterile glass or plastic container by masturbation.
- The sample should not be collected into a condom.
- The sample should be collected within the laboratory premises or should be transported to the laboratory within 30 minutes.

Answer 9.3

a. 39 million spermatozoa per ejaculate or more
b. 40% or more motile sperms (grades a and b)
c. 58% or more live forms
d. >4% normal forms
e. White blood cells: Fewer than 1 million pus cells per ml

QUESTION 10

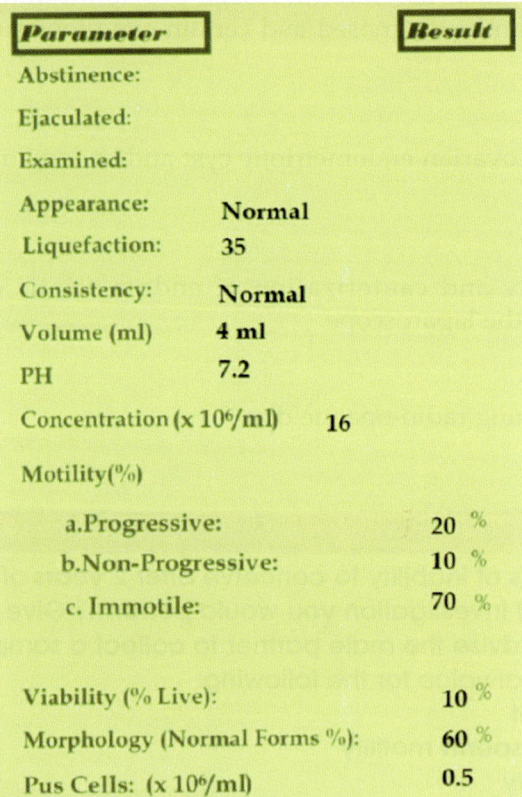

Parameter	Result
Abstinence:	
Ejaculated:	
Examined:	
Appearance:	Normal
Liquefaction:	35
Consistency:	Normal
Volume (ml)	4 ml
PH	7.2
Concentration (x 10⁶/ml)	16
Motility(%)	
a.Progressive:	20 %
b.Non-Progressive:	10 %
c. Immotile:	70 %
Viability (% Live):	10 %
Morphology (Normal Forms %):	60 %
Pus Cells: (x 10⁶/ml)	0.5

This is the seminal fluid analysis report of a 30-year-old male partner of a couple who have been infertile for 2 years.

10.1 Comment on the abnormalities.

10.2 State a specific important question you would ask him regarding the main abnormalities.

10.3 What is the first step in the management?

10.4 What is your management if the abnormalities persist?

Answer 10.1

The sperm motility and vitality are reduced. The sperm concentration is within the low normal range. The other parameters are normal.

Answer 10.2

Was the specimen brought to the laboratory within half an hour of collection?

Answer 10.3

Repeat the test in 3 months.

Answer 10.4

Artificial insemination can be performed with prepared sperms for 6 cycles.
- Ovulation should be induced with clomiphene citrate. Follicular tracking should be performed and 5000 IU of hCG should be given when the follicle reaches 1.8–2 cm.
- IUI is carried out 36 hours after the hCG injection.

QUESTION 11

11.1 Comment on the abnormalities found in the seminal fluid analysis.
11.2 What is the first step in the management?
11.3 What is the first-line management if the abnormalities persist?

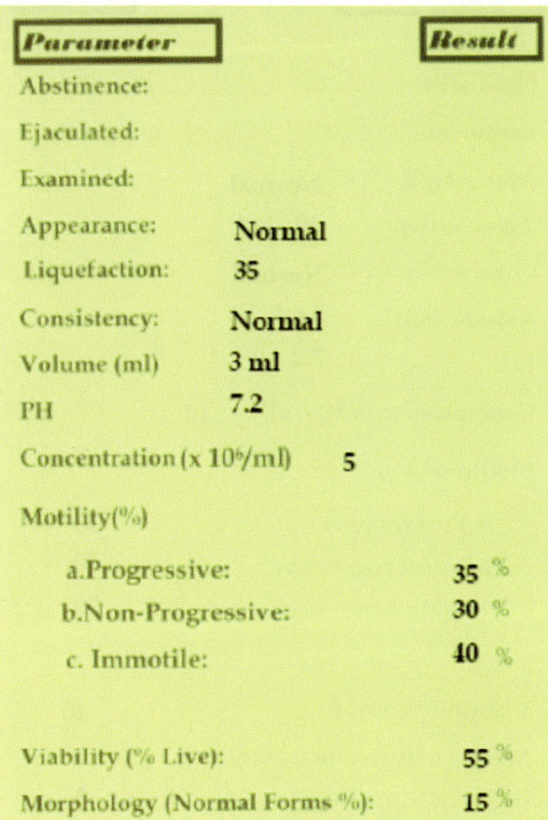

Parameter	Result
Abstinence:	
Ejaculated:	
Examined:	
Appearance:	Normal
Liquefaction:	35
Consistency:	Normal
Volume (ml)	3 ml
PH	7.2
Concentration (x 10^6/ml)	5
Motility(%)	
a.Progressive:	35 %
b.Non-Progressive:	30 %
c. Immotile:	40 %
Viability (% Live):	55 %
Morphology (Normal Forms %):	15 %

Answer 11.1

- Sperm concentration is reduced.
- There is a slight reduction in vitality from 58 to 55%

Answer 11.2

Repeat the seminal fluid analysis in 3 months.

Answer 11.3

Perform artificial insemination with prepared sperms for 6 cycles.
- Ovulation should be induced with clomiphene citrate. Follicular tracking should be performed and 5000 IU of hCG should be given when the follicle reaches 1.8–2 cm.
- IUI is carried out 36 hours after the hCG injection.

QUESTION 12

12.1 Comment on the abnormalities found in the seminal fluid analysis.
12.2 What is the first step in the management?
12.3 What is the definitive management?

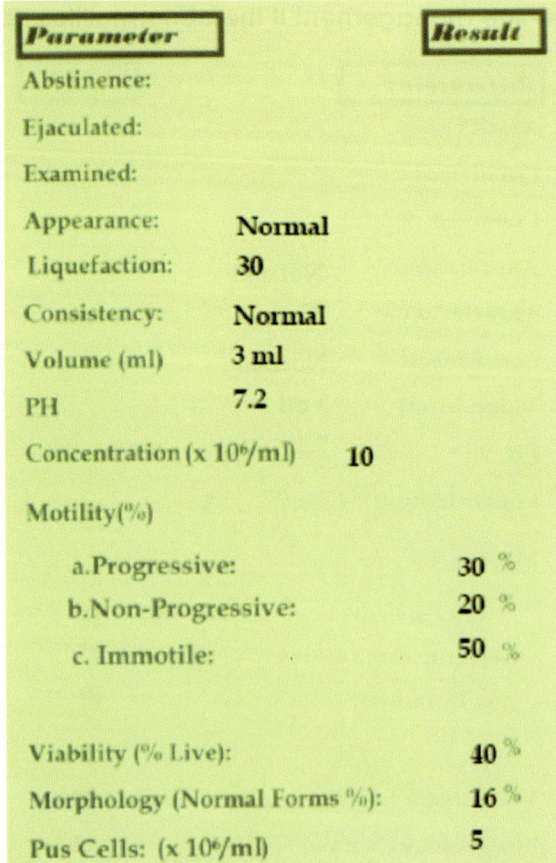

Parameter		Result
Abstinence:		
Ejaculated:		
Examined:		
Appearance:	Normal	
Liquefaction:	30	
Consistency:	Normal	
Volume (ml)	3 ml	
PH	7.2	
Concentration (x 10^6/ml)	10	
Motility(%)		
a. Progressive:		30 %
b. Non-Progressive:		20 %
c. Immotile:		50 %
Viability (% Live):		40 %
Morphology (Normal Forms %):		16 %
Pus Cells: (x 10^6/ml)		5

Answer 12.1

- There are more than 1 million pus cells.
- Sperm concentration and viability are reduced.

Answer 12.2

- Perform a culture and an antibiotic sensitivity test after collecting the ejaculate into a sterile bottle.
- Treat with the appropriate antibiotic for 2 weeks.

Answer 12.3

- Repeat the seminal fluid analysis and culture and ABST after treatment.
- Advise normal regular intercourse if the infection is cured and the sperm concentration and viability are normal.
  If the sperm concentration is still low perform artificial insemination with prepared sperms for 6 cycles.
- Ovulation should be induced with clomiphene citrate. Follicular tracking should be performed and 5000 IU of hCG should be given when the follicle reaches 1.8–2 cm.
- IUI is carried out 36 hours after the hCG injection.

QUESTION 13

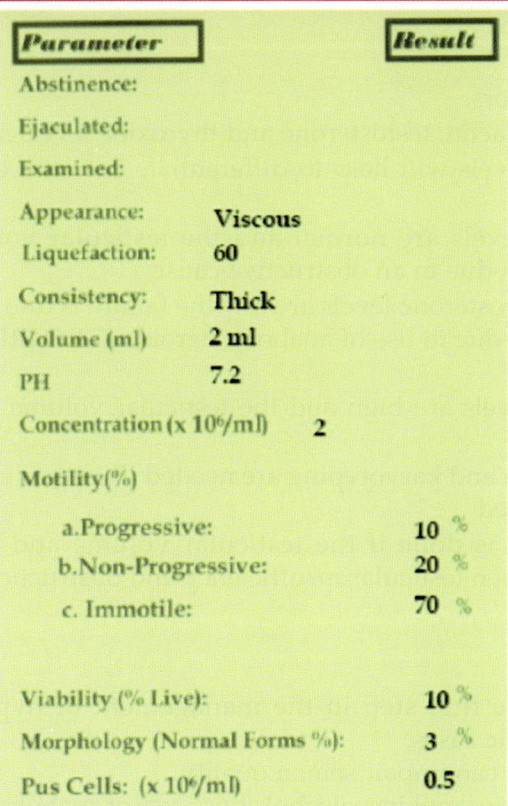

Parameter	Result
Abstinence:	
Ejaculated:	
Examined:	
Appearance:	Viscous
Liquefaction:	60
Consistency:	Thick
Volume (ml)	2 ml
PH	7.2
Concentration (x 10^6/ml)	2
Motility(%)	
a.Progressive:	10 %
b.Non-Progressive:	20 %
c. Immotile:	70 %
Viability (% Live):	10 %
Morphology (Normal Forms %):	3 %
Pus Cells: (x 10^6/ml)	0.5

13.1 Comment on the abnormalities found in this report.

13.2 What is the first step in the management?

13.3 What are the causes of these abnormalities?

13.4 Giving reasons mention the methods you would adopt to diagnose the cause.

13.5 Describe the treatment of each cause you have mentioned.

Answer 13.1

The sperm concentration, motility, normal forms and viability are reduced. The seminal fluid is viscous and thick.

Answer 13.2

Repeat the seminal fluid analysis in 3 months.

Answer 13.3

Abnormalities may be due to:
- Hypothalamic pituitary failure—hypogonadotropic hypogonadism
- Testicular failure due to damage caused by infection, surgery or radiation hypergonadotropic hypogonadism.
- Obstruction of the genital tract.
- Hyperprolactinaemia, thyroid and other endocrine abnormalities.
- Lifestyle factors such as exposure to heat, consumption of prescribed and unprescribed drugs.

Answer 13.4

Exclude lifestyle factors.

Serum FSH, LH, prolactin, testosterone and thyroxine levels should be performed.
- These hormone levels will help to differentiate between obstructive and non-obstructive causes.
- If the hormone levels are normal and the testicular volume is normal, the oligozoospermia is due to an obstructive cause
- If FSH LH and testosterone levels are low the failure is due to a hypothalamic or pituitary cause, or due to use of anabolic steroids. CT/MRI scan of the pituitary may be needed.
- If FSH and LH levels are high and the testicular volume is reduced testicular failure is present.
- Genetic evaluation and karyotyping are needed if congenital causes of testicular failure are suspected
- Testicular biopsy is done if the testicular volume and FSH are normal, to differentiate between testicular insufficiency and obstruction of the male genital tract.

Answer 13.5

- Counselling is the first step in the management of hypogonadotropic and normogonadotropic cases.
  - Lifestyle factors can impair semen quality,
  - Should stop heavy smoking, alcohol abuse, use of anabolic steroids and extreme sports (marathon training, excessive strength sports).

- Should prevent an increase in scrotal temperature through thermal underwear, sauna, hot tub use, or occupational exposure to heat sources.
  - A considerable number of drugs can affect spermatogenesis.
- Hormone treatment can be tried in those with hypogonadotropic hypogonadism.
  - The case should be managed with the help of an endocrinologist
  - Clomiphene citrate 50 mg/day or tamoxifen 20 mg/day may be tried for 3 months in mild cases..
  - In those not responding to treatment commence hCG injections 1500 IU three times a week. If the response is poor add HMG or FSH 75–150 IU intramuscularly 3 times per week, until adequate spermatogenesis occurs.
  - Bromocriptine is used to treat hyperprolactinaemia.
  - Other hormonal disorders should be treated.
- Surgical treatment
  - Microsurgery/vasovasostomy and epididymovasostomy can be performed for obstructive causes. If not successful carry out aspiration of sperms and intrauterine insemination or Intra-cytoplasmic sperm injection.
- Treatment of hypergonadotropic hypogonadism
  - The only option for is intrauterine insemination or IVF using donor sperms.

References
- *Fertility problems: assessment and treatment, NICE Clinical guideline [CG156] Published date: February 2013, Last updated: September 2017*
- *SBA Questions in Gynaecology, Chapter 10.*

Bleeding in Early Pregnancy

1.1 What are the causes of bleeding in early pregnancy?

A 23-year-old woman who has been married for 1 year attends the clinic with a history of mild vaginal bleeding and mild abdominal pain for 1 day at a POA of 7 weeks. She has had a positive urine hCG test 1 week ago.

1.2 What is the likely differential diagnosis? How do you support your diagnosis with the given history?

1.3 How can you exclude other causes of bleeding in early pregnancy with the given information?

1.4 Mention the clinical examinations which will be helpful in the differential diagnosis.

1.5 What is the investigation which will be useful to confirm the diagnosis?

Answer 1.1

- Threatened miscarriage
- Inevitable miscarriage
- Missed miscarriage
- Incomplete miscarriage
- Ectopic pregnancy
- Hydatidiform mole

Answer 1.2

- Threatened miscarriage
- Missed miscarriage
- Hydatidiform mole

The woman is pregnant because she has a POA and the urine hCG test is positive. She has mild bleeding and mild abdominal pain which are the typical symptoms of threatened miscarriage. The same symptoms occur in a missed miscarriage and the urine hCG test remains positive for some time. In a hydatidiform mole the bleeding is mild at first.

Answer 1.3

- An inevitable miscarriage will cause more severe pain and profuse bleeding.
- An incomplete miscarriage will have a longer history with abdominal pain and passage of clots which is followed by continuous or intermittent bleeding and mild pain.
- In an ectopic pregnancy pain will be a prominent feature.

Answer 1.4

- The general condition may be poor with severe bleeding, pallor, low blood pressure and tachycardia in an inevitable miscarriage.
- If there are signs of infection such as fever and purulent vaginal discharge an incomplete miscarriage should be suspected.
- If there is abdominal tenderness and guarding an ectopic pregnancy is a possibility. There may be pallor, low blood pressure and tachycardia.
- The uterus may be large for dates in a hydatidiform mole.
- Speculum examination and bimanual vaginal examination will reveal an open os and there may products or clots at the os in inevitable and incomplete miscarriages.
- The general condition will be satisfactory in threatened and missed miscarriage. The size of the uterus will correspond to the POA in the former while it will be smaller than the POA in the latter. The os will be closed in threatened and missed miscarriage.
- In a hydatidiform mole the general condition is satisfactory at first and the cervical os may be closed.

Answer 1.5

USS should be performed next and will be very useful to diagnose the condition.
- A live pregnancy will be seen in a threatened abortion.
- A live pregnancy may also be seen in an inevitable miscarriage as the fetus is still within the uterus.
- An intrauterine sac with an absent fetal heart beat will be seen in a missed miscarriage.
- A snow storm appearance will be seen in a complete hydatidiform mole. A fetus may be seen with a snowstorm appearance in a partial mole.
- An ectopic pregnancy should be suspected if there is no IUP. It can be confirmed if there is free fluid in the pelvis or an adnexal mass.
- If there is no IUP or other features of an ectopic pregnancy in the USS two serum beta hCG tests are done 48 hours apart.

QUESTION 2

The ultrasound scan image belonging to a primiparous woman who attended the antenatal clinic at a POA of 7 weeks is given below. The gestational sac diameter corresponds to 5 weeks.

2.1 What is the most likely diagnosis?
2.2 Mention the important points you would elicit in the history.
2.3 What is the initial management?
2.4 What is your definitive management if the repeat USS reveals the same findings?

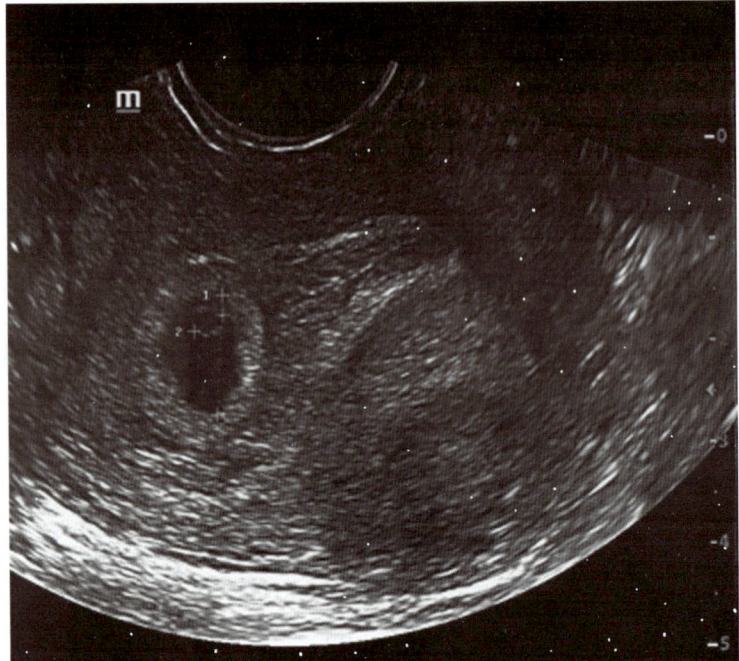

Answer 2.1

A blighted ovum is the most likely diagnosis if her dates are correct. However, the possibility of wrong dates should be considered especially as the yolk sac is seen.

Answer 2.2

- Her dates should be confirmed. Inquire whether she has 28 day regular periods and whether she is sure of dates. Has she conceived while taking hormonal contraceptives? When was the hCG test positive?
- Has she got bleeding and/or abdominal pain?
- Has she been exposed to any febrile illnesses, genital tract infections, prescribed or unprescribed drugs, toxins or smoke (active or passive smoking)
- Has she got chronic illnesses such as diabetes, hypertension, autoimmune diseases or renal disease.
- Is there consanguinity or a family history of genetic or chromosomal abnormalities.

Answer 2.3

Her dates may be wrong. Therefore a repeat scan should be performed after one week.

Reassurance and explanation is essential.

Answer 2.4

A diagnosis of a blighted ovum is made.

Expectant management can be carried out for two weeks if the patient is willing and there is no infection or excessive bleeding. A coagulation profile should be performed.

If expectant management fails, or if the patient is not willing for expectant management insert 800 µg of misoprostol. Give 2 doses 3 hours apart and leave for 1–2 weeks. Perform a transvaginal scan after the products are expelled. If the endometrial thickness is more than 15 mm perform a suction evacuation.

QUESTION 3

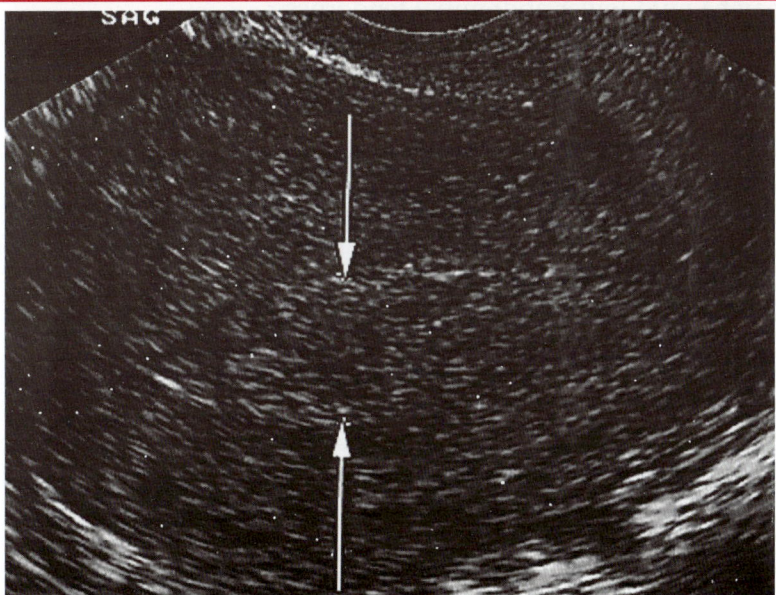

This USS image was obtained from a 28-year-old woman who complained of abdominal pain and bleeding after a POA of 8 weeks. She has passed clots at first and mild bleeding has continued for one week.

3.1 What is the most likely cause?
3.2 Mention another condition which should be considered in the differential diagnosis.
3.3 What are the important aspects in her history which will help in the differential diagnosis?
3.4 What are the physical signs which will help in the diagnosis?
3.5 How can you confirm the diagnosis?
3.6 What is the best management option?

Answer 3.1

Incomplete miscarriage

Answer 3.2

Ectopic pregnancy. A strong decidual reaction which can mimic retained products may be seen in the ultrasound scan in an ectopic pregnancy.

Answer 3.3

• The history is more suggestive of an incomplete miscarriage as she has passed clots at first, followed by prolonged mild bleeding. Pain though present has not been severe. Symptoms were present for a few days.

- In an ectopic pregnancy symptoms are usually of sudden onset. Pain will be the prominent symptom. Bleeding will be mild without passage of clots.

Answer 3.4

In an incomplete miscarriage:
- The general condition will be satisfactory.
- There may be mild lower abdominal tenderness.
- The cervical os is usually open. The products may be felt at the os.
- However, an incomplete miscarriage cannot be excluded if the cervical os is closed.

In an ectopic pregnancy:
- The general condition may be poor. However, it may be satisfactory in an unruptured ectopic pregnancy.
- There may be marked lower abdominal tenderness.
- The cervical os will be closed. There will be adnexal tenderness. There may be cervical motion tenderness.

Answer 3.5

An incomplete miscarriage cannot be diagnosed by USS scanning alone if an IUP has not been seen previously.

If the diagnosis is in doubt perform two serum beta hCG tests 48 hours apart. There will be a reduction of more than 50% in an incomplete miscarriage while there will be an increase of less than 63% in an ectopic pregnancy.

Answer 3.6

Once the diagnosis of an incomplete miscarriage is confirmed give 600 µg of misoprostol orally as a single dose and review in 2 weeks in the absence of heavy bleeding or infection.

QUESTION 4

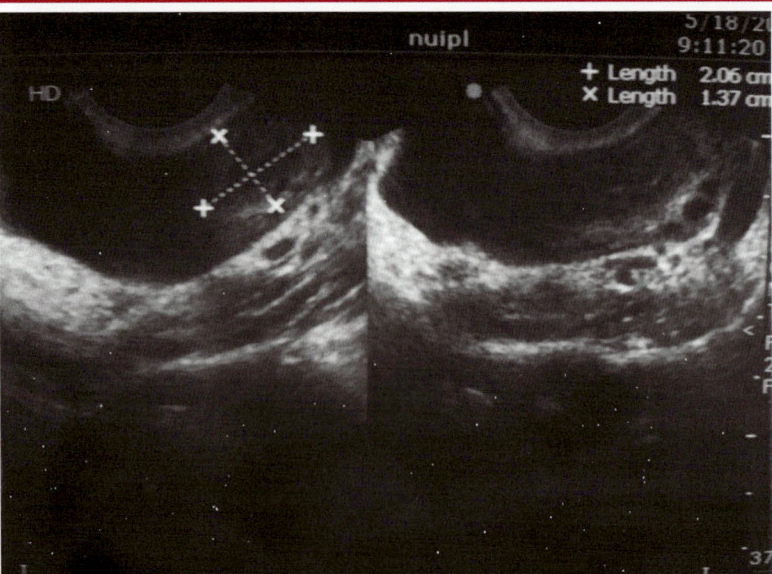

4.1 What are the abnormalities in this ultrasound image obtained on a 27-year-old unmarried woman who has a period of amenorrhoea of 6 weeks and complains of sudden onset of lower abdominal pain? What is the most likely diagnosis?

4.2 List 5 questions you would ask from this patient.

4.3 List 3 investigations you would perform.

4.4 What is the next step in the management?

Answer 4.1

- There is free fluid in the pelvis.
- There is no intrauterine pregnancy. A diagnosis of a ruptured ectopic pregnancy is likely.

Answer 4.2

Is there a history of:
- Vaginal bleeding?
- Fainting episodes?
- Sexual intercourse?
- Previous terminations of pregnancy?
- Pelvic inflammatory disease/sexually transmitted disease?

Answer 4.3

- Urine hCG test/serum beta hCG test.
- Full blood count.
- Crossmatch 3 units of blood.

Answer 4.4

Surgery should be performed as soon as possible.

Salpingectomy by laparoscopy is the best management option for a ruptured ectopic pregnancy. The tube is repaired only if the other tube is damaged.

QUESTION 5

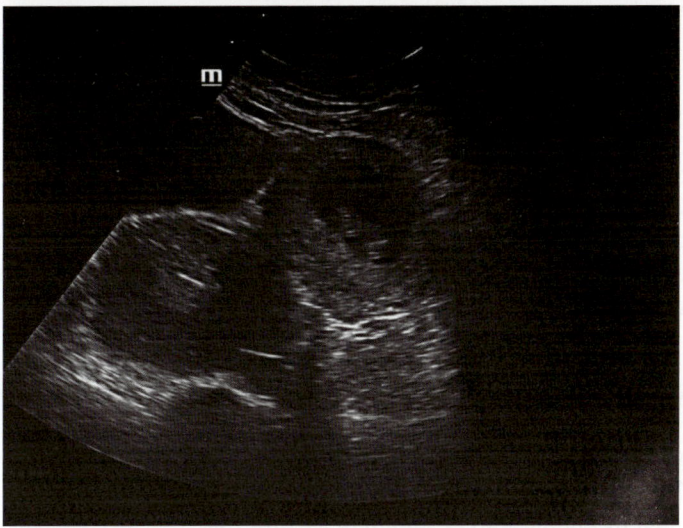

This ultrasound image was obtained from a multiparous woman who complained of sudden onset of lower abdominal pain at a period of amenorrhoea of 9 weeks.

5.1 What are the abnormalities seen in this ultrasound image and what is the probable diagnosis?

5.2 What other ultrasound features will help you to arrive at a diagnosis?

5.3 What other tests can be performed to further confirm the diagnosis?

5.4 What are the methods available to treat her? Give reasons for selecting each method.

Answer 5.1

A well-defined sac is seen in the tube with a ring sign. There appears to be fetal echoes. The appearance is most probably due to an unruptured ectopic pregnancy. The uterus shows a decidual reaction without an intrauterine pregnancy.

Answer 5.2

A ring of fire appearance round the sac can be demonstrated by colour Doppler scan.

Answer 5.3

Urine hCG test. If it is positive the diagnosis is most probably an ectopic pregnancy.

The diagnosis can be confirmed further by performing two serum beta hCG tests 48 hours apart. The rise will be less than 63% in an ectopic pregnancy.

Answer 5.4

Medical treatment with methotrexate is appropriate as the first line treatment for this woman as she has an unruptured ectopic pregnancy if:

- She consents for medical treatment.
- The adnexal mass is smaller than 35 mm with no visible heartbeat.
- The serum B hCG level is less than 1500 IU/liter.
- There is no significant pain.
- She is able to come for regular follow-up.
  All the above criteria should be satisfied.

Surgical treatment is carried out if the:

- Women is not willing for medical treatment.
- Women is unable to return for follow-up.
- Woman has significant pain.
- Adnexal mass is 35 mm or larger.
- Fetal heart beat is visible on the ultrasound scan.
- Serum hCG level is 5000 IU/liter or more.
  Since the ectopic pregnancy is unruptured laparoscopic salpingotomy is an option. However, there is a risk of another ectopic occurring at the same site. Therefore, salpingectomy is a better option in a multiparous woman if the other tube is normal.

References for Questions 1 to 5

- *Ectopic pregnancy and miscarriage: Diagnosis and initial management—NICE guidelines [CG154] December 2012.*
- *The Investigation and Treatment of Couples with Recurrent First trimester and Second-trimester Miscarriage. RCOG Green-top Guideline No. 17 April 2011.*
- *SBA Questions in Gynaecology, Chapters 11 and 12.*

QUESTION 6

A 30-year-old woman in her third pregnancy presents with vaginal bleeding after a period of amenorrhoea of 10 weeks. The urine hCG test is positive.

6.1   What is the next step in the management?

6.2   The following picture is seen on the ultrasound scan. What is the diagnosis?

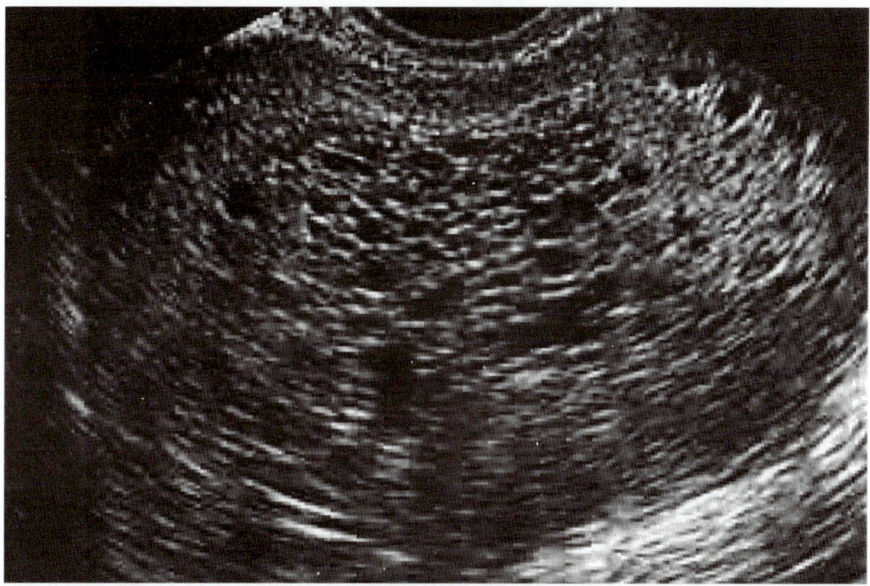

Reproduced with permission from Medscape Drugs & Diseases (https://emedicine. medscape.com)

6.3   What is the most appropriate management?

6.4   What is the most appropriate management if this woman is a 42-year-old grand multipara? Give your reasons.

Answer 6.1

Perform an ultrasound scan.

Answer 6.2

Complete hydatidiform mole.

Answer 6.3

Perform suction evacuation.

Answer 6.4

Total hysterectomy is the best option as she has completed the family and is 42 years of age. Also her advanced age increases the risk of developing gestational trophoblastic neoplasia.

QUESTION 7

A 30-year-old woman in her first pregnancy presents with vaginal bleeding at a period of amenorrhoea of 16 weeks.

7.1 What is the diagnosis if the image given below is seen on the ultrasound scan?

7.2 What is the most appropriate treatment? Give your reasons.

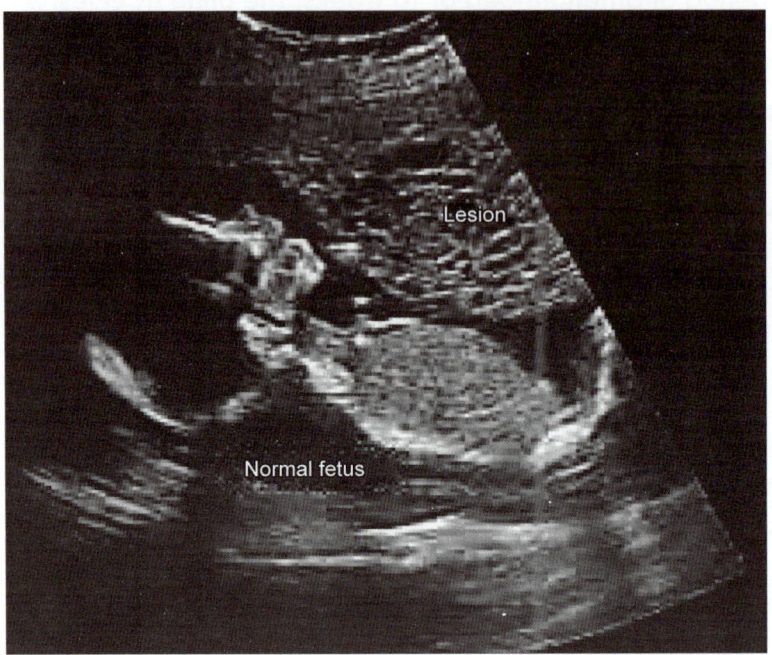

7.3 What is the most appropriate immediate follow up after evacuating a hydatidiform mole?

Answer 7.1

Partial hydatidiform mole.

Answer 7.2

Evacuate the uterus by inserting misoprostol into the vagina. Use of oxytocic drugs is best avoided in the management of a hydatidiform mole because of the risk of trophoblastic embolization. However, in this case the fetus is too big for suction evacuation.

Answer 7.3

- hCG levels are estimated once a week, until the levels return to normal.
- If the hCG levels return to normal within 56 days after evacuation, hCG levels should be checked monthly for 6 months from the day of evacuation.
- If the hCG levels return to normal more than 56 days after evacuation, hCG levels should be checked monthly for 6 months after the values become normal.
- Women should be advised not to conceive till their follow up is complete.

QUESTION 8

8.1 What are the types of gestational trophoblastic neoplasia?

8.2 How can you diagnose gestational trophoblastic neoplasia?

8.3 What are the basic principles of treating gestational trophoblastic neoplasia?

Answer 8.1

- Persistent post-molar gestational trophoblastic disease
- Invasive hydatidiform mole
- Choriocarcinoma
- Placental site trophoblastic tumour (PSTT)
- Epithelioid trophoblastic tumour (ETT).

Answer 8.2

Presence of irregular vaginal bleeding after a pregnancy event should cause suspicion of the possibility of gestational trophoblastic neoplasia.

Diagnosis is made by the following changes in the serum beta hCG levels
- Rising hCG levels.
- hCG plateau in 3 consecutive samples.
- A hCG level of more than 20000 IU/4 weeks after evacuation of a hydatidiform mole or a miscarriage.
- Raised hCG level 6 months after evacuation of a hydatidiform mole or a miscarriage or after a normal pregnancy.

Chest X-ray may reveal metastatic deposits or there may be evidence of distant metastasis.

Histological evidence of choriocarcinoma will be obtained only in cases where the tumour is in the uterus and a curettage or a hysterectomy has been performed.

Answer 8.3

- Patients with a FIGO prognostic score of 6 or less are at low risk. They are treated with a single drug(methotrexate or actinomycin D) together with folinic acid.
- Women with scores of 7 or more are at high risk. They need treatment with multiple chemotherapeutic drugs.
- The drugs which are used include combinations of intravenous methotrexate, dactinomycin, etoposide, cyclophosphamide and vincristine, with folinic acid rescue.
- A hysterectomy should be done if the focus is in the uterus and the woman does not desire further pregnancies. This is preferably performed after chemotherapy is given except in cases with severe bleeding.

QUESTION 9

9.1 Describe how you would treat women with gestational trophoblastic neoplasia whose FIGO prognostic score is 6 or less
9.2 Describe how you would treat women with gestational trophoblastic neoplasia whose FIGO prognostic score is 7 or more.
9.3 How will you follow up these patients?

Answer 9.1

Methotrexate 50 mg intramuscularly (or 1 mg/kg) is given every 48 hours for 4 doses, with folinic acid 15 mg (or 0.1 mg/kg) 24–30 hours after each dose of methotrexate. The course is repeated every 2 weeks till the serum hCG becomes negative.

- During treatment, the serum hCG levels are monitored every week
- Six weeks of maintenance chemotherapy is administered after the serum hCG level becomes normal.
- hCG is monitored monthly for 1 year.
- A switch from methotrexate to actinomycin D is made if the serum hCG levels rise or plateau (actinomycin D pulse 1.25 mg/m^2 intravenously every 2 weeks or actinomycin D 0.5 mg intravenously for 5 days every 2 weeks).

Answer 9.2

Combination chemotherapy is given.

EMA-CO regimen—a combination of etoposide, methotrexate, and actinomycin D are administered in the first week of a 2-week cycle, and cyclophosphamide and vincristine (Oncovin) are administered in the second week.

Week 1

Day 1	Actinomycin-D 0.5 mg IV (intravenous)
	Etoposide 100 mg/m^2 IV
	Methotrexate 300 mg/m^2 IV
Day 2	Actinomycin D 0.5 mg IV
	Etoposide 100 mg/m^2 IV
	Folinic acid 15 mg PO 12 hourly × 4 doses starting 24 hrs after commencing methotrexate

Week 2

Day 8	Vincristine 1.4 mg/m^2 (max 2 mg)
	Cyclophosphamide 600 mg/m^2

EMA-CE regimen—cisplatin and etoposide are substituted for cyclophosphamide and vincristine during the second week. This regimen is sometimes reserved for patients in whom EMA-CO fails

Week 1

Day 1	Actinomycin D 0.5 mg IV
	Etoposide 100 mg/m^2 IV
	Methotrexate 300 mg/m^2 IV
Day 2	Folinic acid 15 mg orally 12 hourly × 4 doses
	Starting 24 hrs after commencing methotrexate

Week 2

Day 8	Etoposide 150 mg/m^2 IV
	Cisplatin 75 mg/m^2 IV

- Treatment is given weekly till serum beta hCG becomes negative, at least 6 weeks of maintenance EMA-CO or EMA-CE are administered after serum hCG level becomes normal.
- Patients with brain metastasis are considered for irradiation. Whole brain irradiation (3000 cGy) is given in combination with chemotherapy. Dexamethasone is administered to reduce brain edema.
- Early neurosurgical intervention for solitary lesions or stereotactic radiotherapy for multiple lesions or solitary lesions in locations at high risk for surgical morbidity, followed by moderate- and high-dose intravenous methotrexate is carried out. At some centres, intrathecal methotrexate is given.

Answer 9.3

Year 1	2-weekly serum hCG for 1–6 months
	2-weekly urine hCG for 7–12 months
Year 2	4-weekly urine hCG
Year 3	8-weekly urine hCG
Year 4	3-monthly urine hCG
Year 5	4-monthly urine hCG
Year 6-life	6-monthly urine hCG

QUESTION 10

What is the best treatment option for:

10.1 A 25-year-old primipara who has a serum beta hCG level of 20000 IU/ml 4 weeks after evacuation of a hydatidiform mole.

10.2 A 25-year-old primipara who has a serum beta hCG level of 20000 IU/ml 4 weeks after evacuation of an invasive mole. There is no evidence of extra-uterine spread.

10.3 A 40-year-old multipara who has irregular bleeding and a serum beta hCG level of 50000 IU/ml 8 months after an abortion.

10.4 A 40-year-old multipara who has irregular bleeding and a serum beta hCG level of 50,000 IU/ml 8 months after a normal delivery who does not respond to first-line chemotherapy.

10.5 A 40-year-old multipara who has a choriocarcinoma with brain metastasis.

Answer 10.1

Methotrexate 50 mg intramuscularly (or 1 mg/kg) is given every 48 hours for 4 doses, with folinic acid 15 mg (or 0.1 mg/kg) 24–30 hours after each dose of methotrexate. The course is repeated every 2 weeks till the serum hCG becomes negative.

Answer 10.2

Methotrexate 50 mg intramuscularly (or 1 mg/kg) is given every 48 hours for 4 doses, with folinic acid 15 mg (or 0.1 mg/kg) 24–30 hours after each dose of methotrexate. The course is repeated every 2 weeks till the serum hCG becomes negative.

Answer 10.3

EMA-CO regimen—a combination of etoposide, methotrexate and actinomycin D are administered with folinic acid rescue in the first week of a 2-week cycle, and cyclophosphamide and vincristine (Oncovin) are administered in the second week.

Answer 10.4

EMA-CE regimen—cisplatin and etoposide are substituted for cyclophosphamide and vincristine during the second week. This is given as EMA-CO has failed.

Answer 10.5

• Patients with brain metastasis are considered for irradiation. Whole brain irradiation (3000 cGy) is given in combination with chemotherapy (EMA-CO regimen). Dexamethasone is administered to reduce cerebral oedema (most common approach in US).

• Early neurosurgical intervention for solitary lesions or stereotactic radiotherapy for multiple lesions or solitary lesions in locations at high risk for surgical morbidity, followed by high-dose intravenous methotrexate is carried out. At some centres, intrathecal methotrexate is given.

References for Questions 6 to 10

• *Gestational Trophoblastic Disease (RCOG Green-top Guideline No. 38). Published: 04/03/2010.*
• *SBA Questions in Gynaecology, Chapter 13.*

Benign Ovarian Tumours

The following pictures were obtained when an USS scan was performed on a 30-year-old woman attending the infertility clinic.

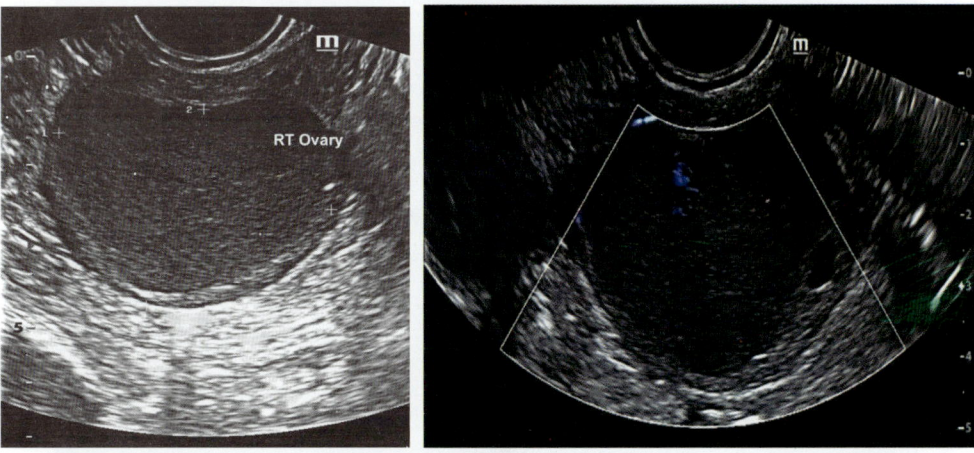

1.1 What is the most likely diagnosis? Give reasons for your diagnosis.
1.2 What are the other symptoms of this condition?
1.3 What is the best treatment option?
1.4 What is the best treatment option in a woman who does not desire early fertility?

Answer 1.1

An endometrial cyst of the right ovary.

   The cyst is well circumscribed with a thin wall and a ground glass appearance and low vascularity.

Answer 1.2

- Dysmenorrhea
- Dyspareunia

- Frequent menstrual cycles
- Backache
- Dyschezia

Answer 1.3

Laparoscopic cystectomy should be performed. Any other endometriotic deposits should be cauterized and adhesiolysis should be performed, if required. Medical management is best avoided as it prevents conception during and for some time after treatment.

Answer 1.4

Medical management can be tried for 3–6 months as the first line option because the cyst is small. GnRH analogues 3.75 mg IM once a month for 3–6 months or DMPA 150 mg IM once a month for the same duration are the drugs of choice.

QUESTION 2

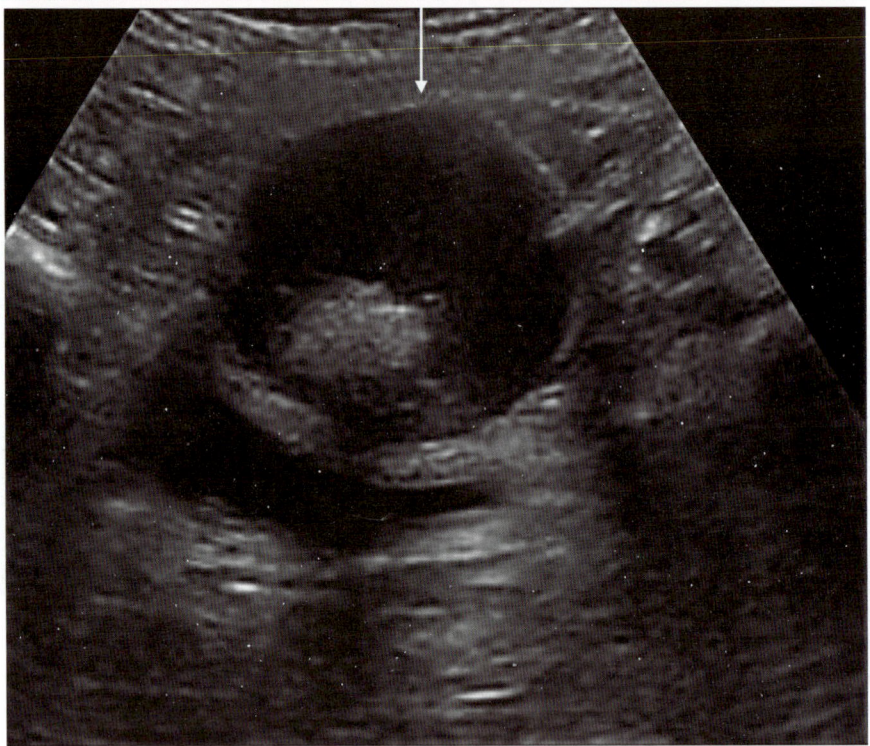

Reproduced with permission from ultrasoundcases.info

The following picture was obtained when an USS scan was performed on a woman who is complaining of abdominal pain.

2.1   What is the most likely diagnosis? Give reasons for your diagnosis.
2.2   What is the best management option if this woman is 25 years of age?
2.3   What is the best management option if this woman is 45 years of age?
2.4   What is the best management option if torsion is suspected?

Answer 2.1

A dermoid cyst is the most likely diagnosis.

The cyst is thin walled and unilocular with a well circumscribed small solid nodule.

Answer 2.2

Laparoscopic cystectomy

Answer 2.3

Laparoscopic cystectomy is the treatment of choice as the cyst appears to be benign.

Answer 2.4

Surgery should be performed immediately to prevent the ovary from becoming gangrenous. Laparoscopic cystectomy is performed if the ovary is not gangrenous. Oophorectomy has to be performed if gangrene has occurred.

QUESTION 3

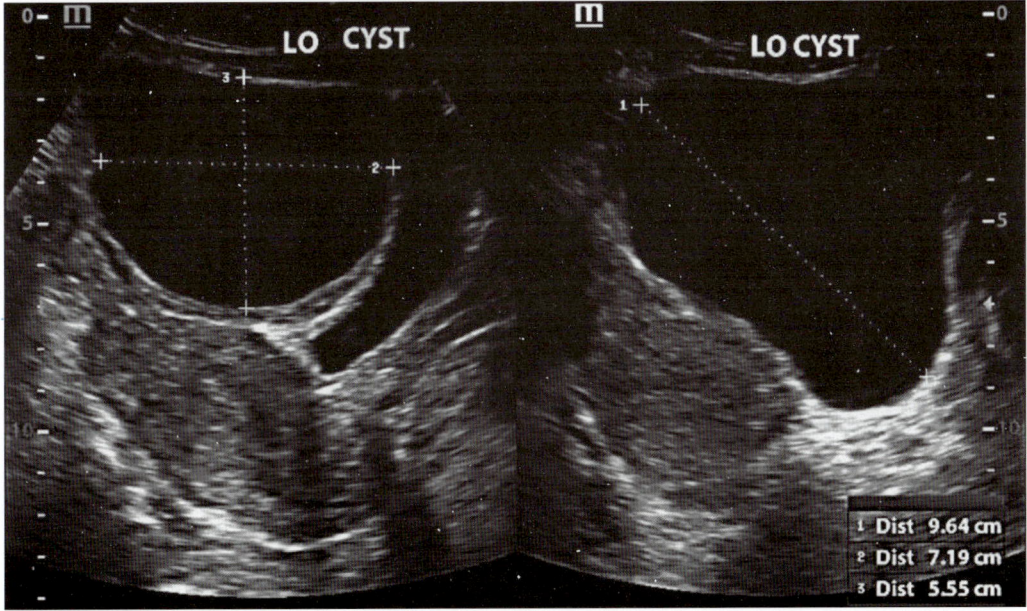

The following pictures were obtained when an USS scan was performed on a 40-year-old woman who is complaining of abdominal discomfort.

3.1   What is the most likely diagnosis? Give reasons for your diagnosis.

3.2   What is the best management option?

3.3   What is the best management option if this woman is 60 years of age?

Answer 3.1

She has a benign ovarian cyst. The tumour is thin walled. There are no solid areas or septa and the capsule is intact.

Answer 3.2

Perform a laparoscopic cystectomy.

Answer 3.3

- Perform CA 125 levels.
- If CA 125 is below 30 IU/ml and the RMI is below 200 perform laparoscopic salpingo-oophorectomy.
- If CA 125 level is elevated and the RMI is equal to or more than 200, perform a MRI scan followed by TAH, BSO and infracolic omentectomy and full surgical staging of the tumour in a specialized centre.

QUESTION 4

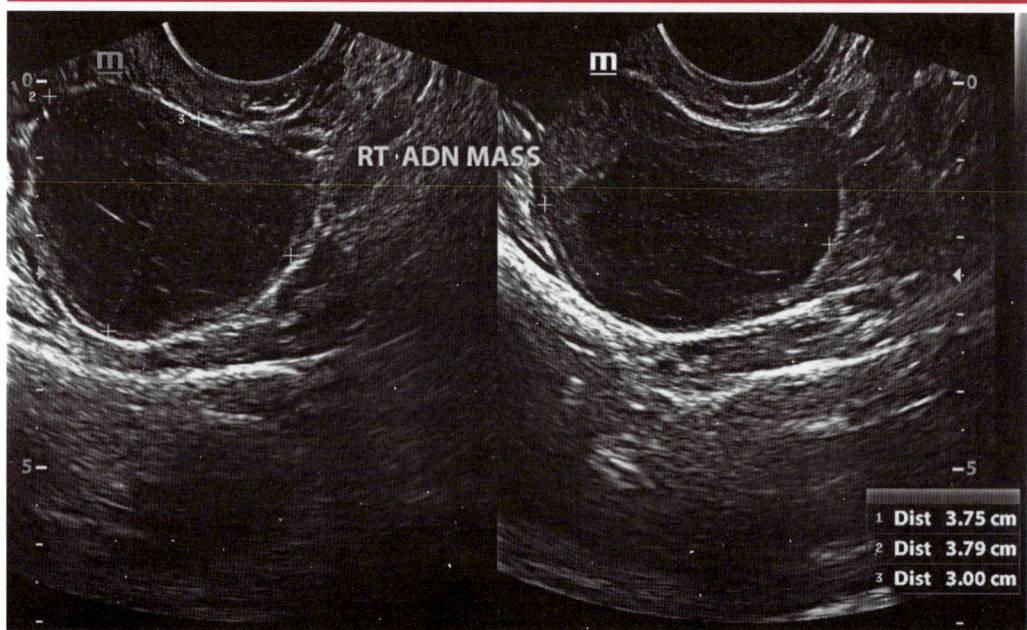

The following picture was obtained when an USS scan was performed on a 40-year-old woman who is complaining of abdominal discomfort.

4.1   What is the most likely diagnosis? Give reasons for your diagnosis.

4.2   What is the best management option?

4.3   What is the best management option if the diameter of this tumour is 7 cm?

4.4   What is the best management option if this woman is 60 years of age?

Answer 4.1

A physiological ovarian cyst.

It is a thin walled unilocular small cyst measuring less than 5 cm without solid areas.

Answer 4.2

As the woman is young and the cyst is 3 cm, unilocular and thin walled (simple cyst) reassure the woman. Follow up is not necessary.

Answer 4.3

Reassure and review after 1 year with an ultrasound scan.

Answer 4.4

Perform CA 125 levels. If CA 125 is below 30 IU/ml and the RMI is below 200 review with an ultrasound scan in 4 months. Laparoscopic oophorectomy has to be done if the cyst is larger than 5 cm.

QUESTION 5

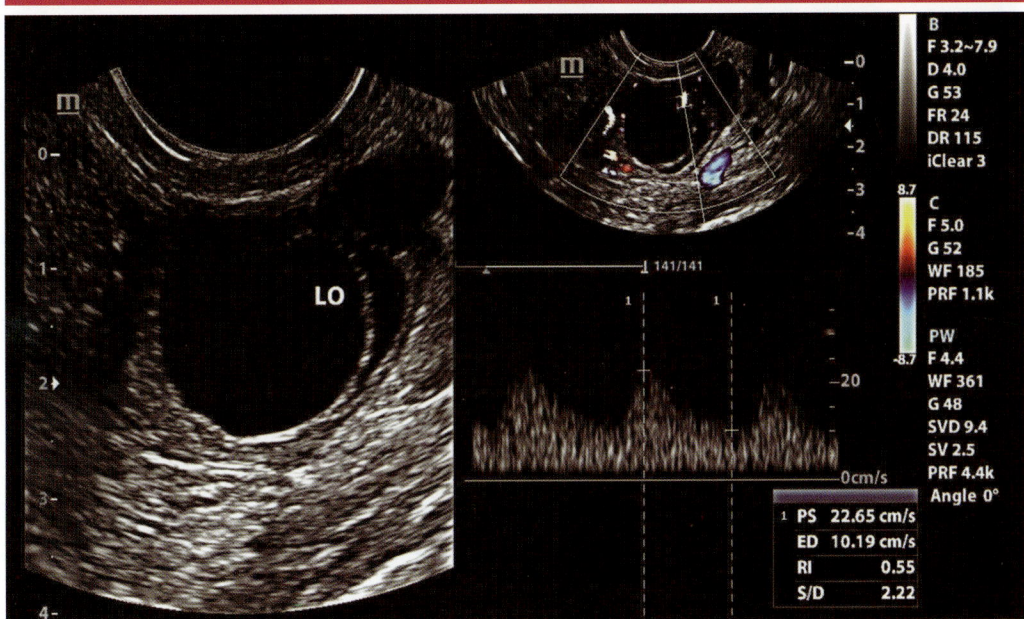

5.1 Describe this USS image. What is your diagnosis?
5.2 What is the next investigation which should be performed?
5.3 What is the best management option if this woman is 45 years of age?
5.4 What is the best management option if this woman is 65 years of age?

Answer 5.1

It is an image of a multilocular ovarian cyst with thin septa without solid areas.

Answer 5.2

Perform CA 125 levels

Answer 5.3

- If CA 125 is below 30 IU/ml perform laparoscopic cystectomy.
- If CA 125 level is elevated perform a MRI scan followed by TAH, BSO and infra-colic omentectomy and full surgical staging of the tumour in a specialized centre.

Answer 5.4

- If CA 125 is below 30 IU/ml and the RMI is below 200 perform laparoscopic salpingo-oophorectomy.

- If CA 125 level is elevated and the RMI is above 200 perform a MRI scan. Perform TAH, BSO and infracolic omentectomy and full surgical staging of the tumour in a specialized center.

References:
- *Ovarian Cysts in Postmenopausal Women RCOG Guideline No. 34, October 2003 Reviewed 2010.*
- *Management of Suspected Ovarian Masses in Premenopausal Women Green–top Guideline No. 62 RCOG/BSGE Joint Guideline November 2011.*
- *SBA Questions in Gynaecology, Chapter 6.*

Malignant Ovarian Tumours

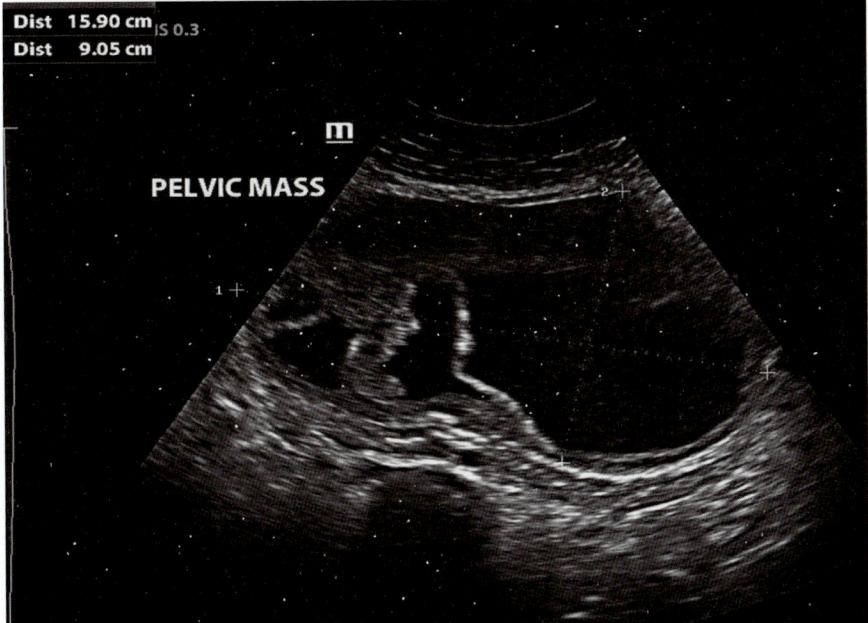

Dist 15.90 cm IS 0.3
Dist 9.05 cm

m

PELVIC MASS

1.1 This is the ultrasound image obtained from a 32-year-old woman with one child who complained of abdominal discomfort. State your diagnosis and give your reasons.

1.2 State the investigations you would perform to determine the nature of the tumour.

1.3 Explain how you can determine the risk of malignancy of an ovarian tumour before performing surgery.

1.4 What are the ultrasound features of benign and malignant tumours?

1.5 What is the best management option for this woman?

Answer 1.1

It is most probably a malignant ovarian tumour because there is a solid area and multiple septa.

Answer 1.2

- Perform CA 125, LDH and alpha fetoprotein levels
- Perform a MRI scan to determine the extent of spread

Answer 1.3

This is done by calculating the risk of malignancy index.
Calculation of the RMI is based on:
- Serum cancer antigen (CA 125)
- Menopausal status (M)
- Ultrasound score (U)
  RMI = U × M × CA 125 (units/ml).

The ultrasound score is calculated by awarding 1 point each for:
- Multilocular cysts
- Solid areas
- Metastases
- Ascites
- Bilateral lesions
  U = 0 (for an ultrasound score of 0), U = 1 (for an ultrasound score of 1), U = 3 (for an ultrasound score of 2–5)

The following score is calculated for menopausal status.
  1 = premenopausal and 3 = postmenopausal.
  Women who have had no period for more than one year or women over the age of 50 who have had a hysterectomy are regarded as postmenopausal.
  Serum CA 125 can vary between zero and hundreds or even thousands of units/ml.

RMI	Risk of malignancy
Low <25	<3%
Moderate 25–250	20%
High >250	75%

Answer 1.4

B rules for benign cysts:
- Unilocular cysts.
- Presence of solid components where the largest solid component is less than 7 mm.
- Presence of acoustic shadowing.
- No blood flow.
- Smooth multilocular tumour with the largest diameter less than 100 mm

M rules for malignant cysts:
- Irregular solid tumour.
- Ascites.
- Presence of at least 4 papillary structures.
- Irregular, multilocular, solid tumour with the largest diameter greater than 100 mm.
- Very strong blood flow.

Answer 1.5

- A laparotomy is performed after calculating the RMI.
- This woman is young and nulliparous. Therefore, if the tumour has not breached the capsule, the other ovary appears to be normal and there is no macroscopic evidence of spread, the best surgical option would be unilateral salpingo-oophorectomy, infracolic omentectomy and biopsy of the other ovary and to await histology report.
- If the surgical stage is 1B or higher TAH and BSO and infracolic omentectomy should be done.

QUESTION 2

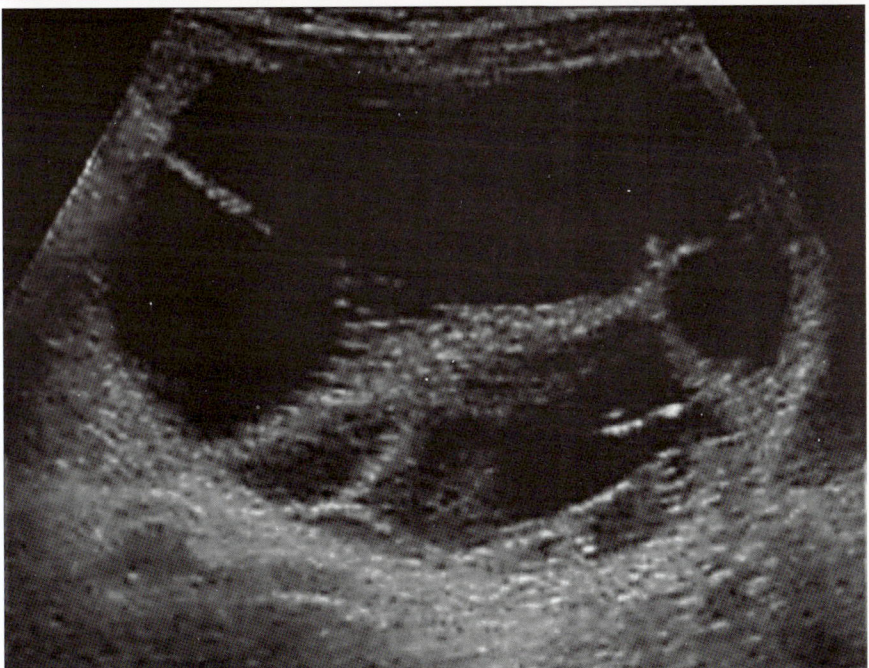

Reproduced with permission from http://www.ultrasoundcases.info/

2.1 This is the ultrasound image obtained from a 45-year-old multiparous woman. State your diagnosis and give your reasons.

2.2 What is the best treatment option?

2.3 What are the features of a malignant ovarian tumour at surgery?

2.4 How will you stage an ovarian tumour?

2.5 Who are the patients who will need adjuvant chemotherapy?

Answer 2.1

It is a large ovarian tumour which is most probably malignant because it has multiple thick septa and a thick wall.

Answer 2.2

Perform CA 125 levels and calculate the RMI.

Total abdominal hysterectomy, bilateral salpingo-oophorectomy, infracolic omentectomy and removal of any deposits and full surgical staging should be performed.

Answer 2.3

Malignancy is suspected at surgery, if:
- The tumour has breached the capsule,
- There are large blood vessels on the surface,
- The tumour has solid areas,
- There are bilateral tumours,
- There is ascites,
- There are peritoneal or omental deposits.

Answer 2.4

USS scanning and MRI scanning may be helpful in assessing the spread, but the stage is confirmed at surgery.

The following should be done at surgery to stage the tumour accurately:
- Cytology of ascetic fluid or peritoneal washings.
- Multiple peritoneal biopsies.
- Biopsies from adhesions and suspicious areas.
- Omentectomy and histology.
- Bilateral pelvic and para-aortic lymph node sampling.
- Diaphragmatic scraping or biopsy for histology.

Answer 2.5

- Only patients with stage IA grade 1 and stage IB grade 1, serous, mucinous, endometrioid and Brenner tumours can be treated with surgery alone. Others need adjuvant chemotherapy.
- Clear-cell carcinomas have a worse prognosis in stage I and should be considered for chemotherapy at all stages
- First-line chemotherapy is cisplatin which can be used alone or with pacitaxel in advanced disease.

References
- *Ovarian cancer: recognition and initial management, NICE guidelines [CG122] Published date: April 2011.*
- *SBA Questions in Gynaecology, Chapter 6*

Surgical Instruments and Procedures

QUESTION 1

Name the instruments.

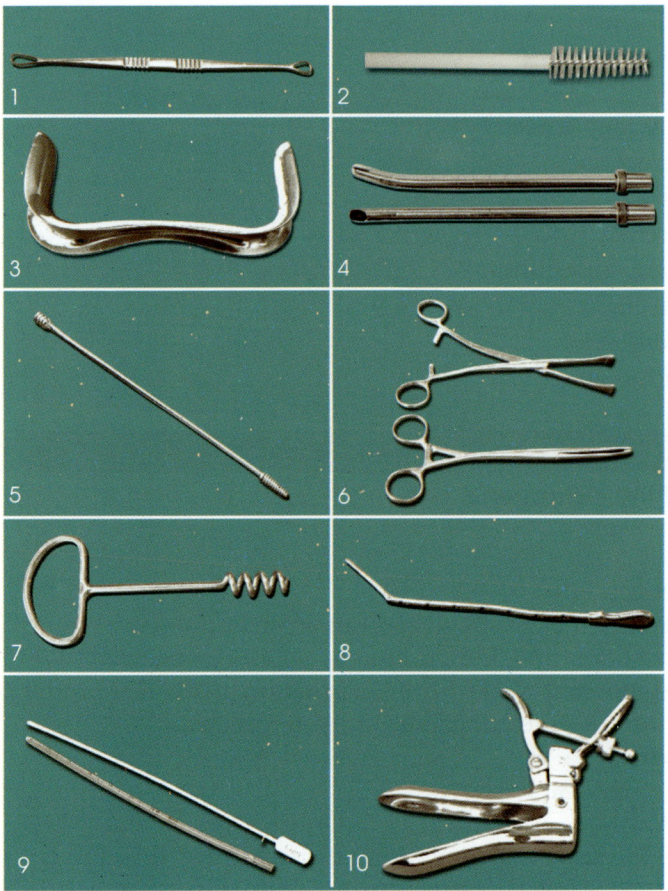

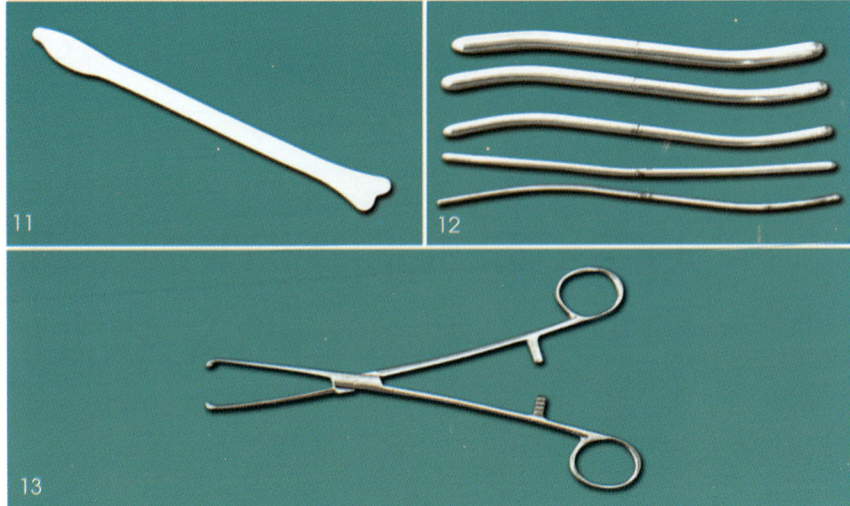

Answer

1. Uterine curette
2. Cervical brush
3. Sim's speculum
4. Suction curette
5. Leech Wilkinson cannula
6. Green-Armytage forceps
7. Myoma screw
8. Uterine sound
9. Pipelle curette
10. Cusco bi-valve speculum
11. Ayre's spatula
12. Hegar's dilators
13. Vulsellum forceps

QUESTION 2

List the uses of the instruments 1–7.

Answer

1. Uterine curette
   - To perform uterine curettage and obtain an endometrial sample for diagnostic purposes at dilatation and curettage
   - To remove adherent tissue during evacuation of retained products of conception.
   - To break intrauterine adhesions at hysteroscopy.
2. Cervical brush
   - To obtain a cervical smear.
3. Sim's speculum
   - To expose the cervix during surgeries performed through the vaginal route.
   - To inspect for urinary fistulae during vaginal examination.

- To examine an uterovaginal prolapse at the clinic.
- To inspect the genital tract for tears after instrumental deliveries.

4. Suction curette
   - To remove retained products of conception.
   - To evacuate a hydatidiform mole.
   - To perform termination of pregnancy.

5. Leech Wilkinson cannula
   - This instrument is screwed into the cervix to insert the dye while performing a HSG.

6. Green-Armytage forceps
   - To hold the pregnant cervix when inspecting for tears after delivery and when inserting a cervical circlage.
   - To hold the flaps of the uterus at caesarean section.
   - To control bleeding from uterine sinuses at caesarean section.

7. Myoma screw
   - To hold and stabilize a fibroid at myomectomy
   - To hold a large uterus at hysterectomy

QUESTION 3

List the uses of the instruments 8–13.

8. Uterine sound
   - To assess the length of the uterine cavity and to determine the direction of the uterus before inserting other instruments into the uterus.

9. Pipelle curette
   - To obtain an endometrial sample at the clinic. This procedure is carried out without anaesthesia.

10. Cusco's bi-valve speculum is used to:
    - Inspect the cervix.
    - Obtain a cervical smear.
    - Obtain an endocervical and a high vaginal swab.
    - Perform colposcopic examination.
    - Perform a hysterosalpingogram.
    - Perform pipelle endometrial sampling.
    - Insert an IUCD.
    - Diagnose the presence of dribbling.
    - Remove a cervical circlage.
    - Remove products of conception from the cervical canal in the ward in an inevitable or incomplete miscarriage.

11. Ayre's spatula
    - To obtain a cervical smear.

12. Hegar's dilators
    - To dilate the cervical canal at dilatation and curettage and dilatation and evacuation.

13. Vulsellum forceps
    - To hold the uterus at hysterectomy for non-malignant conditions.
    - To hold the non-pregnant cervix during surgical procedures performed through the vaginal route. To hold the cervix during insertion of an IUCD, Pipelle aspiration and when performing a hysterosalpingogram.
    - To hold the cervix during evacuation of retained products of conception during the first trimester.

QUESTION 4

4.1 Pick the instruments required to perform a dilatation and curettage and place them in the correct order of use during the procedure.

4.2 Pick the instruments required to inspect the genital tract for tears after delivery and place them in the correct order of use during the procedure.

4.3 Pick the instruments required to perform a hysterosalpingogram and place them in the correct order of use during the procedure.

4.4 Pick the instruments required to obtain a cervical smear and place them in the correct order of use during the procedure. What else is needed to complete the procedure?

4.5 Pick the instruments required to perform a Pipelle aspiration and place them in the correct order of use during the procedure. What else is needed to complete the procedure?

4.6 Pick the instruments required to perform a suction evacuation and place them in the correct order of use during the procedure. What else is needed to complete the procedure?

Answer 4.1

3, 13, 8, 12 and 1

Answer 4.2

3 and 6

Answer 4.3

10, 13, 8, and 5

Answer 4.4

10 and 2 or 11

Two glass slides and a container of 95% alcohol to fix the slides are needed to complete procedure.

Answer 4.5

10, 13 and 9

A small bottle containing formalin is required to place the curettings.

Answer 4.6

3, 13, 8, 12, 4 and 1

A suction apparatus should be connected to the suction curette to apply negative pressure to suck out the products.

QUESTION 5

Describe in detail how you would ripen the cervix prior to induction of labour.

Answer

- The procedure should be explained to the patient. Informed consent is obtained.
- The procedure is carried out in the morning in the antenatal ward.
- A CTG is performed.
- The woman should empty the bladder.
- The operator should scrub and wear sterile gloves.
- The patient is placed in the dorsal position.
- The vulva is cleaned with an antiseptic solution using the five swab technique.
- A vaginal examination should be performed to assess the Bishop score.
- Cervical ripening is needed if the Bishop score is less than 7.
- There are two methods of ripening the cervix.
  - Dinoprostone (PGE 2) 3 mg is inserted to the posterior fornix. A CTG is performed after 2 hours. The patient is kept under observation for contractions. If the woman does not go into labour insert a second dose after 6 hours. Perform an amniotomy when the cervical dilatation reaches 5–6 cm.
  - The cervix is exposed after inserting a Cusco's bivalve speculum. A Foley catheter with a 30 cc bulb is inserted through the cervical canal. The bulb should be at the level of the internal os. The bulb is inflated with distilled water. Care should be taken not to rupture the membranes. The catheter will fall off once the cervix is dilated. The Bishop score is assessed the next morning. If the Bishop score is more than 6 an amniotomy can be performed. This may be followed by an infusion of oxytocin after 2 hours. This is a safe method and is preferred for women with a scarred uterus or cardiac disease.

QUESTION 6

Describe in detail how you would insert an urinary catheter to a patient in the second stage of labour.

Answer

- Catheterization should be performed only if the patient is unable to pass urine.
- A rubber catheter should be used. A Foley catheter is preferable.
- The procedure should be explained to the patient. Informed consent is obtained.
- The operator should scrub and wear sterile gloves.
- The patient is placed in the dorsal position.
- The vulva is cleaned with an antiseptic solution using the five swab technique.
- The catheter should be taken out from the sterile package.
- An antiseptic gel is applied to the tip of the catheter.
- The urethral orifice is identified and the catheter is gently inserted.
- This should be done in-between contractions and the patient should be prevented from straining.
- It may be necessary to gently push the urethra upwards with a finger placed in the vagina, especially if the head has descended.
- The catheter is connected to a sterile urine bag.

- The bulb should be inflated with the appropriate volume of distilled water.
- Observe for the free flow of urine into the bag.

QUESTION 7

Describe in detail how you would perform the following procedures.
7.1 Commencing an intravenous infusion
7.2 Commencing a blood transfusion

Answer

All procedures should be explained to the patient and informed consent should be taken.

Answer 7.1

- A tourniquet, antiseptic solution, cotton swabs, an intravenous cannula, the infusion solution and a drip set are required.
- The drip set should be connected to the infusion bottle.
- The drip set should be opened and the tubing should be filled with fluid to expel air from the tubing. The drip set should be clamped and the needle cover should be applied.
- The procedure should be explained to the patient and informed consent should be obtained.
- A suitable vein is identified. It is facilitated by asking the patient to clench the fist.
- The area is cleaned with the antiseptic solution. A tourniquet is applied to make the vein more prominent.
- The vein is punctured with the metal tip of the cannula.
- Once blood flows into the cannula the trocar is removed and the cannula is inserted into the vein.
- The needle of the drip set is removed and it should be quickly connected to the cannula.
- The cap should be placed on the cannula.
- A plaster should be applied to secure the cannula in place.
- The flow should be adjusted to the required rate.

Answer 7.2

Check and compare the following information on the tag attached to the blood pack and the stamp placed on the patient's BHT by the blood bank when the blood is issued.

- The name of the patient.
- The name of the donor.
- The BHT number of the patient.
- The bottle number
- Expiry date of the pack.

Check and exclude the following:
- Check for hemolysis by looking at the plasma portion of the pack and noticing any pink discoloration.

- Check whether the injection ports are open.
- Check whether there are any leaks in the pack.
- Check whether the tube sealing is intact without any leaks.
- Check the expiry date of the pack.

Perform a venepuncture:
- A tourniquet, antiseptic solution, cotton swabs, an intravenous cannula, the blood pack and blood set are required.
- The blood set should be connected to the blood pack.
- The set should be opened and the tubing should be filled with blood to expel air from the tubing. The set should be clamped.
- Venepuncture is performed as described in 7.1 and blood transfusion is commenced.

The following should be documented in the bed head ticket.
- Start blood transfusion.
- Observe pulse, BP and the respiratory rate every 5 minutes for 15 minutes and every 15 minutes for 2 hours.
- Look for any rash, itching, breathing difficulty, confusion, fever and chills.
- Inform the house officer immediately if a reaction occurs.

QUESTION 8

8.1 Pick the instruments required to remove a cervical circlage.
8.2 Describe in detail the method of removing a cervical circlage

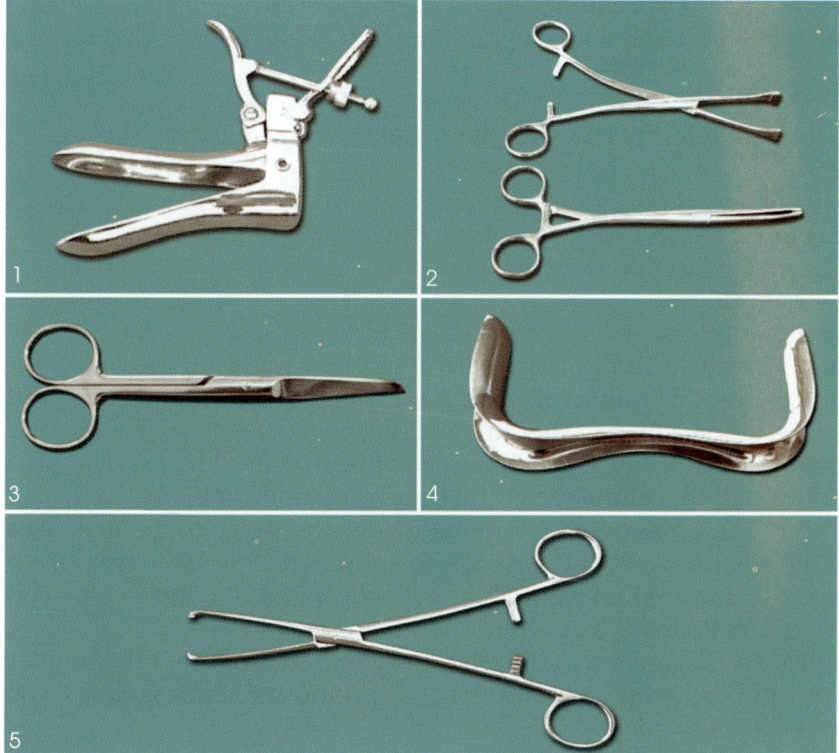

Answer 8.1

1 and 3. A pair of long artery forceps may be needed to hold the ends of the thread.

Answer 8.2

- It is carried out at 37 weeks or earlier if the patient develops labour pains.
- It is carried out in the ward.
- Informed consent should be obtained.
- Read the diagnosis card to find out the position of the knot of the circlage.
- Place the patient in the dorsal position.
- Wear sterile gloves.
- Clean the vulva using an antiseptic solution.
- Insert a Cusco's speculum and visualize the knot. The end of the suture is usually kept long.
- Grasp the end of the thread with a pair of long artery forceps, expose the knot and cut it with a pair of long scissors.
- Remove the entire stitch. Close and withdraw the speculum.
- Perform a vaginal examination to confirm that the entire stitch has been removed.

QUESTION 9

9.1 **List the equipment required to perform a cervical smear.**
9.2 **Describe in detail the method of performing a cervical smear.**

Answer 9.1

- A Cusco's bivalve speculum, Ayer's spatula/cervical brush, two glass slides, a container of 95% alcohol and a good light are needed.

Answer 9.2

- The patient should not be menstruating at the time of the procedure.
- Informed consent should be obtained.
- The bladder should be empty.
- This is performed in the gynaecology clinic.
- The patient is placed in the dorsal position.
- Wear sterile gloves.
- Antiseptic solutions or lubricating cream are not used.
- A Cusco's bivalve speculum is inserted and the cervix is exposed.
- The procedure is continued if there is no visible ulcer on the cervix. If there is a suspicious lesion a biopsy should be performed.
- The pointed end of the Ayer's spatula is inserted into the cervical canal and is rotated by 360° to include the entire transformation zone.
- It is smeared on a glass slide and immediately dropped into the alcohol container.
- Using the other flat end of the Ayer's spatula a smear is taken from the posterior fornix and is smeared on a glass slide. It is dropped into the alcohol container.
- The speculum is closed and withdrawn.
- The slides are dispatched to the laboratory with a properly filled request form.
- The woman is advised to attend the clinic at the appropriate time to obtain the report.

Important Documents

Mention the mistakes in this operation list.

Health] 288
(F 6 S. & E.) 4/65

NOTICE OF OPERATIONS

The following Operations will be performed by Doctor _E. Samarakoon_

_____on _16/8_ 20 _17_ at _8_ a. m.

1. _____
2. _Kusumawathie ward 3 15697_
3. _- Abdominal hysterectomy_
4. _____
5. _Manel Silva ward 3 15693_
6. _- laparotomy_
7. _____
8. _Premawathie ward 3 15485_
9. _Laparascopy_
10. _____
11. _____
12. _____

S. perera

House Surgeon.

Date _____

H 040321 – 5,000,000 (2012/06) P

Answer

- The names of Kusumawathie and Premawathie are incomplete as there are no initials or a surname.
- The indication for laparotomy should be mentioned.
- The indication or the surgical procedure for laparoscopy should be mentioned (ex: laparoscopy and dye test, diagnostic laparoscopy, ovarian cystectomy, etc.)
- The designation of the surgeon has not been mentioned. An operation list can be sent only under the name of a Board Certified Consultant.
- The date of writing the list is not mentioned at the bottom.
- It is better to mention at the top whether it is a routine or a casualty list.
- It is better to mention at the top the designation of the officer receiving the list or the place to which the list should be sent (ex: theater or the ward).

QUESTION 2

List 10 faults in this diagnosis card.

Blood group A(+)ve

Take this card when you visit the Doctor

Health 383A
(Card* S.T. & E. 7 3/4" x 7 3/4")

DIAGNOSIS TICKET

Name of Patient } Kusumawathie   Age } 45yrs

Ward } 10.   Reg. No. } 13698 /17

Date of Admission } 10/1/17   Date of Discharge }

Investigations and Treatments

Investigations
full blood count
urine full report.
fasting blood sugar
ECG, CXR
Serum creatinine
(all the above
results are
normal)

TAH + BSO.
Indication   by Dr P Samaraweera
multiple fibroids   Asst - Dr S Bandara.
                              under GA.
procedure - Pfannenstiel incision
              uterus enlarged to 16/52 with
multiple fibroids. other pelvic and abdominal
viscera - normal.
TAH + BSO done. Skin closed with
absorbable sutures. Uneventful recovery

Referred to ___94n___ Clinic

M. TU. WD. TH. / FR. SA. Physician/Surgeon } _____

8.00a.m./2.00 p.m. _____ { Hospital

Date : _____   [Turn Over]

H 038067 – 1,250,000 (2011/05) P

Answer

- The name is written without initials.
- The name of the operation is not written fully.
- The following details are not mentioned.
  - The designation of the surgeon.
  - The date of the operation.
  - The time of the clinic.
  - The date of clinic attendance.
  - The date of discharge.
  - The name of the consultant.
  - The name and designation of the anaesthetist
  - The name of the hospital.
- It is not indicated whether:
  - Blood was transfused.
  - The specimen was sent for histology.
  - Antibiotics were given after surgery.
  - She was discharged on any drugs.

QUESTION 3

What are the mistakes in this pathology request form?

·Health | 350
(F O S. & B.) 7/64

DEPARTMENT OF HEALTH SERVICES
REQUEST FORM

To : **The Pathologist, General Hospital, Colombo.**

Please examine specimen of...... Cuvettings ....with regard to...... histology ....

Signature] ... S. Perera ....

Date] .... Designation] ....

Particulars of Patient

Name] ...... Karunawathie .... Age] ... 50.yrs..

Case No.] 159246 Sex ....

Ward] ... 03 .... District] ....

Short clinical history with probable diagnosis.

This patient presented with heavy menstrual bleeding

(For Pathologist's use)

Answer

- The specimen should be mentioned as uterine curettings.
- The following details have not been documented.
  - The designation of the person who signed the form.
  - The date of collection of the sample.
  - The sex of the patient.
- The name should be written with initials and the surname.
- The history is inadequate as the following details have not been mentioned.
  - Duration of the illness.
  - Use of hormones.
  - Whether the illness was preceded by a period of amenorrhoea.
  - USS findings.
  - Findings of the examination under anaesthesia.
  - Macroscopic nature of the curettings.

Preoperative and Postoperative Care

QUESTION 1

A 35-year-old otherwise healthy woman who underwent an uncomplicated total hysterectomy for uterine fibroids is found to be restless 4 hours after the surgery.

1.1 List the possible causes for her condition.

1.2 How will you arrive at a diagosis?

Answer 1.1

- Pain
- Retention of urine
- Intraperitoneal haemorrhage
- Myocardial infarction
- Aspiration
- Hypoglycaemia
- Dehydration

Answer 1.2

- *Question her regarding:*
  - Abdominal pain/chest pain/shoulder tip pain.
  - Passage of urine.
  - Difficulty in breathing.
  - Sweating.
  - Vaginal bleeding.
- *Perform a general and systemic examination for:*
  - Pallor of mucous membranes.
  - Pulse rate/respiratory rate/blood pressure.
  - Basal crepitations.
- *Perform an abdominal examination for:*
  - Distension.
  - Tenderness/guarding/rigidity.
  - Presence of free fluid.
  - Distension of the bladder.

- *Perform:*
  - An USS to exclude free fluid in the peritoneal cavity.
  - A full blood count.
  - Random blood sugar
  - An ECG and troponin T levels if a myocardial infarction is suspected.
  - A chest X-ray if aspiration is suspected.

If the catheter is draining and patient is complaining of abdominal pain and her general condition is satisfactory with no abdominal distension or free fluid the restlessness is most probably due to post-operative pain.

If there is no indwelling catheter and the patient has not passed urine and her general condition is satisfactory with no abdominal distension or free fluid the restlessness is most probably caused by pain due to urinary retention. Distended bladder can be detected by percussion.

If the patient has severe abdominal pain shoulder tip pain and chest pain, intraperitoneal bleeding should be suspected. There will be pallor, low blood pressure and tachycardia. The abdomen will be distended with tenderness, guarding and flank dullness on percussion. Intraperitoneal bleeding is a clinical diagnosis based on vital signs. However, an USS can be performed to detect the presence of free fluid and the full blood count may reveal a low haemoglobin level.

If chestpain, dyspnoea and sweating are present an acute myocardial infarction should be suspected. Diagnosis can be confirmed by occurrence of ECG changes and high treponin T levels.

If dyspnoea is the prominent symptom and crepitations are found in the lungs aspiration is suspected and confirmed by performing a chest X-ray.

QUESTION 2

A woman develops abdominal distension and vomitting 36 hours after a total hysterectomy and bilateral salpingo-oophorectomy for extensive endometriosis.
2.1 List the causes
2.2 List the investigations you would perform to confirm the diagnosis. Give your reasons.
2.3 What is the first-line management ?
2.4 What are the indications for immediate surgery?

Answer 2.1

- Paralytic ileus
- Peritonitis
- Bowel damage
- Retained foreign body
- Urinary leak due to damage to the ureter/bladder

Answer 2.2

- WBCDC, procalcitonin and C-reactive protein levels should be performed to exclude severe infection. The levels will be grossly elevated in peritonitis, bowel damage and in retained foreign body.
- Ultrasound scanning will reveal:
  - Only dilated bowel loops in paralytic ileus

– Free fluid in bowel damage and in ureteric damage. Small solid particles may be identified in bowel damage. A small amount of pus/free fluid may be seen in peritonitis.
– A retained foreign body.
- Serum electrolytes should be performed. Low potassium levels can cause paralytic ileus or the electrolytes can be deranged due to vomitting.

Answer 2.3

- Keep the patient nil orally.
- Commence intravenous fluids and nasogastric suction.
- Send blood for culture and ABST
- Commence intravenous broad spectrum antibiotics.

Maintain a temerature chart.
- Perform C-reactive protein and WBCDC daily.
- Perform serum electrolytes daily.
- Perform USS daily.

Answer 2.4

Immediate surgery is indicated if there is even a suspicion of bowel damage, ureteric damage or the presence of a retained foreign body.

QUESTION 3

A woman develops abdominal distension and vomitting 36 hours after a total hysterectomy and bilateral salpingo-oophorectomy. USS reveals mild distension of the bowel loops without any other abnormalities.
3.1 According to the above clinical picture, what are the causes?
3.2 List the steps in your first-line management.
3.3 What are the indications to perform surgery.

Answer 3.1

- Paralytic ileus
- Peritonitis

Answer 3.2

- Keep the patient nil orally.
- Commence intravenous fluids and nasogastric suction.
- Send blood for culture and ABST
- Commence intravenous broad spectrum antibiotics.
- Maintain a temerature chart.
- Perform C-reactive protein and WBCDC daily.
- Perform serum electrolytes daily.
- Perform USS daily.

Answer 3.3

- Failure to improve within 48 hours.
- Appearance of free fluid in the peritoneal cavity.
- Suspicion of bowel damage or presence of a retained foreign body.

QUESTION 4

A woman who had undergone a hysterectomy in the morning is found to be restless at 2 pm. She complains of abdominal pain. There is no vaginal bleeding. On examination she is pale. Her blood pressure is 80/60 mmHg and the pulse rate is 130 bpm.

4.1 What is the most likely cause?
4.2 How will you confirm the diagnosis?
4.3 List the steps in your management in the appropriate order during the next 48 hours.

Answer 4.1

Intraperitoneal haemorrhage due to a slip ligature.

Answer 4.2

On abdominal examination there will be distension and guarding with flank dullness. There will be evidence of haemodynamic compromise with tachycardia and low blood pressure.

USS will reveal echogenic fluid in the peritoneal cavity.

Answer 4.3

- Insert two 14 gauge cannulae and commence intravenous crystalloids.
- Crossmatch five units of blood.
- Inform the consultant gynaecologist and the anaethetist .
- The condition should be explained to the patient and she should be reassured. Informed consent should be obtained for laparotomy.
- Commence blood transfusion.
- Prepare for immediate laparotomy.
- At laparotomy the slipped vessel should be ligated.
- It may be safer to ligate the internal iliac arteries as well.
- She should be commenced on intravenous broad spectrum antibiotics.
- A drain should be inserted.
- Blood transfusion should be continued till she is haemodynamically stable.
- An indwelling catheter should be inserted and intake output should be charted.
- She should be monitored in the ICU for 24–48 hours till her condition is stable.
- Once the patient recovers she should be debriefed.

QUESTION 5

A woman develops profuse vaginal bleeding 7 days after vaginal hysterectomy. This was preceded by fever and offensive vaginal discharge for three days.

5.1 What is the most likely cause?
5.2 What are the investigations you would perform?
5.3 List the steps in your management in the appropriate order during the next 48 hours.

Answer 5.1

Secondary haemorrhage

Answer 5.2

- Blood and a high vaginal swab for culture and ABST
- Full blood count
- C-reactive protein and procalcitonin levels.

Answer 5.3

- Insert two 14 gauge cannulae and commence intravenous crystalloids.
- Commence intravenous broad spectrum antibiotics after sending blood and high vaginal swabs for culture and ABST.
- Crossmatch five units of blood.
- Inform the consultant gynaecologist and the anaethetist .
- The condition should be explained to the patient and she should be reassured. The management should be explained to her.
- Commence blood transfusion if necessary.
- An indwelling catheter should be inserted and intake output should be charted.
- Insert a tight vaginal pack to control bleeding.
- The vital parameters should be monitored and she should be observed for bleeding till her condition stabilises. She should be observed in the ICU.
- The pack should be removed in 24 hours.
- Change the antibiotics if necessary once the ABST report is available. Give oral antibiotics for 2 weeks.

QUESTION 6

A woman develops swinging fever rising up to 39°C and a pulse rate of 130 beats per minute, with abdominal pain, diarrhoea and vomiting, 5 days after an uncomplicated hysterectomy.

6.1   What is the most likely diagnosis?
6.2   What are the investigations you would perform? Give your reasons.
6.3   List the steps in your management in the appropriate order during the next 48 hours.
6.4   What are the indications to perform a laparotomy?

Answer 6.1

Pelvic abscess with severe sepsis

Answer 6.2

- Ultrasound scan to confirm the pelvic abscess.
- Blood and high vaginal swab for culture and ABST to identify the causative organism/s and to determine the appropriate antibiotic.
- WBCDC, C-reactive protein levels and serum lactate levels to determine the severity of the infection.

Answer 6.3

- Insert two 14 gauge cannulae and commence IV crystalloids.
- Commence broad spectrum intravenous antibiotics after sending blood and high vaginal swabs for culture and ABST
- Aspirate the abscess under ultrasound guidance.

- The vital parameters and the urine output should be monitored in the ICU till her condition stabilises.
- Maintain a temperature chart.
- Perform USS daily to exclude refilling.
- Monitor WBCDC, C-reactive protein levels and serum lactate levels daily to assess progress.
- Continue intravenous antibiotics till her condition improves. Change the antibiotics, if necessary once the ABST report is available. Give oral antibiotics for 2 weeks.

Answer 6.4

Indications to perform a laparotomy include:
- Inability to aspirate the abscess under ultrasound guidance due inaccessibility or due to increased thickness of the pus.
- Presence of free pus in the peritoneal cavity.
- Refilling of the abscess after aspiration.

QUESTION 7

What is your immediate management of the following postoperative complications?

7.1 A woman who underwent vaginal hysterectomy is on catheter drainage. The urine bag is found to be empty 6 hours after the surgery.

7.2 A woman who underwent abdominal hysterectomy complains of throbbing pain at the wound on the fourth postoperative day. On inspection there is redness, swelling and discharge from one end of the wound.

7.3 A woman who complains of abdominal pain 24 hours after laparotomy.

Answer 7.1

- Inquire whether the bag was emptied by an attendant without making an entry in the output chart.
- Assess the level of hydration and the vital parameters.
- Percuss to assess whether the bladder is distended.
- Check whether the catheter is in the proper place.
- Syringe the catheter with distilled water to flush out any blocks. Change the catheter if necessary.
- Improve her hydration with intravenous fluids.
- Measure the urine output after one hour.

Answer 7.2

- Open the swollen area of the wound under local anaesthesia and drain the pus.
- Send the pus for culture and ABST.
- Commence broad spectrum antibiotics.
- Clean and dress the wound with normal saline twice daily. Remove any slough.
- Resuture if necessary when the wound is clean.

Answer 7.3

- Examine the abdomen for distension, guarding, rigidity and flank dullness. If these are absent and the abomen is soft relieve pain with mild analgesics at first.

- Give parcetamol 2 tablets 6 hourly.
- Insert diclophenac sodium rectal suppositories 75 mg twice daily.
- Opioids will be necessary only if the pain is not relieved by the above methods.

QUESTION 8

8.1 What are the clinical features of bowel damage?
8.2 How do you confirm bowel damage?
8.3 How will you treat bowel damage?

Answer 8.1

- Abdominal distension and vomitting will occur 24–48 hours after surgery. Fever is usually present and there will be signs of sepsis.
- The abdomen will be distended with marked tenderness and guarding.
- Flank dullness will be elicited due to the presence of free fluid.
- The patient will be ill.

Answer 8.2

- An erect X-ray abdomen may show gas under the diaphragm.
- USS will show free fluid with solid particles.
- A CT scan could be performed immediately to determine the site of damage.

Answer 8.3

A laparotomy should be performed immediately to repair the damage. Help should be sought from te surgical team.

QUESTION 9

9.1 List 4 steps you would carry out in the preoperative preparation for major surgery in the clinic.
9.2 List 10 steps in the preparation of a patient awaiting major surgery after admission to the ward.
9.3 What is your check list immediately before sending the patient to the theatre?

Answer 9.1

- Take a full history and do a complete general and systemic examination.
- Do the following investigations—blood group, full blood count, urine full report, serum creatinine, fasting blood sugar, chest X-ray and ECG.
- Treat any intercurrent illness such as anaemia, urinary tract infection, hypertension, diabetes, heart disease, respiratory disease or any other major illness. Refer to a physician if necessary. Treat dental caries.
- Once the investigations and necessary treatment is completed, give a date for admission. Ask the consultant and refer the operation register.
  Patients awaiting major surgery are admitted 1–2 days before surgery.

Answer 9.2

- Re asses the indication.
- Take a complete history and do a full examination.

- Re-scrutinize the investigation reports
- Advice patient to bathe, explain procedure and reassure.
- Obtain informed consent using a prescribed form.
- Send blood for crossmatching before 9 am on the previous day.
- Send the operation list before 12 noon the previous day.
- Give premedication prescribed by the anaesthetist.
- Keep fasting for six hours.
- Shave the area of the incision .
- Dress in clean clothes. Be ready before the time for surgery.

Answer 9.3

Check whether
- The patient is sent for the appropriate surgery.
- The patient is fasting.
- The patient has given consent.
- Blood is available.
- All the investigation reports are available.
- Dentures and jewelry have been removed.
- The area is properly shaved.

QUESTION 10

List the steps in the postoperative management of a woman who has undergone major surgery:
10.1 During the afternoon round
10.2 On day 2: Next day
10.3 On day 3
10.4 List the steps you would follow when discharging a patient after major surgery.

Answer 10.1

- Respiratory rate, pulse rate, blood pressure, level of consciousness, colour, bleeding and urine output should be checked.
- Relieve pain with intramuscular pethidine 75 mg 6 hourly and/or diclophenac sodium suppositories 75 mg 12 hourly.
- Oral sips can be given in 6 hours if bowel sounds are present.

Answer 10.2

- Inquire regarding complaints.
- Check the vital parameters.
- Check temperature.
- Perform abdominal examination to exclude guarding and distension. Auscultate for bowel sounds
- Examine the respiratory system
- Remove the intravenous line and commence light solids, if bowel sounds are present. All drugs can be given orally.
- Remove the urinary catheter.
- Get the patient to walk.
- Give diclophenac sodium suppositories and paracetamol for pain relief.

Answer 10.3

- Inquire regarding complaints.
- Perform a full examination.
- Continue the same treatment as on day 2. The patient should be ambulant.
- Normal diet can be given.

Answer 10.4

- Make sure the patient is well and the wound has commenced healing.
- Patient is usually discharged on the 4th day. However, the date of discharge will vary in different units. If accelerated recovery is practiced the woman can be discharged in 48 hours if there are no complications.
- Give a detailed diagnosis card.
- Give medical leave for one month after major surgery.
- Advise her to take a normal diet and to gradually commence her day-to-day activities. She can have a bath. Sexual intercourse should be avoided for one month after abdominal hysterectomy and for 6 weeks after vaginal surgery.
- She should attend the clinic in one month. The histology report should be available by this time.

QUESTION 11

What is the mandatory WHO check list you would carry out in the operating theater before:

11.1 Induction of anaesthesia?

Answer 11.1

Before induction of anaesthesia ▶▶▶

❖ Has the patient confirmed his/her identity, procedure, site and consent?
☐ Yes   ☐ Not applicable

❖ Is the ward preparation completed?
☐ Yes   ☐ Not applicable

❖ Is the surgical site marked?
☐ Yes   ☐ Not applicable

❖ Are the anaesthesia machine, pulse oximeter and other relevant monitors, defibrillator and drugs checked?
☐ Yes   ☐ Not applicable

❖ Does the patient have a:
  ▪ Known allergy?
    ☐ Yes
    ☐ No
  ▪ Difficult airway/aspiration risk?
    ☐ Yes, equipment and assistance available
    ☐ No
  ▪ Risk of > 500ml blood loss (in children >7ml/kg)?
    ☐ Yes, adequate IV access and fluids planned
    ☐ No

❖ Are there any known infection risks which will affect the safety of the team (Hep B, MRSA, etc.)?
☐ Yes   ☐ No

11.2 Commencing the surgical intervention?

Answer 11.2

❯❯ Before start of surgical intervention ❯❯❯

❖ Confirm introduction of team members by name and role to each other? ☐ Yes ☐ No
❖ Reconfirm patient identity, procedure and site? ☐ Yes ☐ No
❖ Has DVT prophylaxis been undertaken? ☐ Yes ☐ Not applicable
❖ **Blood** ☐ Cross matched ☐ Grouped & Saved ☐ Not applicable
❖ Has the SSI bundle been undertaken? Antibiotic prophylaxis ☐ Yes ☐ Not applicable Patient warming ☐ Yes ☐ Not applicable Hair removal ☐ Yes ☐ Not applicable Glycaemic control ☐ Yes ☐ Not applicable
❖ Is essential imaging displayed /reviewed? ☐ Yes ☐ Not applicable
❖ **Anticipated Critical Events** ▪ **To Surgeon:** Way the patient is to be positioned? .... What are the critical or non-routine steps? .... Any special investigations/instruments needed during surgery?.................................. ▪ **To Anaesthetist:** Any patient specific concerns? .... ▪ **To Nursing Team:** Has sterility of instruments been confirmed? ☐ Yes ☐ No Are there any equipment issues or concerns? ☐ Yes .... ☐ No

11.3 The patient leaves the theatre?

Answer 11.3

❯❯❯ Before patient leaves the theatre

❖ **Nurse verbally confirms:** ☐ The name of the procedure ☐ Completion of instrument, sponge and needle counts ☐ Specimen labeling & completion of request forms ☐ Any equipment problems to be addressed
❖ **Confirm recording of following on the BHT** ☐ Level of consciousness ☐ Vital signs ☐ Splints/Prosthesis/Vascular lines attached ☐ Operative notes and significant events ☐ Management guide for next 24hours

Reference: SBA Questions in Gynaecology, Chapter 4.

Cervical Intraepithelial Neoplasia

From Colposcopy and Treatment of Cervical Intraepithelial Neoplasia: A Beginners' Manual by J W Sellors and R Sankaranarayanan

This cervical smear was obtained from a 36-year-old multiparous woman.

1.1   Name the above cytological abnormality.

1.2   Give reasons for your diagnosis.

1.3   What is the next step in the management?

1.4   What is your management if this woman was 22 years old?

Answer 1.1

Atypical squamous cells of unknown significance.

Answer 1.2

There are cells with mild nuclear enlargement, slight nuclear membrane irregularity and mild hyperchromasia in a clean background.

Answer 1.3

- Test for high-risk HPV types. If the test is positive colposcopy is done.
- If the HPV test is negative the risk of having CIN 2–3 + is less than 2% and they can be referred for follow up.
- Follow up include repeat cytology and HPV testing in 1 year.
- Colposcopy is done if HPV testing is positive or cytology is ASC-US or greater on follow up. If the results are negative they are routinely screened in 3 years.

Answer 1.4

- Test for high risk HPV types.
- Adolescents have a very low risk of invasive cancer and the likelihood of HPV clearance is very high. Therefore, cytology testing is performed at 6 and 12 months or a single HPV test is performed at 12 months in adolescents with ASC and HPV positive test results. Colposcopy is performed only for an abnormal cytology result or positive HPV test result during follow up.

QUESTION 2

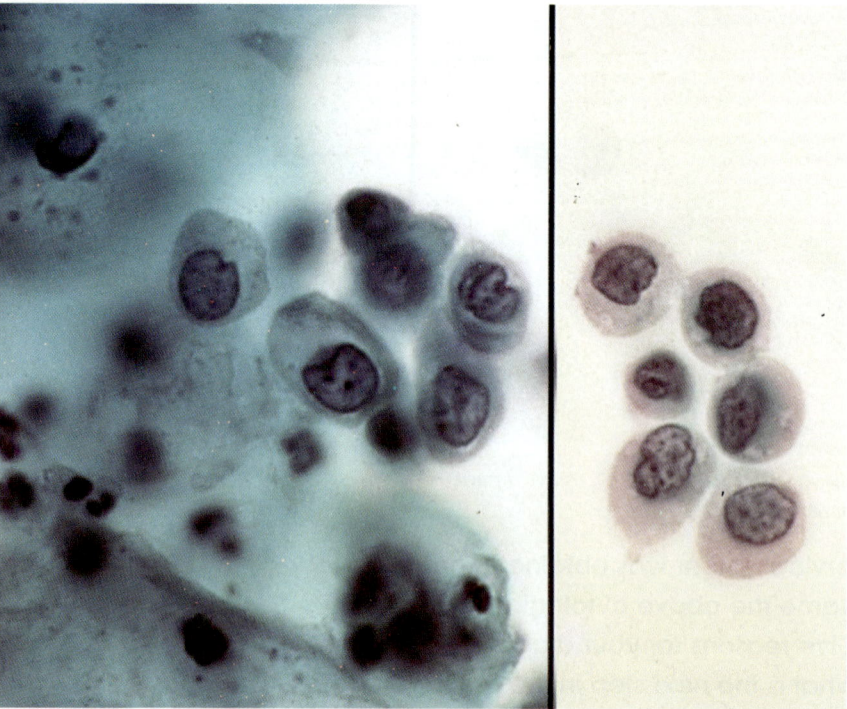

From the Bethesda System of Reporting Cervical Cytology, third edition, by Ritu Nayar and David C Wilbur

This cervical smear was obtained from a 40-year-old multiparous woman.
2.1   Name the above cytological abnormality.
2.2   Give reasons for your diagnosis.
2.3   What is the next step in the management?

Answer 2.1

Atypical squamous cells cannot exclude a high-grade squamous intraepithelial lesion (ASC-H).

Answer 2.2

Isolated cells are seen with enlarged irregular nuclei and reduced nuclear/cytoplasmic ratios.

Answer 2.3

- The incidence of CIN 2, 3 is as high as 50%.
- Therefore, colposcopy is recommended.
- HPV testing for women with ASC-H is not included in the guideline but a negative test is reassuring.
- Cytology testing at six and 12 months or an HPV DNA test at 12 months is performed if colposcopy reveals CIN 1 or normal results. Excision is not indicated for these women.

QUESTION 3

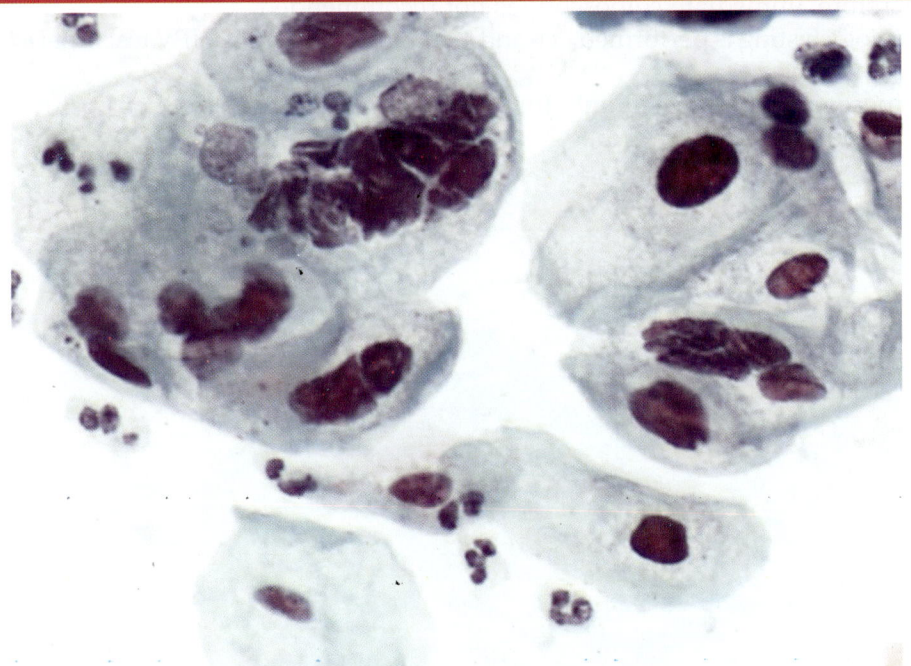

From the Bethesda System of Reporting Cervical Cytology, third edition, by Ritu Nayar and David C Wilbur

This cervical smear was obtained from a 35-year-old multiparous woman.
3.1   Name the above cytological abnormality.

3.2   Give reasons for your diagnosis.
3.3   What is the next step in the management?
3.4   What is your management if this woman was 22 years old?

Answer 3.1

Low grade squamous intraepithelial lesion.

Answer 3.2

Cells are enlarged with enlarged irregular nuclei and smudged appearance of nuclear chromatin. There is increased nuclear/cytoplasmic ratio. There are multinucleate cells.

Answer 3.3

- The risk of CIN 2–3+ at initial colposcopy following a LSIL result is between 15 and 30%.
- Therefore, colposcopy is performed for further investigation of LSIL.
- Cytology testing at six and 12 months or an HPV DNA test at 12 months is performed if colposcopy reveals CIN 1 or normal results. Excision is not indicated for these women.

Answer 3.4

- Adolescents with LSIL have a very low risk of invasive cancer and the likelihood of HPV clearance is very high.
- Therefore, immediate colposcopy is not recommended.
- Cytology testing is performed at 6 and 12 months or a single HPV test is performed at 12 months.
- Colposcopy is performed only for an abnormal cytology result or positive HPV test result during follow up.

QUESTION 4

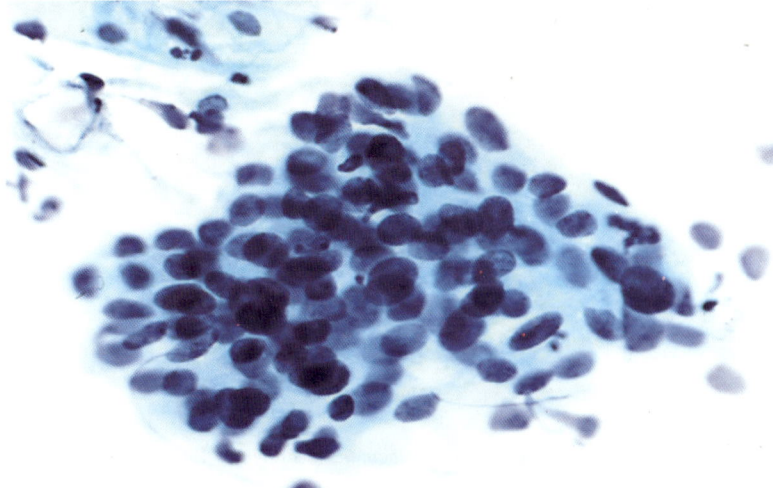

From the Bethesda System of Reporting Cervical Cytology, third edition, by Ritu Nayar and David C Wilbur

This cervical smear was obtained from a 35-year-old multiparous woman.
4.1   Name the above cytological abnormality.
4.2   Give reasons for your diagnosis.
4.3   What is the next step in the management?

Answer 4.1

High-grade squamous intraepithelial lesion.

Answer 4.2

The cells are in a syncytial sheet. They have hyperchromatic nuclei. There is a marked increase in the nuclear cytoplasmic ratio. The nuclei appear irregular and there are no nucleoli. The cells are smaller than in LSIL.

Answer 4.3

- CIN 2 or CIN 3 occurs in about 70% of women with high-grade squamous intraepithelial lesions (HSIL), and 1 to 2% have invasive cancer.
- Colposcopy and biopsy of visible lesions are recommended. Biopsy may be performed from an abnormal area detected on colposcopy. Biopsy is essential when a visual diagnosis of CIN 2 or CIN 3 is made
- CIN 2 and CIN 3 are potential cancer precursors, although CIN 2 can undergo spontaneous regression.
- Non-pregnant patients with CIN 2 and CIN 3 require immediate treatment with excision.

QUESTION 5

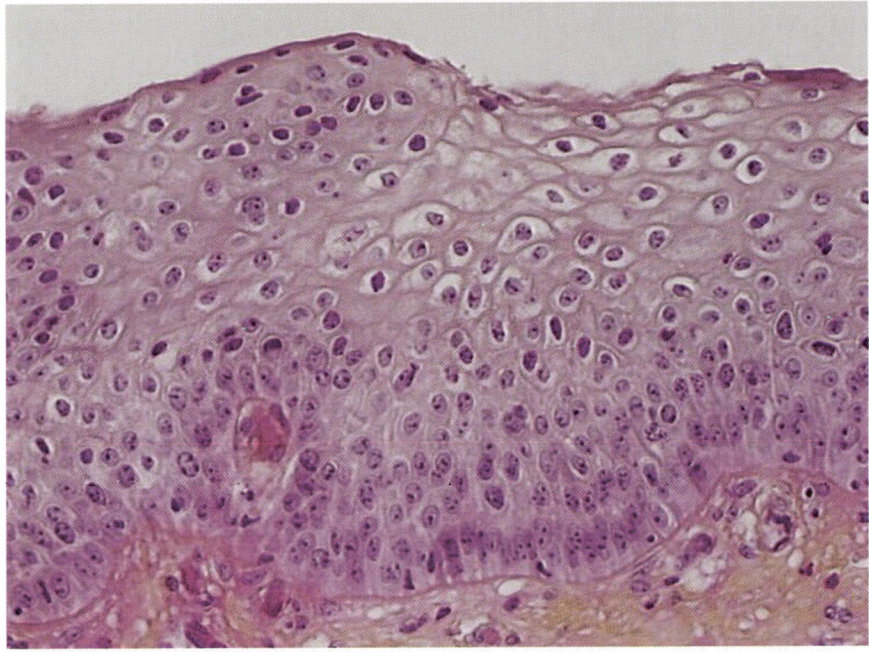

5.1   What is the abnormality seen in the above biopsy obtained from a 35-year-old woman? Give reasons for your diagnosis.

5.2   What is the best management option?

Answer 5.1

CIN 1: Enlarged nuclei, increased nuclear-cytoplasmic ratio and increased intensity of nuclear staining are seen. Abnormal cells are confined to the lower third of the epithelium. Mitotic figures are present, but not very numerous.

Answer 5.2

Excision is not indicated for these women.

Cytology and an HPV DNA test is performed at 12 and 24 months. If HPV is positive or if there are cytological abnormalities repeat colposcopy is performed. If HPV and cytology is negative routine follow up is done in 3 years.

QUESTION 6

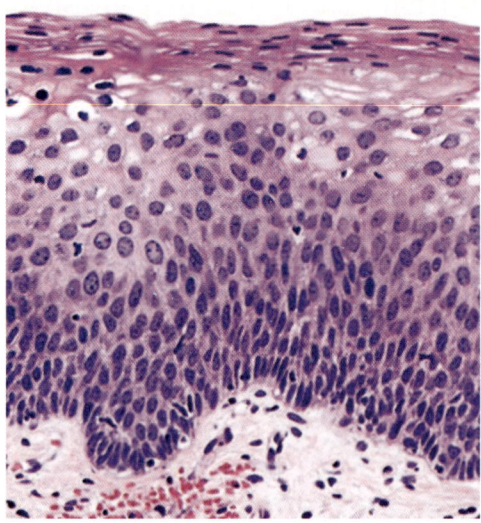

6.1   What is the abnormality seen in the above colposcopic image obtained from a 35-year-old woman? Give reasons for your diagnosis.
6.2   What is the best management option?
6.3   How do you treat a 20-year-old woman with the above abnormality?
6.4   How do you treat a pregnant woman with the above abnormality?

Answer 6.1

CIN 2. Dysplastic cellular changes are mostly restricted to the lower two-thirds of the epithelium, with marked nuclear abnormalities. Mitotic figures are seen throughout the lower half of the epithelium.

Answer 6.2

Carry out excision.

Cytology and an HPV DNA test is performed at 12 and 24 months after excision. If HPV is positive or if there are cytological abnormalities repeat colposcopy is performed. If HPV and cytology is negative routine follow up is done in 3 years.

Answer 6.3

Excision is not indicated for these women. Cytology and colposcopy is performed at 12 and 24 months. If both are normal co-testing is performed in 1 year. If the results are normal co-testing is performed again in 3 years. If any abnormality is detected colposcopy and biopsy is performed. Excision is recommended if CIN 2 persists for 2 years.

Answer 6.4

Excision is performed after 6 weeks of delivery.

QUESTION 7

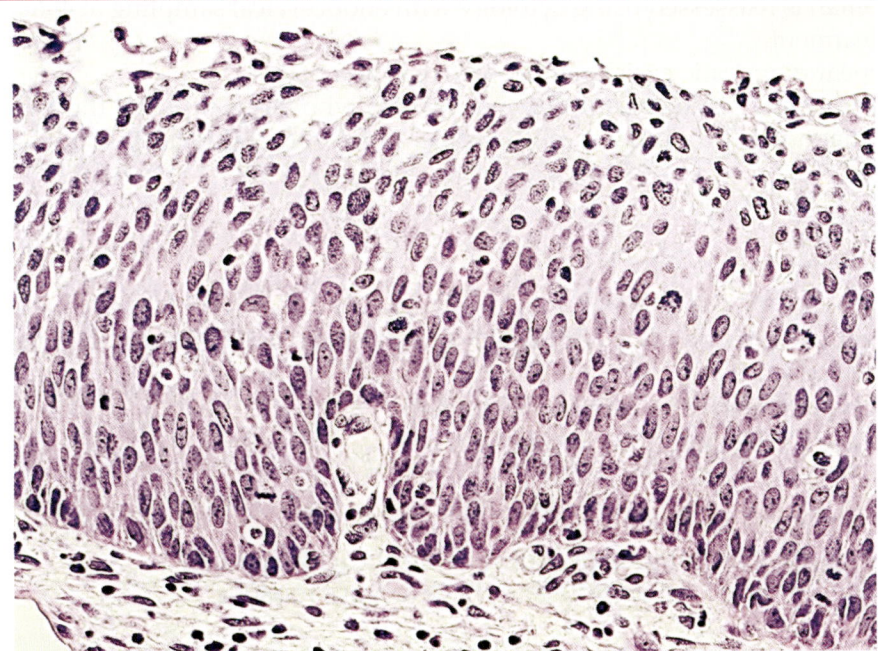

From The Bethesda System for Reporting Cervical Cytology, third edition, edited by Ritu Nayar and David C Wilbur

7.1 **What is the abnormality seen in the above colposcopic image obtained from a 35-year-old woman? Give reasons for your diagnosis.**

7.2 **What is the best management option?**

7.3 **How do you treat a 20-year-old woman with the above abnormality?**

7.4 **What is your management option if the abnormality is found at the margins of the excised tissue?**

7.5 **What are the indications for hysterectomy in a woman with cervical intra-epithelial neoplasia?**

Answer 7.1

CIN3. Maturation is absent. Nuclear abnormalities extend throughout the thickness of the epithelium. There are numerous mitotic figures. Many mitotic figures have abnormal forms. The nuclei are hyperchromatic and there is increased nuclear/cytoplasmic ratio.

Answer 7.2

Carry-out excision.

Answer 7.3

Excision is not indicated for these women.

Cytology and colposcopy is performed at 12 and 24 months. If both are normal co-testing is performed in 1 year. If normal, co-testing is performed in 3 years.

If any abnormality is detected colposcopy and biopsy is performed.

Excision is recommended if CIN 3 persists for 2 years.

Answer 7.4

The woman is reassessed using cytology with endocervical sampling at 4–6 months after treatment.

A repeat diagnostic excisional procedure is acceptable.

Hysterectomy can be performed in a woman who has completed the family if a repeat diagnostic procedure is not feasible. However, malignancy should be first excluded.

Answer 7.5

- Persistent CIN 2 or CIN 3
- Recurrent CIN 2 or CIN 3
- Incomplete excision of CIN 2 or CIN 3 with the abnormality present in the margins of the excised tissue.

Malignancy should be carefully excluded.

It is better if the family is completed.

QUESTION 8

8.1 What are the methods available to treat CIN 2 and CIN 3
8.2 Which method would you select? Give your reasons.

Answer 8.1

- Cryotherapy
- Loop electrosurgical excision
- Cold knife conisation

Answer 8.2

Loop electrosurgical excision is the best method.

This method is preferred for CIN2 and CIN 3 because histological examination is possible.

It is also possible to determine whether the entire lesion has been removed. It can be done as an out-patient procedure. Bleeding is minimal.

Cold knife conization is carried out if the above procedure is not available. This procedure has the disadvantages of needing hospital admission and bleeding. However, histological examination is possible.

Cryotherapy can be performed if the entire lesion and the squamocolumnar junction are visible, and the lesion does not cover more than three quarters of the ectocervix. It cannot be performed if the lesion extends beyond the cryoprobe or into the endocervical canal or when there is suspicion of malignancy. Histological examination is not possible.

References for Questions 1 to 8
- *ACOG Releases Guidelines for Management of Abnormal Cervical Cytology and Histology Carrie A. Morantz Am Fam Physician. 2006 Feb 15;73(4):719–729.*
- *2012 Updated ASCCP Consensus Guidelines for the Management of Abnormal Cervical Cancer Screening Tests and Cancer Precursors.*
- *SBA Questions in Gynaecology, Chapter 7.*

QUESTION 9

9.1 Identify the stages of cervical carcinoma shown in each diagram. Give your reasons.

9.2 State the management of each stage of the disease you have identified.

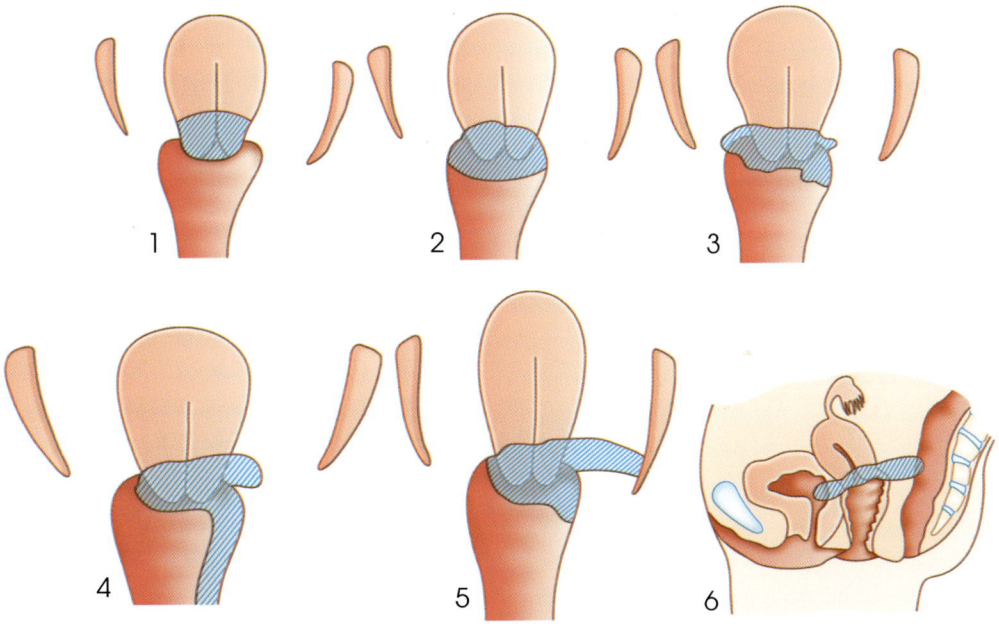

Answer 9.1

1. Stage IB	Carcinoma (a visible lesion) confined to the cervix.	
2. Stage IIA	Carcinoma has spread to the upper two-thirds of the vagina but the parametrium is not involved.	
3. Stage IIB	Carcinoma has spread to the upper two-thirds of the vagina and the parametrium but the lateral pelvic wall is not involved	
4. Stage IIIA	The lateral pelvic wall is not involved but the tumour has spread to the lower third of the vagina.	
5. Stage IIIB	Extension into the lateral pelvic wall.	
6. Stage IVA	Tumour has spread to the rectum and the bladder.	

Answer 9.2

(1) If the lesion is smaller than 4 cm (Stage 1B: 1) type 3 radical hysterectomy is performed.

If the nodes contain cancer cells postoperative radiotherapy and chemotherapy with cisplatin is necessary. If the lesion is larger than 4 cm (stage 1B: 2) the standard treatment is chemotherapy with cisplatin or cisplatin and 5 fluorouracil with radiation therapy (chemoradiotherapy). Both external beam radiation and brachytherapy are used.

2, 3, 4, 5 and 6—Chemoradiotherapy is used to treat women with FIGO IB2, IIA, IIB, IIIA, IIIB and IVA diseases. Surgery is not offered because of the significant risk of positive margins and positive nodes.

References

- *Staging classifications and clinical practice guidelines of gynaecologic cancers FIGO Committee on Gynaecologic Oncology JL Benedet, H Bender, H Jones III, HYS Ngan, S Pecorelli*
- *SBA Questions in Gynaecology, Chapter 8.*

Examination Paper 1

QUESTION 1

This is a blood pack received from the blood bank for transfusion to a patient.

1.1 List the criteria you would check to confirm whether it is the correct pack.

(0.5 × 4 = 2 marks)

1.2 List five features you would check in the blood pack to confirm that it is safe for transfusion. (5 marks)

1.3 Write the instructions you would document in the bed head ticket before commencing the transfusion. (0.5 × 6 =3 marks)

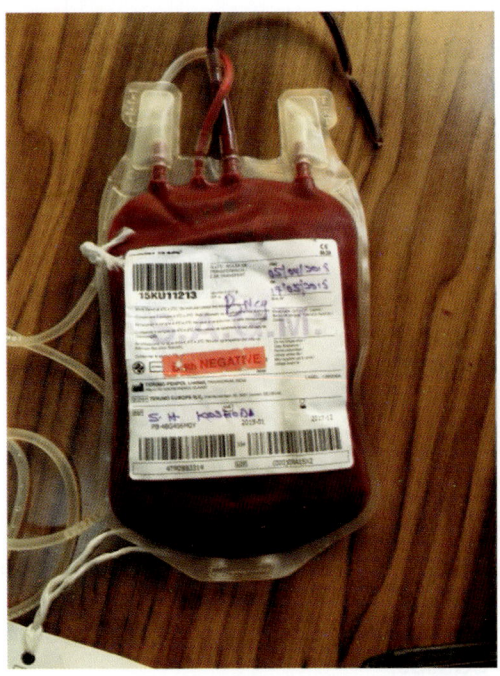

QUESTION 2

Identify the following instruments.   (2 × 5 =10 marks)

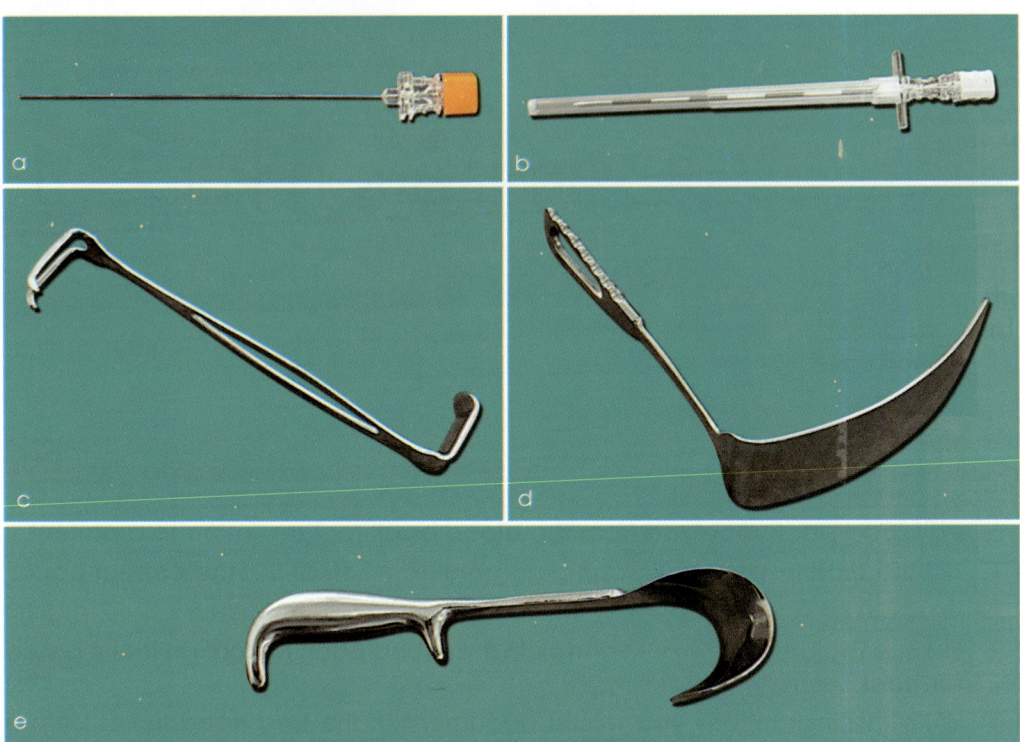

QUESTION 3

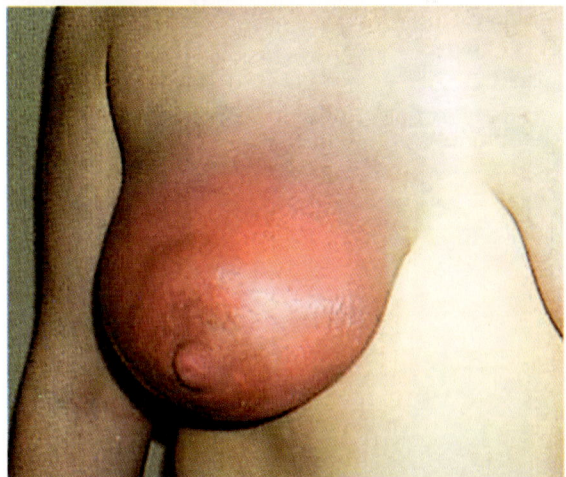

This is a breast of a woman who complained of severe pain in the breast on the 5th postpartum day.

3.1   List 2 clinical conditions which can cause this appearance. (0.5 × 2 = 1 mark)

3.2   List two possible causes.   (2 marks)

3.3   List 5 steps in the management of this patient.   (5 marks)
3.4   List two advices you would you give this mother to prevent recurrence of this complication.   (2 marks)

QUESTION 4

You are the house officer in the labour ward. You are present when an uterine inversion occurs while the midwife is trying to deliver the placenta. You have observed the management of this complication on a previous occasion.
4.1   What is your immediate management?   (5 marks)
4.2   What is the subsequent management if the first-line management fails?
          (5 marks)

QUESTION 5

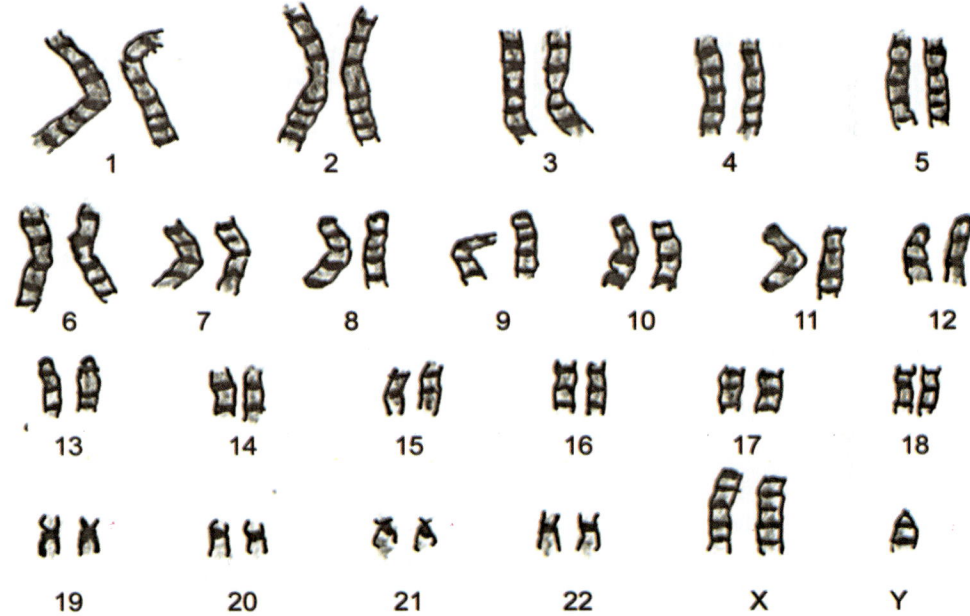

This is the karyotype of a male with azoospermia.
5.1   What is the diagnosis?   (1 mark)
5.2   List five clinical features you would expect to see in this patient.   (5 marks)
5.3   What advice would you give this couple regarding fertility wishes?   (4 marks)

QUESTION 6

6.1   List 4 indications for performing anti-müllerian hormone levels.   (4 marks)
6.2   List the methods of assessing the ovarian reserve.   (3 marks)
6.3   Mention a drug which can cause lowering of anti-müllerian hormone levels.
          (1 mark)
6.4   List 4 factors which increase success at IVF.   (0.5 × 4 = 2 marks)

QUESTION 7

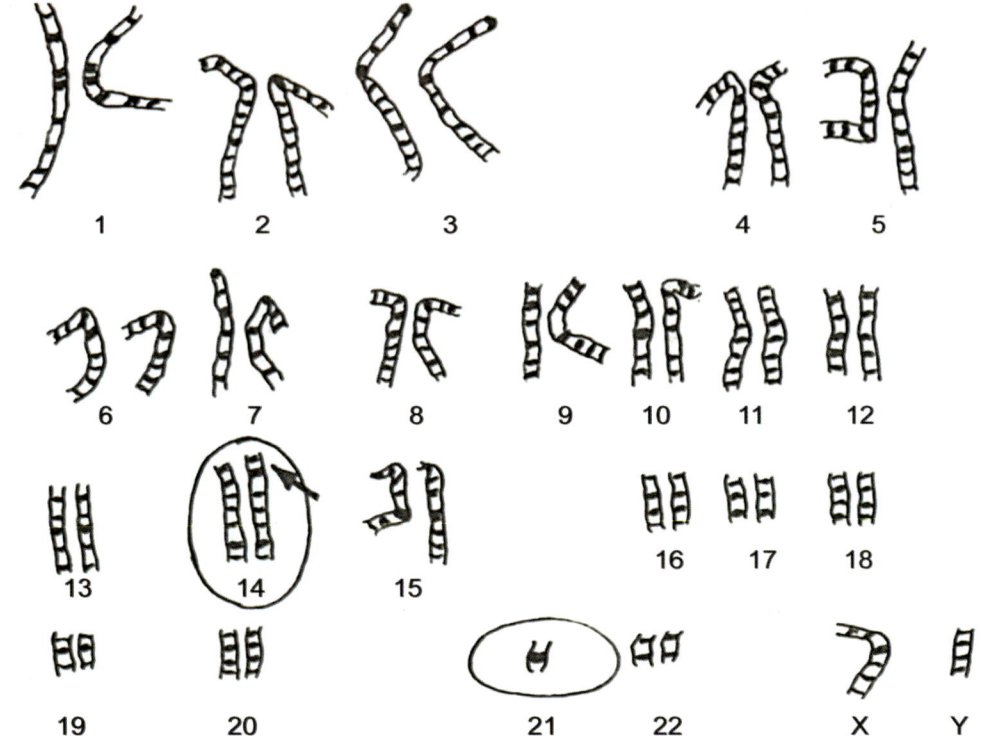

This is the karyotype of a father who has an abnormal baby.

7.1   What is the diagnosis?   (1 mark)
7.2   What advice would you give this couple regarding future fertility? (9 marks)

QUESTION 8

This is a contraceptive method we use in our clinic.

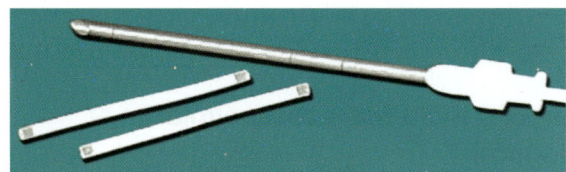

8.1   Name the hormone and the total dose contained in this contraceptive
       device.   (1 mark)
8.2   List the steps in inserting this implant.   (9 marks)

QUESTION 9

This is a partogram of a woman in the first stage of labour.

9.1   What is the abnormality of labour shown in the chart?   (3 marks)
9.2   What is the primary cause of this condition?   (1 mark)
9.3   List 2 contributory factors.   (0.5 × 2 = 1 mark)
9.4   What is your management?   (5 marks)

National Partogram

H. 1255

Name: Age: BHT. No:

Gravida: Parity: Blood Group: Date and Time:

Special Problems: Special Instructions:

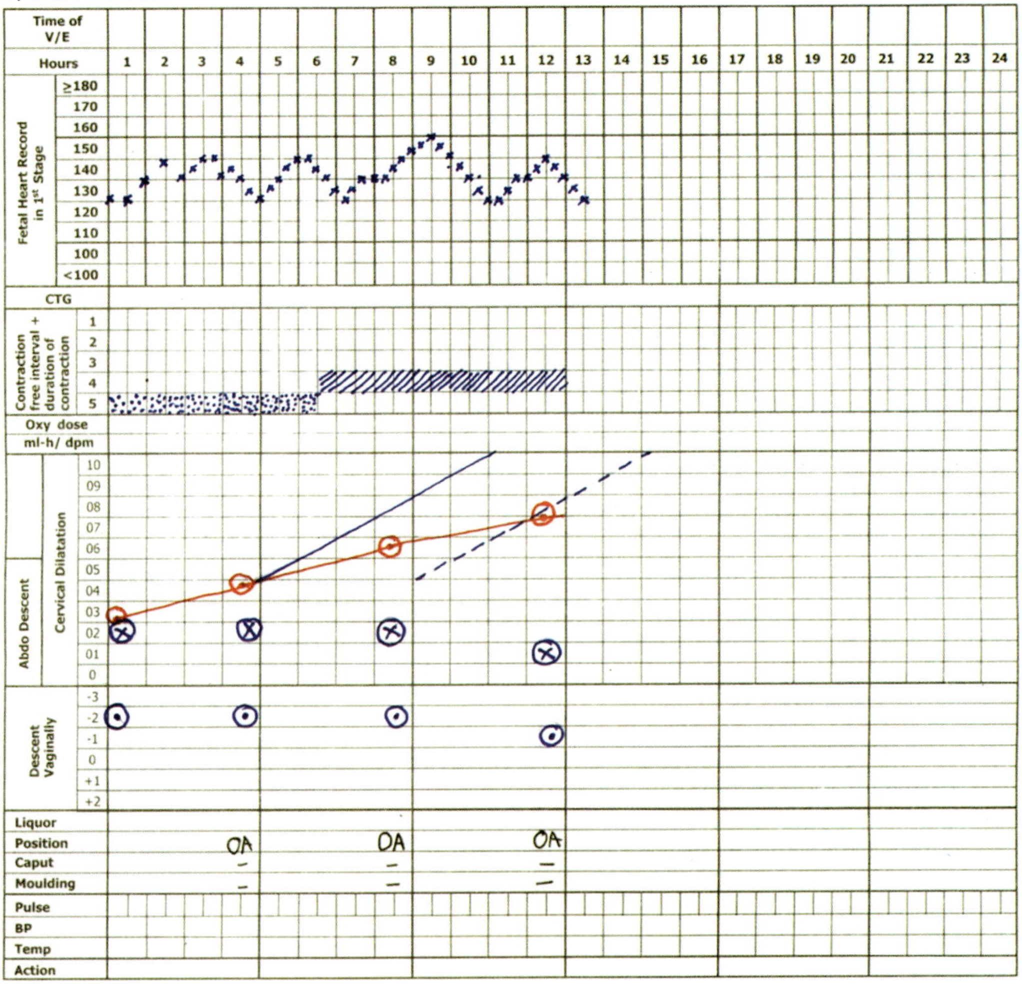

Time of V/E																									
Hours	1	2	3	4	5	6	7	8	9	10	11	12	13	14	15	16	17	18	19	20	21	22	23	24

Fetal Heart Record in 1st Stage: ≥180, 170, 160, 150, 140, 130, 120, 110, 100, <100

CTG

Contraction free interval + duration of contraction: 1, 2, 3, 4, 5

Oxy dose ml-h/ dpm

Abdo Descent / Cervical Dilatation: 10, 09, 08, 07, 06, 05, 04, 03, 02, 01, 0

Descent Vaginally: -3, -2, -1, 0, +1, +2

Liquor																								
Position			OA		OA		OA																		
Caput			–		–		–																		
Moulding			–		–		–																		
Pulse																									
BP																									
Temp																									
Action																									

2nd Stage Fetal Heart Rate Record   Time: Fully dilated:.................... Commenced pushing:. .... (Mark ▼▼)

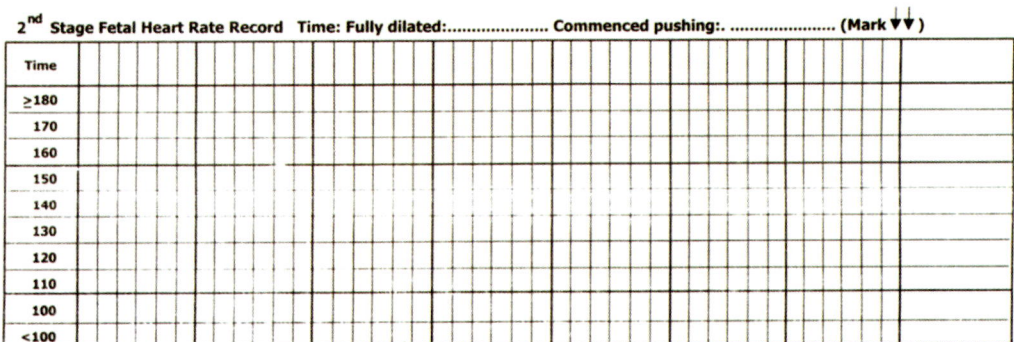

QUESTION 10

This is the temperature chart of a patient after caesarean section.

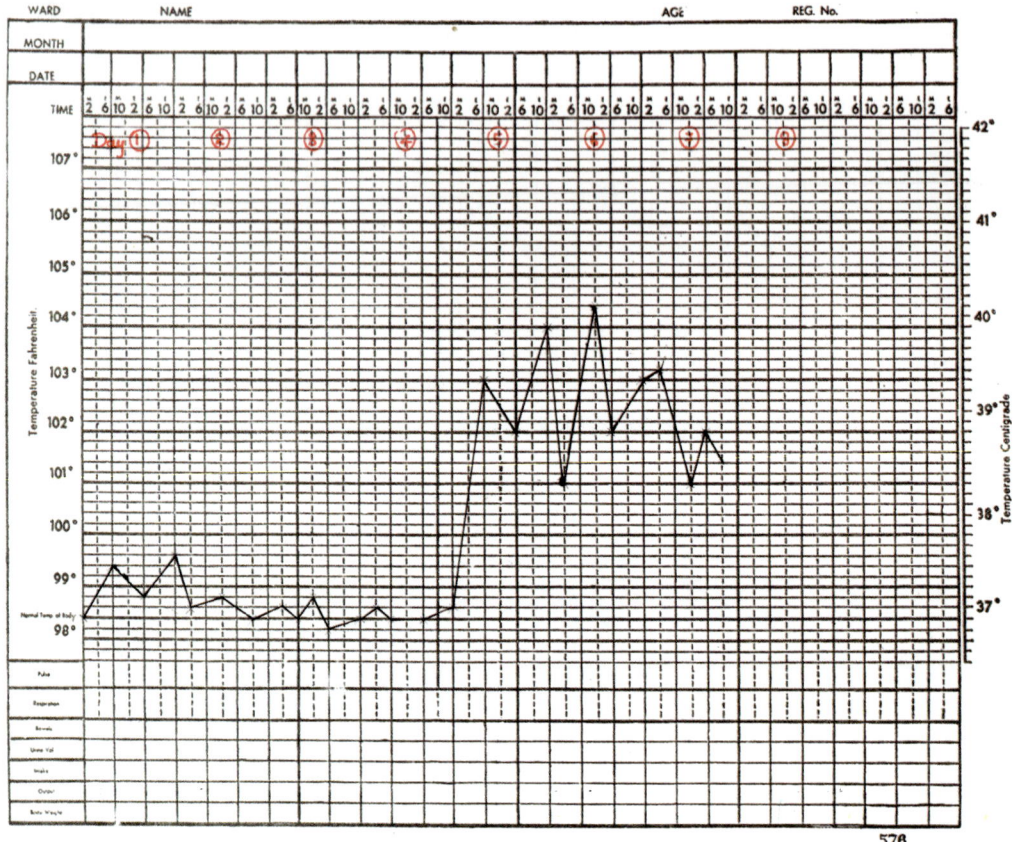

576

10.1 List 5 causes for this presentation. (5 marks)

10.2 List 4 investigations you would perform. (0.5 × 4 = 2 marks)

10.3 List 3 steps in your first line management. (3 marks)

ANSWERS FOR EXAMINATION PAPER 1

Answer 1.1

Check and compare the following information on the tag attached to the blood pack and the stamp placed on the patient's BHT by the blood bank when the blood is issued.

- The name of the patient.
- The name of the donor.
- The BHT number of the patient.
- The bottle number
- Expiry date of the pack.

Answer 1.2

- Check for hemolysis by looking at the plasma portion of the pack and noticing any pink discoloration.

- Check whether the injection ports are open
- Check whether there are any leaks in the pack
- Check whether the tube sealing is intact without any leaks
- Check the expiry date of the pack.

Answer 1.3

- Start blood transfusion.
- Observe pulse, BP and the respiratory rate every 5 minutes for 15 minutes and every15 minutes for 2 hours.
- Look for any rash, itching, breathing difficulty, confusion, fever and chills.
- Inform the house officer immediately if a reaction occurs.

Answer 2

a. Spinal needle
b. Epidural needle
c. Czerny retractor
d. Kelly retractor
e. Doyen retractor

Answer 3.1

- Mastitis
- Breast abscess

Answer 3.2

- Infection following a cracked nipple.
- Infection following milk retention (breast engorgement).

Answer 3.3

- Encourage feeding from this breast and express the remaining breast milk.
- Commence analgesics such as paracetamol or NSAIDs.
- Commence broad spectrum antibiotics.
- Watch for signs of abscess formation such as high fever, purulent discharge from the nipple, throbbing pain and localization of pus with increased redness and fluctuation.
- Obtain surgical opinion to carry out incision and drainage, if an abscess is suspected.

Answer 3.4

- The baby should not be allowed to suck only on the nipple. Part of the areola should be introduced into the mouth.
- The breasts should be emptied after each feed.
- The baby should be fed from both breasts at each feed and should be allowed to suck for 10 minutes from each nipple.
- Baby should not be allowed to keep the nipple in the mouth if he is not sucking.
- Use proper feeding techniques to prevent the baby demanding for frequent feeds as this can result in cracked nipples.
- Wash with water after each feed.

Answer 4.1

- Call for help.
- Do not attempt removal of the placenta, if it is still attached. Do not give oxytocic drugs.

- Insert two 14 gauge cannulae and commence crystalloids. Give intravenous glyceryl trinitrate, ritodrine or subcutaneous terbutaline.
- Attempt manual reduction of the inversion immediately since you have previously observed the management of this complication.
- Assess vital signs.
- Assess blood loss.
- Request for five units of blood.

Answer 4.2

- Inform the senior consultant and the anaesthetist.
- Commence blood transfusion if bleeding is present.
- Commence intravenous uterine relaxants—glyceryl trinitrate or ritodrine.
- Take to the theatre immediately.
- Perform O'Sullivan's hydrostatic method of reduction under GA. Perform manual removal, if the placenta is attached. Give oxytocic drugs once the reduction is complete.
- The above procedure is usually successful. If it fails perform laparotomy and reduction.
- Hysterectomy is performed only as the last resort
- Correct anaemia by blood transfusion.

Answer 5.1

Klinefelter's syndrome

Answer 5.2

- Less facial and pubic hair
- Reduced muscle mass
- Small atrophic testis
- Small penis
- Gynaecomastia

Answer 5.3

Since there is no treatment to improve the sperm count they should be advised to resort to adoption or donor insemination.

Answer 6.1

- Assessment of ovarian reserve.
- Prediction of success of ovarian stimulation.
- Prediction of success at IVF.
- Prediction of the time to reach menopause.
- To assess the response to treatment in granulosa cell tumours.

Answer 6.2

- Total antral follicle count of less than or equal to 4 for a low response and greater than 16 for a high response.
- Anti-müllerian hormone level of less than or equal to 5.4 pmol/L for a low response and greater than or equal to 25.0 pmol/L for a high response.
- Follicle stimulating hormone level greater than 8.9 IU/L for a low response and less than 4 IU/L for a high response.

Answer 6.3
Combined oral contraceptive pills

Answer 6.4
- Age below 35 years
- Good ovarian reserve
- BMI between 19 and 30
- Shorter duration of infertility

Answer 7.1
There is an unbalanced translocation of 21–>14 chromosomes.

Answer 7.2
Father is the carrier of this translocation. Therefore, there is a 3% risk of transmission.

They can embark on a pregnancy and perform chorionic villous sampling at 11–13 weeks.

Adoption and donor insemination are other options.

Answer 8.1
Levonorgestrel 150 mg

Answer 8.2
- It is inserted into the medial aspect of forearm of the non-dominant hand.
- The skin is cleaned with an antiseptic solution and sterile towels are laid.
- 1% lignocaine is infiltrated subcutaneously in the shape of a V.
- The skin is punctured with the trocar.
- The trocar is inserted under the skin in the shape of a V till the second mark is reached.
- The introducer is removed.
- A contraceptive rod is loaded into the trocar.
- The introducer is re-inserted and the rod is pushed in till a resistance is felt.
- The introducer is removed.
- Palpate to make sure that the rod is just under the skin.
- The trocar is withdrawn up to the first mark.
- Reinsert the trocar under the skin in a direction to complete the V.
- Introduce the second rod in the same manner.
- Withdraw the introducer and then the trocar.
- Apply a sterile adhesive strip to the wound.

Answer 9.1
Primary dysfunctional labour

Answer 9.2
Occurrence of inadequate uterine contractions, less than 4 per 10 minutes in the first stage of labour.

Answer 9.3
- Occipito-posterior position

- Mento-anterior face presentation
- Uterine over distension due to twins or hydramnios

Answer 9.4

- Exclude fetal distress, cephalo-pelvic disproportion and maternal distress.
- An amniotomy should be performed and an oxytocin infusion should be commenced.
- The patient should be well hydrated. Adequate pain relief should be provided preferably with epidural analgesia. Continuous fetal heart rate monitoring should be commenced.
- The progress of labour should be assessed by performing a vaginal examination in 2 hours.
- Perform a caesarean section if there is no progress or if there is maternal or fetal distress.

Answer 10.1

- Urinary tract infection
- Pelvic infection/pelvic abscess
- Respiratory tract infection
- Wound infection
- Breast abscess

Answer 10.2

Perform

- C-reactive protein/procalcitonin levels.
- Full blood count.
- Urine full report and urine culture.
- Blood culture.
- Chest X-ray if there are signs of chest infection.
- Culture of vaginal discharge.
- US scan and other imaging.

Answer 10.3

- Identify the site of infection. Insert a 14 gauge cannula and commence an infusion of Hartman's solution.
- Look for signs of severe sepsis such as tachypnea, hypotension and altered mental state.
- Send blood and other secretions for culture and ABST.
- Commence intravenous broad spectrum antibiotics and change the drug once the ABST report is available.
- Maintain hydration with intravenous crystalloids.
- ICU monitoring is necessary if severe sepsis is present.
- Ultrasound guided aspiration should be performed if there is pelvic abscess formation. The wound should be explored if wound infection is present.

Examination Paper 2

This is an ultrasound image of a 25-year-old married nulliparous woman admitted to the ward with left lower abdominal pain for 2 days. Size of the cyst is 7 cm × 8 cm. The pain had commenced at the end of her menstrual period.

Abdominal examination showed a left sided tender mass on deep palpation.

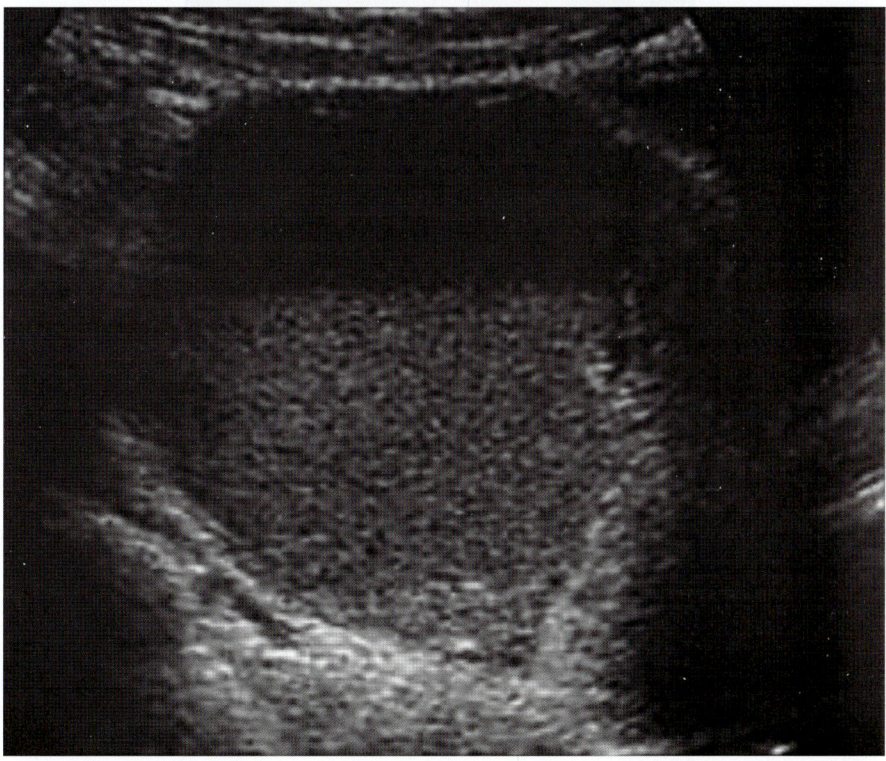

Reproduced with permission from: Ultrasoundcases.info

1.1 What is the most likely diagnosis? (2 marks)
1.2 Give 3 reasons for your diagnosis. (3 marks)
1.3 List 4 issues you will discuss with her. (0.5 × 4 = 2 marks)
1.4 What is the management option you would choose for this patient? (1 mark)
1.5 List 2 aspects in the follow up of this patient. (2 marks)

QUESTION 2

A woman presented with a temperature of 38°C and moderate vaginal bleeding 7 days after vaginal hysterectomy and repair.

2.1 What is the diagnosis? (2 marks)
2.2 What is the cause of bleeding? (2 marks)
2.3 What further investigations would you perform? (3 marks)
2.4 List 3 important steps in treating her condition. (3 marks)

QUESTION 3

This image is from a 28-year-old married woman who presented with vaginal discharge and pelvic pain for 1 week.

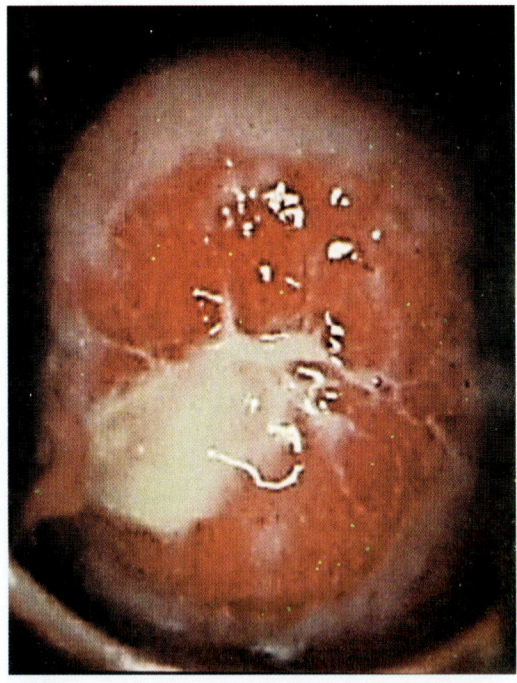

3.1 List 2 infective agents which can cause this condition. (0.5 × 2 = 1 mark)
3.2 List the questions you would ask from this patient in the history. (3 marks)
3.3 Mention a single investigation which will confirm the cause. (1 mark)
3.4 Write down the treatment you are going to provide for each cause you have given with dosage and duration. (2 marks)
3.5 What advice would you give this patient? (3 marks)

QUESTION 4

This is a picture of a procedure used in pregnancy.

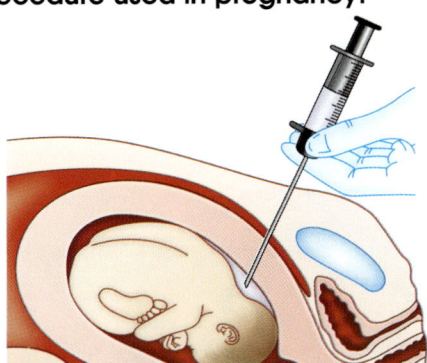

4.1   Mention four indications for this procedure.   (4 marks)
4.2   Mention the POA after which it can be performed.   (1 mark)
4.3   Mention three possible complications of this procedure.   (3 marks)
4.4   Mention an advantage and an disadvantage of this procedure over chorionic villous sampling.   (2 marks)

QUESTION 5

This is a partogram of a multiparous woman in the active phase of the first stage of labour.

National Partogram   **H. 1255**

Name: Age: BHT. No:

Gravida: Parity: Blood Group: Date and Time:

Special Problems: Special Instructions:

5.1   Name the abnormality of cervical dilatation shown in the chart. (2 marks)
5.2   List four causative factors.   (0.5 × 4 = 2 marks)
5.3   List three complications which can occur in this patient.   (3 marks)
5.4   What is your management?   (3 marks)

QUESTION 6

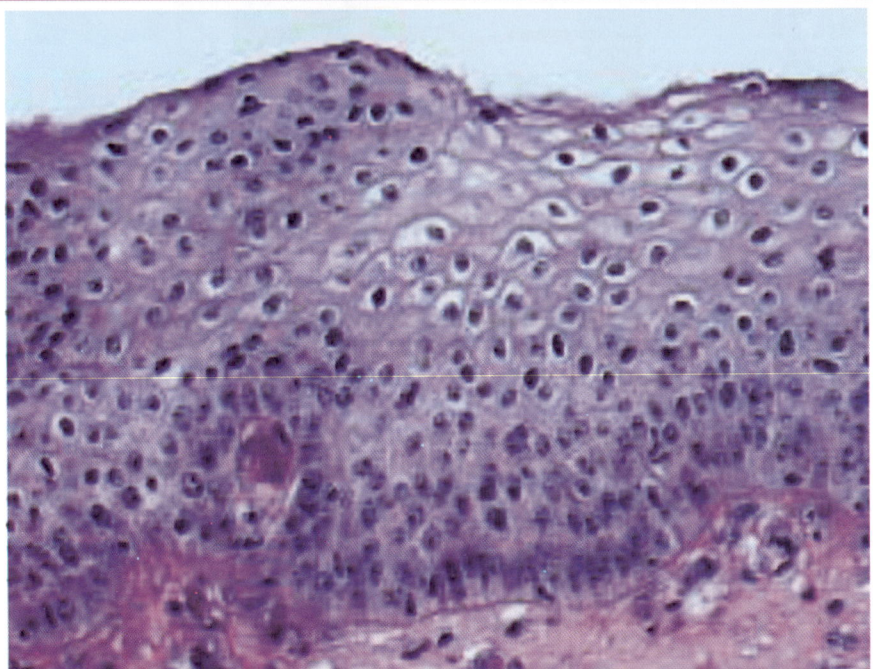

This is a microscopic image of a cervical biopsy of a 35-year-old woman with an abnormal smear report.
6.1   List three abnormalities you see in this slide.   (3 marks)
6.2   What is the most likely diagnosis?   (2 marks)
6.3   What is the next action you would take as the house officer receiving a
      report with the above diagnosis?   (5 marks)

QUESTION 7

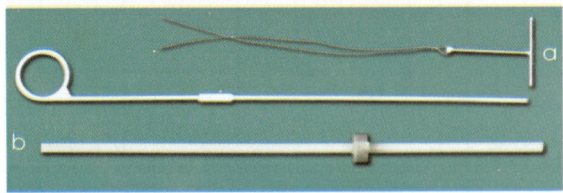

This is a contraceptive method we use in our clinic.
7.1   Name the parts.   (3 marks)
7.2   Write four (4) advices you would give the client before using this method.
                                                                     (4 marks)
7.3   From the picture given below select the instruments required to insert this
      device and place them in the correct order of use.   (3 marks)

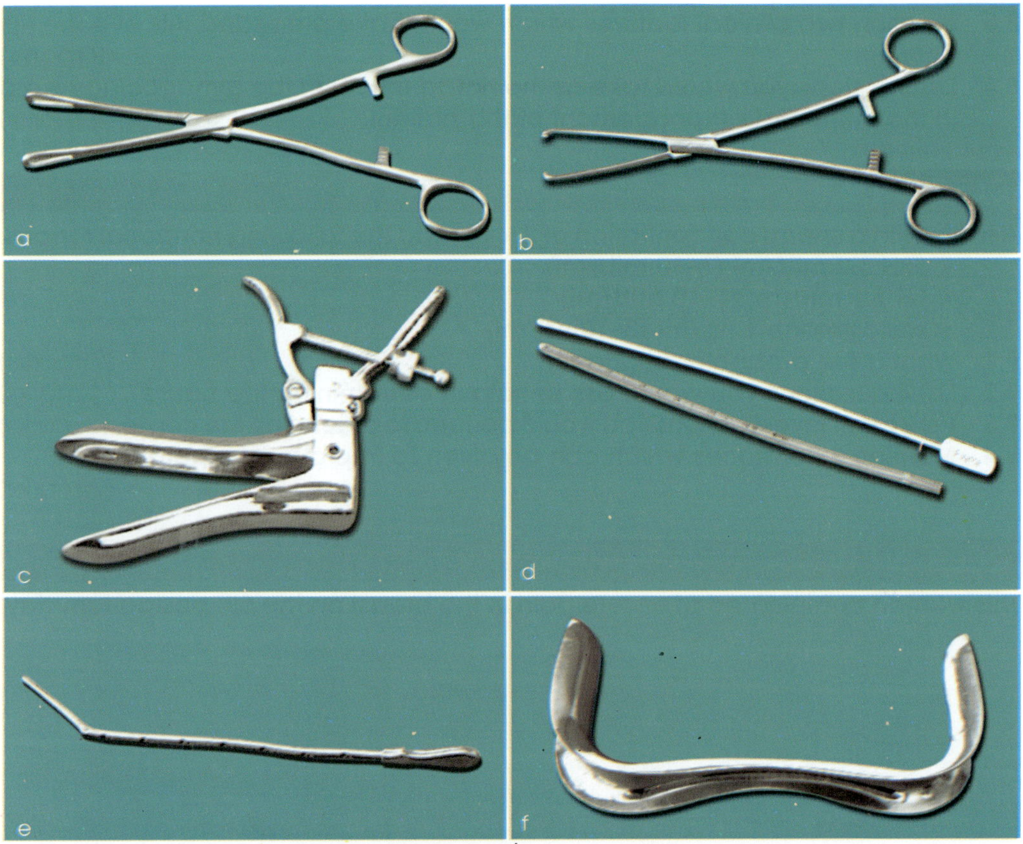

QUESTION 8

This complication occurred on the 7th postoperative day in a woman who underwent laparotomy for stage 3 ovarian cancer.

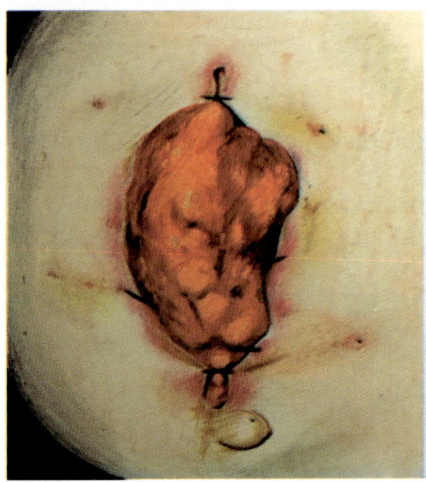

8.1   What is this complication?   (1 mark)

8.2   List 3 causes for this complication.   (3 marks)

8.3 Mention two clinical features which would have preceded this event.

(2 marks)

8.4 List the steps you would take as the house officer in the gynaecology ward in the immediate management of this patient. (4 marks)

QUESTION 9

A male with a sperm concentration of 2×10^6 had the following hormonal reports.
- FSH 1.2 mIU/ml (1–10 mIU/ml)
- LH 1.1 mIU/ml (1–10 mIU/ml)
- Testosterone 1 ng/ml (3–10 ng/ml)

9.1 What is the probable diagnosis? (2 marks)

9.2 List 4 questions you would ask to help in determining the cause. (4 marks)

9.3 List 2 other investigations you would perform to determine the cause. (2 marks)

9.4 Mention 2 hormones which can be given to improve the sperm count.

(2 marks)

QUESTION 10

This woman complained of severe pain in the breast on the 5th postpartum day.

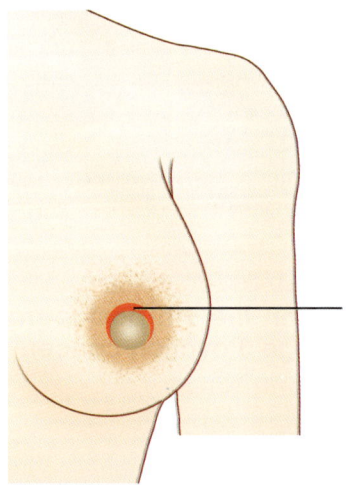

10.1 List a clinical conditions which can cause this appearance. (1 mark)

10.2 List two causes. (2 marks)

10.3 List 5 steps in the management of this patient. (5 marks)

10.4 List two advices you would you give this mother to prevent recurrence of this complication. (2 marks)

ANSWERS FOR EXAMINATION PAPER 2

Answer 1.1

Haemorrhage into an endometrioma

Answer 1.2

- The cyst is most probably a benign endometrioma because it has a ground glass appearance and a thin intact capsule without solid areas.

- The echogenic area is due to bleeding into the cyst.
- The diagnosis is more likely because symptoms occurred towards the end of her menstrual period.

Answer 1.3

She should be informed that:
- There is a cyst in her ovary and her symptoms are most probably due to bleeding into the cyst. If not treated more blood can collect and the viability of ovary may be damaged.
- She needs surgery to drain it. Surgery will be laparoscopic cystectomy and all attempts will be made to preserve her ovary. However, there is a slight risk that oophorectomy may be needed if the ovary is damaged or if bleeding cannot be controlled.
- Final diagnosis is made only after surgery and histological examination.
- If it is an endometrioma, it is benign, but further treatment may be needed to prevent recurrence and subfertility.

Answer 1.4

- Laparoscopic cystectomy and repair of the ovary.
- The specimen is sent for histology.
- The pelvis should be explored for any evidence of malignancy and endometriosis. Any pelvic endometriotic deposits should be cauterized.

Answer 1.5

- Follow up depends on her fertility wishes.
- If she wishes to conceive, she should be advised to try to conceive soon. If natural conception fails early referral should be carried out for IVF.
- If severe symptoms recur medical management should be considered.

Answer 2.1

Secondary haemorrhage

Answer 2.2

Bleeding occurs due to infection of the wound in the vagina and sloughing of the infected tissue, exposing and damaging the underlying blood vessels.

Answer 2.3

- Blood and high vaginal swab for culture and ABST
- Full blood count and clotting profile
- C-reactive protein and serum lactate levels
- Crossmatch blood

Answer 2.4

- Resuscitate with intravenous fluids and blood transfusion if there is haemodynamic compromise.
- Commence intravenous broad spectrum antibiotics after sending blood and high vaginal swab for culture and ABST.
- Insert a tight vaginal pack to control bleeding.

Answer 3.1

- *Chlamydia trachomatis*
- *Neisseria gonorrhoeae*

Answer 3.2

Question her regarding
- Fever
- Dyspareunia
- Dysuria
- Nature of the discharge: whether it is purulent, white and mucoid or bloodstained.
- Multiple sexual partners/history of sexually transmitted diseases.
- Pruritus
- Infertility
- Recent instrumentation of the uterus including miscarriage/delivery.

Answer 3.3

Perform a DNA amplification test on an endocervical swab.

Answer 3.4

- Treatment depends on the infecting organism.
- If chlamydia is isolated treat with doxycycline 100 mg twice daily for 14 days.
- If gonococcus is isolated treat with ceftriaxone 500 mg IM as a single dose plus azithromycin 1 g orally as a single dose.
- Metronidazole 400 mg 8 hourly for 14 days should be added to these regimes, if PID is present.

Answer 3.5

- Educate about safe sex with the use of condoms.
- Trace and treat partners.
- Counsel about the possibility of future impairment of fertility due to PID.
- Counsel about the possibility of future occurrence of an ectopic pregnancy and the need for early scanning if she conceives.

Answer 4.1

Amniocentesis is used to:
- Karyotype the fetus to confirm genetic diseases.
- Perform intrauterine transfusion in severe fetal anaemia.
- Perform amnio-reduction.
- Place a stent for in utero therapy.
- To assess the severity of haemolysis by measuring the amniotic fluid bilirubin levels in rhesus isoimmunisation.

Answer 4.2

15 weeks.

Answer 4.3

- Infection
- Miscarriage

- Preterm delivery
- Rhesus isoimmunization

Answer 4.4

Amniocentesis carries a lower risk of miscarriage than chorionic villous sampling. Placental mosaicism may interfere with accurate diagnosis in chorionic villous sampling.

Fetal abnormalities can be diagnosed earlier with chorionic villous biopsy as it is performed at 10 weeks. Also it takes 2–3 weeks and 1–2 weeks respectively for culturing of cells obtained by amniocentesis and chorionic villus sampling. Therefore, diagnosis is delayed till about 18 weeks with amniocentesis.

Answer 5.1

Secondary arrest

Answer 5.2

- Occipito-posterior position if the pelvis is narrow and android in type.
- Brow presentation
- Mento-posterior face presentation
- Cephalo-pelvic disproportion

Answer 5.3

- Fetal hypoxia, fetal distress and fetal death.
- Obstructed labour
- Uterine rupture
- Sepsis

Answer 5.4

A caesarean section should be performed immediately.

Answer 6.1

- Enlarged nuclei, increased nuclear-cytoplasmic ratio and increased intensity of nuclear staining are seen.
- However, nuclear abnormalities are minimal. Abnormal cells are confined to the deeper layers (lower third) of the epithelium.
- Mitotic figures are present, but not very numerous.

Answer 6.2

CIN 1

Answer 6.3

- Excision is not indicated for these women.
- Cytology and HPV DNA tests are performed at 12 and 24 months. If HPV is positive or if there are cytological abnormalities repeat colposcopy is performed.
- The patient should be advised regarding the future risk of invasive carcinoma and the need for regular follow up.
- If HPV DNA and cytology are negative routine follow up is done in 3 years.

Answer 7.1

a. Copper IUCD
b. Solid rod
c. Introducer

Answer 7.2

- If there is fever or severe pain after insertion advise her to seek medical attention. However, mild pain and mild bleeding may be present for 1–2 days.
- She should feel for the thread frequently, especially after a menstrual period, to make sure that the IUCD is *in situ*.
- The IUCD can be retained for 10 years.
- There may be heavy menstrual bleeding and dysmenorrhea for about 3 months after insertion. However, she should seek medical advice if the symptoms are severe.
- She should attend the clinic after the first menstrual period to confirm that the IUCD is in place.

Answer 7.3

c Cusco's speculum
b Vulsellum
e Uterine sound

Answer 8.1

Burst abdomen

Answer 8.2

- Infection
- Use of poor quality suture material
- Poor surgical technique during closure of the wound
- Use of a vertical incision
- Obesity
- Low immunity due to malignancy

Answer 8.3

- Pain over the wound
- Fever
- Pinkish watery discharge from the wound

Answer 8.4

- Reassure the patient and explain regarding the condition
- Make an attempt to reduce the exposed bowel back into the abdomen and cover the wound with a sterile gauze towel soaked in saline. Inform seniors.
- Provide adequate analgesia and sedation.
- Commence fluid resuscitation as the exposed bowel tends to lose large amounts of fluid rapidly.
- Take a swab from the wound for culture and ABST and commence broad-spectrum antibiotics.

- As the bowel is eviscerating make arrangements for immediate repair of the wound under anaesthesia to prevent bowel injury or strangulation. Surgical opinion should be obtained.

Answer 9.1

Hypogonadotropic hypogonadism.

Answer 9.2

Inquire regarding a history of:
- Headache and visual disturbances.
- Long-standing loss of smell.
- Taking anabolic steroids or psychiatric drugs.
- Weight gain or weight loss.
- Severe stress.
- History of meningitis, head injuries, tuberculosis.

Answer 9.3

- Assess other pituitary hormone levels—ACTH, TSH and prolactin levels.
- Assess the visual fields.
- Perform CT/MRI scan of the brain.

Answer 9.4

- Give hCG 1500 IU intramuscularly 3 times per week, until spermatogenesis occurs.
- If the response is poor add FSH 75–150 IU intramuscularly 3 times per week and reduce the hCG dose. (Treatment with HMG is an alternative method of treatment as it contains both FSH and LH).
- Perform a sperm count after treating for 1 month.

Answer 10.1

Cracked and infected nipple.

Answer 10.2

- Incorrect technique of feeding by allowing the baby to suck on the nipple.
- Monilial infection.

Answer 10.3

- Check whether the baby has oral thrush.
- Breastfeeding can be continued if the pain is not severe. In most cases breast feeding should be stopped till the crack heals. A nipple shield can be used or breast milk can be expressed.
- Apply a little breast milk on the crack and allow it to dry.
- Application of an antibiotic cream such as fucidine may be helpful if infection is present. Oral antibiotics are given if there is severe infection.
- Apply an antifungal cream if monilial infection is present.

Answer 10.4

- Do not allow the baby to suck on the nipple. Admit the nipple and part of the areola into the mouth so that the nipple will be at the back of the mouth.
- The baby should be fed from both breasts at each feed and should be allowed to suck for 10 minutes from each nipple.
- Proper technique of feeding and burping should be used to prevent the baby from demanding frequent feeds.
- The baby should not be allowed to remain on the nipple when not feeding.
- Wash the breasts gently with water without using strong soap.

Examination Paper 3

QUESTION 1

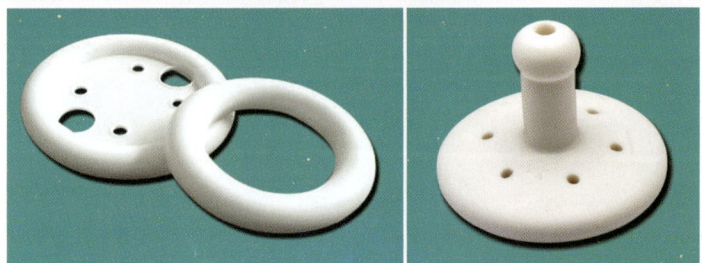

1.1 Name the pessaries shown in the picture. (3 marks)
1.2 List 4 indications for inserting a pessary to treat uterovaginal prolapse.
(4 marks)
1.3 What are the specific indications for the use of A, B and C? (3 marks)

QUESTION 2

2.1 What is this complication?
(1 mark)
2.2 What is the cause for it in this patient?
(1 mark)
2.3 What action could have been taken to prevent this complication in this patient?
(2 marks)
2.4 If you are the house officer what is your immediate management? (3 marks)
2.5 What is the best method of delivery if the cervix is fully dilated?
(2 marks)
2.6 What is your management if the fetus is dead?
(1 mark)

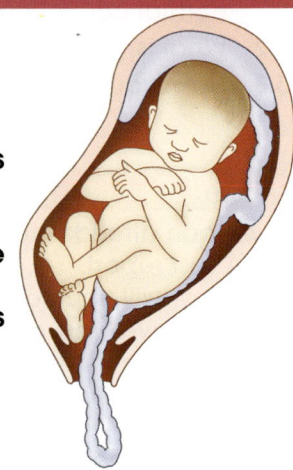

QUESTION 3

a

TEACHING HOSPITAL PERADENIYA - BC6800

First Name: Last Name: Sample ID:
Gender: Age: Patient ID:
Department: Bed No: Date of Analysis:
Mode:
Diagnosis :

Para		Result	Unit	Ref. Ranges	Para		Result	Unit	Ref. Ranges
1 WBC	H	11.06	10^3/UL	4.00-10.00	16 MCH	L	18.9	pg	27.0-34.0
2 New	R	4.22	10^3/UL	2.00-7.00	17 MCHC	L	30.7	g/dL	32.0-36.0
3 Lyn	RH	5.76	10^3/UL	0.80-1.00	18 RDW-CV	H	20.1	%	11.0-16.0
4 Mon	R	1.02	10^3/UL	0.12-1.20	19 RDW-SD	H	44.6	IL	35.0-56.0
5 Eos	L	0.01	10^3/UL	0.02-0.50	20 PLT	H	629	10^3/L	100-300
6 Bas		0.05	10^3/UL	0.00-0.10	21 MPV		7.3	IL	6.5-12.0
7 Neu%	RL	38.2	%	50.0-70.0	22 PDW		15.0		15.0-17.0
8 Lym%	RH	52.1	%	20.0-40.0	23 PCT	H	0.458	%	0.108-0.282
9 Mon%	R	0.2	%	3.0-12.0	24 P-LCC		66	10^9/L	30-90
10 Lios%	L	0.1	%	0.5-5.0	25 P-LCR	L	10.6	%	11.0-45.0
11 Bas%		0.4	%	0.0-1.0	26 IMG		0.04	10^3/UL	0.00-999.99
12 RBC		4.86		3.50-5.50	27 IMG%		0.4	%	0.0-100.0
13 HGB	L	9.2	g/dL	1.0-16.0	*28 HEC	R	0.17	10^9/UL	
14 UGT	L	30.0	%	37.0-54.0	*29 UFC%	R	1.5	%	
15 MCV	L	61.8	IL	80.0-100.0					

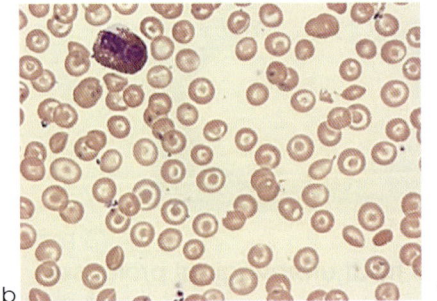

b

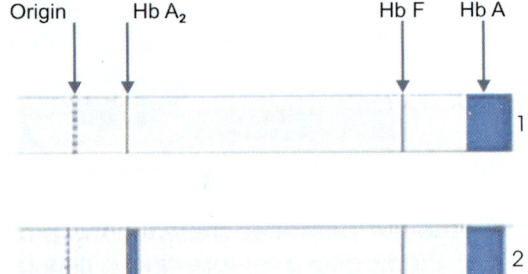

c

These are the blood investigations which were performed in a woman who attended the antenatal clinic at a POA of 16 weeks.

3.1 Mention 2 abnormalities in each of these reports. In the report C (1) is the normal control and (2) is the patient's report.   (6 marks)

3.2 What is your diagnosis?   (2 marks)

3.3 How would you advise this woman regarding the prognosis for her baby?
                                                                             (2 marks)

QUESTION 4

A woman attends the antenatal clinic at a POA of 16 weeks with a positive HIV ELISA test report.

4.1 How will you confirm the diagnosis?   (1 mark)

4.2 How will you commence her on drug treatment? (It is not necessary to mention individual drugs.   (2 marks)

4.3 List 3 other aspects in treating her. (1 mark will be awarded each for any 3 correct responses. (3 marks)

4.4 List the measures you would take to prevent vertical transmission. (4 marks)

QUESTION 5

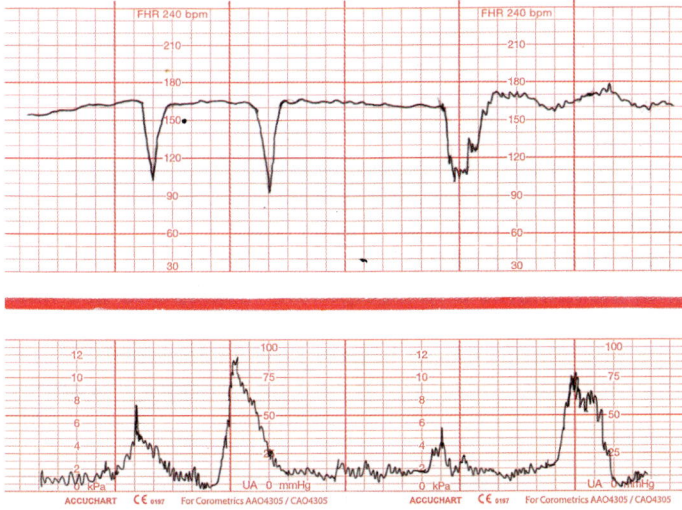

This is a CTG of a primigravid patient in labour. Vaginal examination performed 3 hours ago showed a cervical dilatation of 6 cm.

5.1   List 2 abnormalities seen in this CTG.   (2 marks)

5.2   What is your fist line management if you are the house officer in the labour ward?   (4 marks)

5.3   What is your definitive management if the first line management fails?
                                                                              (2 marks)

5.4   List two conditions where you would see a CTG like this.   (2 marks)

QUESTION 6

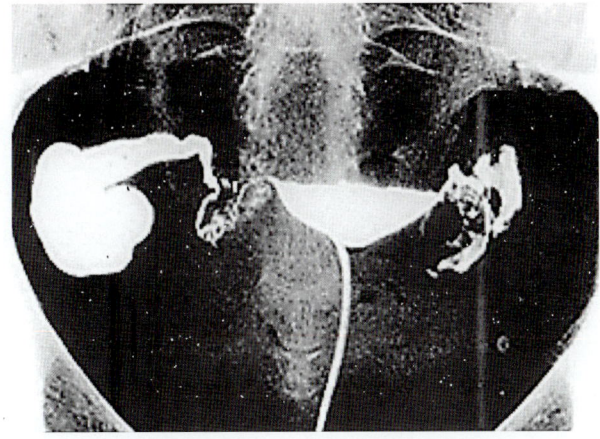

This is a picture of an HSG of a sub-fertile woman.

6.1   Describe the abnormalities seen in this image.   (2 marks)

6.2   Mention 2 causes for this abnormality.   (2 marks)

6.3   What is the first line management?   (2 marks)

6.4   What is the next step in the management if the first line management fails?
                                                                              (2 marks)

6.5 What is the period of the menstrual cycle during which a HSG can be performed? Give your reasons. (2 marks)

QUESTION 7

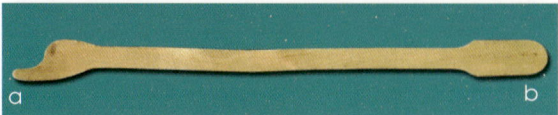

7.1 Identify the instrument and mention its use. (2 marks)
7.2 Write the uses of ends a and b. (0.5 × 2 = 1 mark)
7.3 List the other instruments and equipment required to use this instrument. (0.5 × 4 = 2 marks)
7.4 List the steps you would follow in using this instrument. (4 marks)
7.5 Mention another instrument which can be used for the same purpose. (1 mark)

QUESTION 8

List 2 drugs which can be used safely in each of these clinical conditions in a pregnant woman. (2 × 5 =10 marks)
8.1 Allergic rhinitis
8.2 Heart burn
8.3 Chlamydial infection
8.4 Typhoid fever
8.5 Vaginal candidiasis

QUESTION 9

This is an ultrasound image of a woman who was admitted with a complaint of abdominal pain and fever of 102°F, 5 days after caesarean section for prolonged labour.

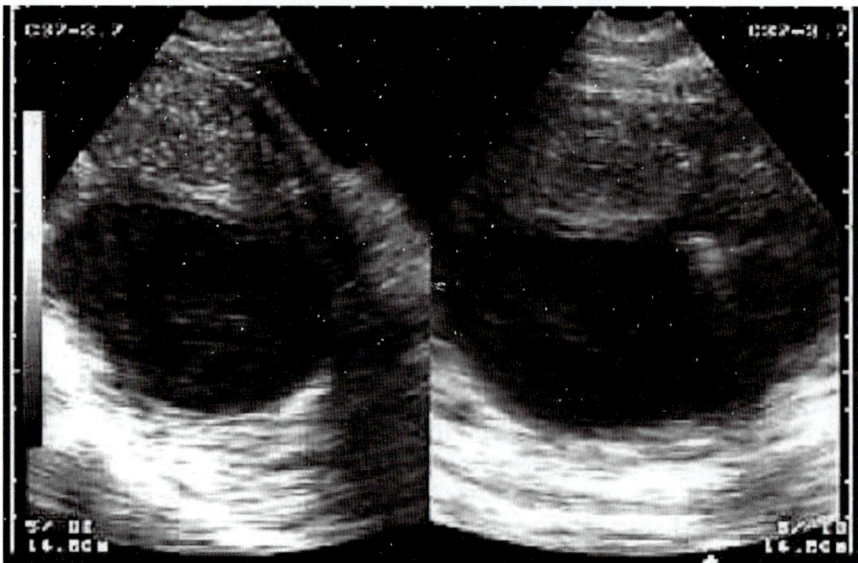

9.1   What is the most likely diagnosis?   (1 mark)
9.2   Give reasons for your diagnosis.   (2 marks)
9.3   Mention another condition which could give a similar appearance on
      ultrasound scanning.   (1 mark)
9.4   List 3 investigations you would perform to confirm your diagnosis. (3 marks)
9.5   What is the first line management?   (2 marks)
9.6   Mention an indication for laparotomy/laparoscopy.   (1 mark)

QUESTION 10

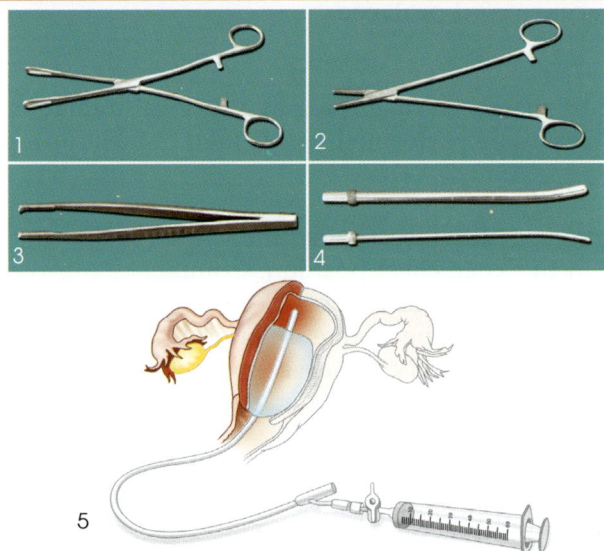

Identify these instruments and mention one of their uses.   (2 marks for each)

ANSWERS FOR EXAMINATION PAPER 3

Answer 1.1

a. Ring pessary with support
b. Ring pessary
c. Gelhorn pessary

Answer 1.2

A pessary is inserted to:
• Keep the prolapse reduced during pregnancy
• Keep the prolapse reduced for a decubitus ulcer to heal
• Treat a patient who is unfit for surgery due to a serious untreatable medical
  condition or as a temporary measure till the medical condition is treated.
• Treat a patient who wishes to conceive soon.

Answer 1.3

a. For a woman with a large 3rd or 4th degree prolapse who is unable to retain a
   ring pessary and is actively engaged in sex.
b. This is more suitable for a 1st or 2nd degree prolapse.

c. For a woman with a large 3rd or 4th degree prolapse who is unable to retain a ring pessary and is not actively engaged in sex. It is difficult to insert and remove this pessary.

Answer 2.1

Cord prolapse.

Answer 2.2

Since this woman has a footling breech presentation spontaneous or artificial rupture of membranes can cause cord prolapse.

Answer 2.3

The malpresentation should be diagnosed at a cervical dilatation of 4–5 cm and a caesarean section should be performed before membranes rupture.

Answer 2.4

- If the cord is outside gently insert it into the vagina but not into the uterus.
- Put the patient in the knee chest position. Commence intravenous tocolytics if there are frequent strong contractions.
- Commence continuous fetal heart rate monitoring.
- Arrange for immediate delivery by caesarean section.

Answer 2.5

A caesarean section should be performed. Breech extraction is best avoided for a singleton breech presentation because of the risk of cephalopelvic disproportion and subsequent head entrapment.

Answer 2.6

Allow spontaneous vaginal delivery.

Answer 3.1

a. • The haemoglobin percentage is low.
   • The red cell count is normal.
   • MCH and MCV are reduced.
b. • It is a hypochromic microcytic blood picture.
   • There are target cells and tear drop shaped cells.
c. • The HbA is reduced.
   • HbA2 is present

Answer 3.2

Beta thalassemia trait. There is only a small amount of HbA2.

Answer 3.3

- Haemoglobin electrophoresis should be carried out on her partner's blood to determine if he is also a thalassemia carrier.
- If both are carriers the baby is at risk of having thalassemia major.
- If both are carriers amniocentesis or cell free fetal DNA testing should be performed to confirm/exclude occurrence of thalassemia in the baby.

- If only she is the carrier the baby has a 50% chance of being a thalassemia trait.
- Baby may need further testing after delivery.

Answer 4.1
Refer to the STD clinic to perform a Western blot test.

Answer 4.2
- A multi-disciplinary team approach is necessary with the STD team.
- Women who do not require treatment for their own health should commence temporary cART at the beginning of the second trimester if the baseline viral load(VL) is >30 000 HIV RNA copies/ml (consider starting earlier if VL >100 000 HIV RNA copies/ml.)
- Women whose plasma viral load is less than 10,000 copies per ml and planning to deliver by caesarean section could be treated with Zidovudine (ZDV) mono-therapy from 20 to 28 weeks onwards.

Answer 4.3
- Management plan should be discussed with the patient.
- Test for other sexually transmitted infections.
- She should also be tested for antibodies against rubella measles and varicella zoster. If she has no antibodies she should be advised to avoid exposure to these conditions.
- She should be vaccinated against hepatitis B, pneumococcus and influenza. Killed vaccines should be given.
- Her sexual contacts should be traced, tested and treated.
- She should be advised regarding safe sex with the use of condoms.

Answer 4.4
Vertical transmission is prevented by:
- Giving anti-retroviral therapy for the mother.
- Performing an elective caesarean section.
- Avoiding breastfeeding.
- Giving anti-retroviral therapy for the baby.

Answer 5.1
The abnormalities seen in this CTG include:
- Recurrent variable decelerations with reduced baseline variability.
- Moderately strong, in coordinate, irregular uterine contractions.

Answer 5.2
- Stop the oxytocin infusion.
- Turn to the left lateral position.
- Give oxygen by face mask.
- Insert an IV cannula, take blood for cross-matching and commence an infusion of normal saline
- Perform a vaginal examination to assess the cervical dilatation and to exclude cord prolapse.

- Inform seniors.
- Perform scalp blood sampling to confirm fetal acidosis (if available).

Answer 5.3

A caesarean section should be performed immediately.

Answer 5.4

- Cord compression
- Nuchal cord
- Over stimulation with oxytocin.

Answer 6.1

- The right tube has a hydrosalpnix with no spill.
- Scanty spill is seen from the other side indicating partial block of the tube.

Answer 6.2

- Endometriosis
- Pelvic inflammatory disease.

Answer 6.3

- Perform tubal reconstruction.
- Treat endometriosis or pelvic inflammatory disease, if present.

Answer 6.4

- In vitro fertilization is the best management option.
- Salpingectomy should be performed before IVF because a hydrosalpinx is present.

Answer 6.5

It is best performed between the 7th and 10th day of the menstrual cycle to ensure the absence of a fertilized ovum.

Answer 7.1

Ayer's spatula. It is used to perform a cervical smear.

Answer 7.2

a. It is inserted into the cervical canal and rotated by 360° to obtain a smear from the junctional zone of the cervix.
b. It is used to obtain a smear from the surface of the cervix and the posterior fornix.

Answer 7.3

- Cusco's bivalve speculum.
- Two glass slides.
- A small glass container of 95% alcohol to fix the slides.
- A good light.

Answer 7.4

- Place the patient in the dorsal position.
- Do not use antiseptic solutions or lubricants.

- Insert the Cusco's bivalve speculum and visualize the cervix using a good light.
- Continue the procedure if there is no visible lesion or active bleeding.
- Insert the A side of the spatula into the cervical canal and rotate 360 degrees.
- Smear on a dry slide and dip into 95% alcohol.
- Obtain a smear from the surface of the cervix and the posterior fornix using the B end and smear on a dry slide and dip into 95% alcohol.
- Dispatch the specimen to the laboratory with a properly filled request form.

Answer 7.5
Cervical brush.

Answer 8.1
- Diphenhydramine
- Loretidine.

Answer 8.2
- Cimetidine
- Famotidine

Answer 8.3
- Erythromycin
- Azithromycin.

Answer 8.4
- Intramuscular ceftriaxone
- Oral cefixime.

Answer 8.5
Nystatin vaginal tablets or clotrimazole vaginal tablets.

Answer 9.1
A pelvic abscess.

Answer 9.2
Occurrence of typical symptoms of abdominal pain and fever of 102°F, 5 days after caesarean section for prolonged labour.

   Ultrasound scan appearance of a heterogeneous cyst with fluid levels.

Answer 9.3
Haemorrhage into an ovarian cyst or an endometrioma.

Answer 9.4
- WBCDC
- C-reactive protein or procalcitonin levels
- Blood and high vaginal and endocervical swabs for culture and ABST.

Answer 9.5

Commence intravenous broad spectrum antibiotics after sending blood and high vaginal and endocervical swabs for culture and ABST and drain the abscess under ultrasound guidance.

Answer 9.6

Open drainage through laparotomy/laparoscopy is needed, if there is:
- Increased thickness of the fluid.
- Presence of free fluid in the peritoneal cavity.
- Inaccessibility of the abscess for ultrasound drainage.

Answer 10

1: Sponge holding forceps.

It is used to:
- To hold the pregnant cervix when inspecting for tears.
- To remove the products of conception when performing an ERPC.

2: Needle holder is used to hold the needle when suturing a tissue.

3: Catch forceps is used to hold the tissues while suturing.

4: Suction curette is used to connect to the suction apparatus, to apply negative pressure when performing a suction evacuation of retained products or a hydatidiform mole.

5: Bakry balloon is used for uterine tamponade in the treatment of PPH.

Examination Paper 4

The following CTG was obtained at a cervical dilatation of 4 cm in a primigravid woman who is in spontaneous labour.

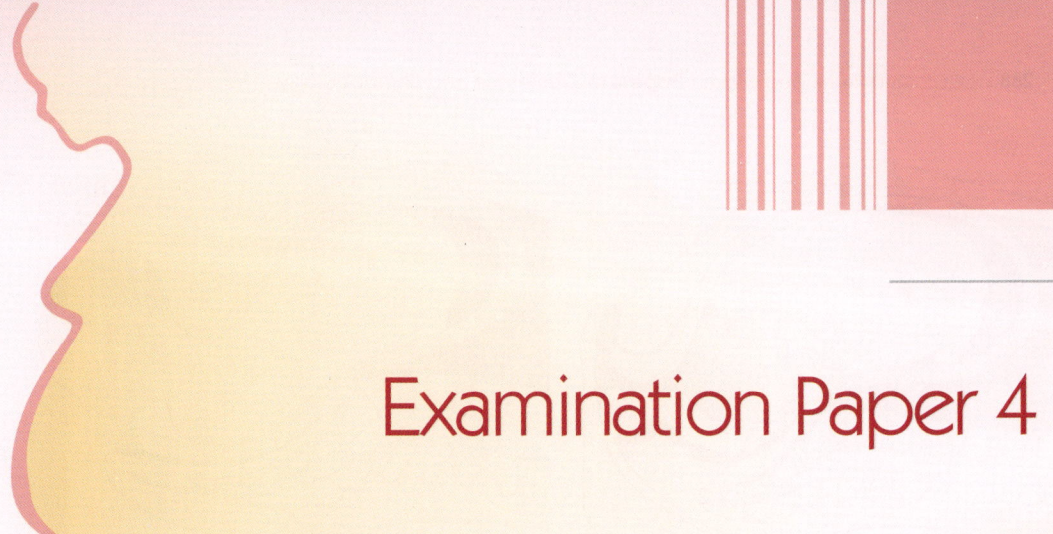

1.1   What is the abnormality seen in this CTG?   (2 marks)
1.2   List 4 causes for this abnormality.   (4 marks)
1.3   What is your management?   (4 marks)

QUESTION 2

The following images show different stages in the mechanism of normal labour.
2.1   Mention the changes which occur in each image.   (6 marks)
2.2   Place them in the appropriate order in which they occur during labour.

                                                                            (4 marks)

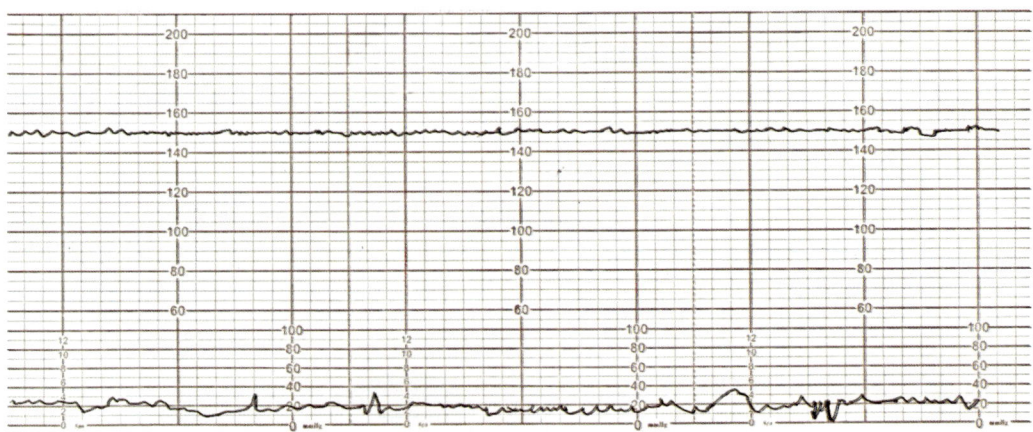

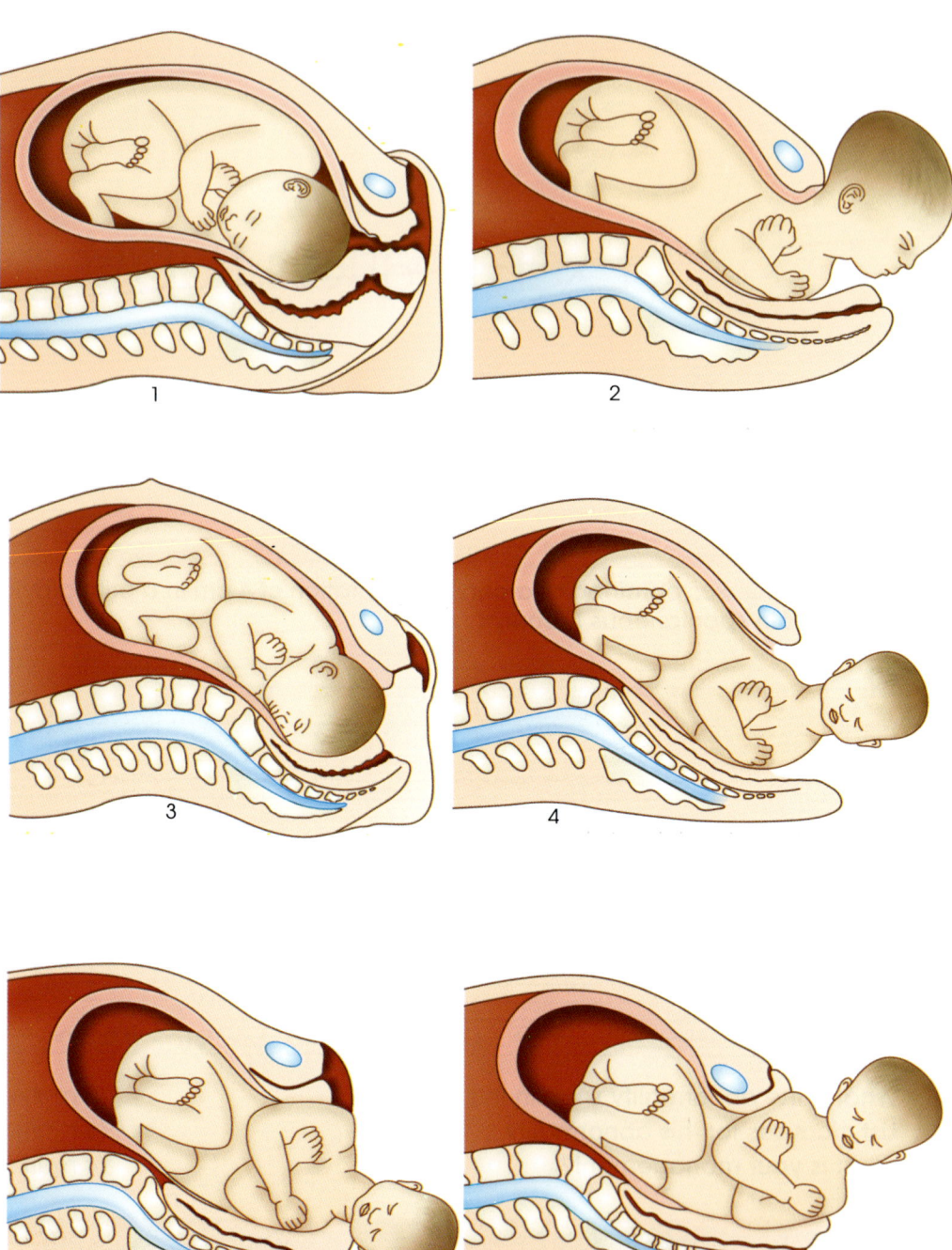

This is a picture of a 14-year-old girl with primary amenorrhea.

3.1   List 4 abnormalities seen in this picture.   (0.5 × 4 = 2 marks)

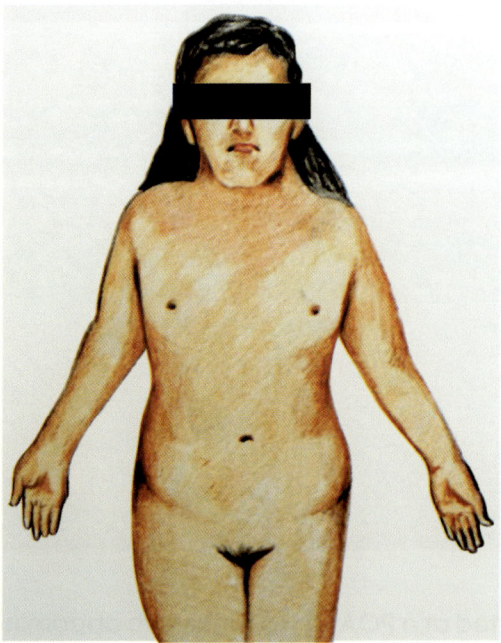

3.2   What is the likely diagnosis?   (1 mark)
3.3   Mention a single investigation you would perform to confirm the diagnosis.
                                                                     (1 mark)
3.4   List 3 steps in the treatment of this girl.   (3 marks)
3.5   She attends the clinic at the age of 18 years and wishes to know the further
      management and the prognosis. How would you advise her?   (3 marks)

QUESTION 4

4.1   Mention 4 absolute contraindications for hormone replacement therapy.
                                                          (0.5 × 4 = 2 marks)
4.2   List 6 investigations you would perform before prescribing hormone
      replacement therapy.   (0.5 × 6 = 3 marks)
4.3   List 5 important aspects of counseling a woman before commencing HRT.
                                                                     (5 marks)

QUESTION 5

Tetanus toxoid is routinely administered at the antenatal clinic.
5.1   What is the reason for its administration?   (4 marks)
5.2   What is the POA at which it is usually given?   (1 mark)
5.3   What is the dose, mode and frequency of administration in a primigravida?
                                                                     (3 marks)
5.4   What is your recommendation for a woman in her second pregnancy with
      a 2-year-old child?   (2 marks)

QUESTION 6

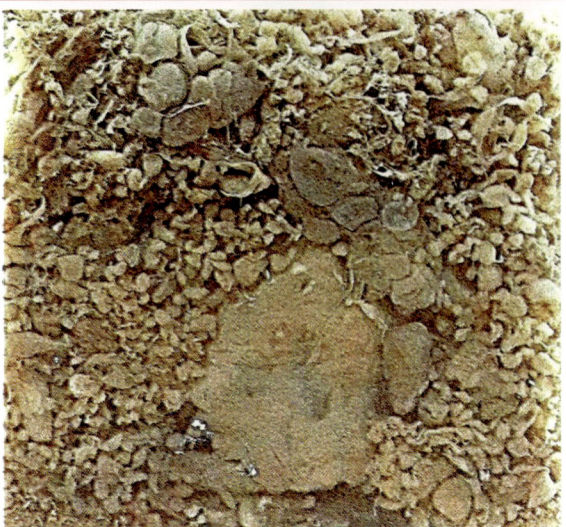

From Wikipedia commons

A patient who presented at a POA of 16 weeks with abdominal pain and bleeding per vagina aborted the above specimen soon after admission.

6.1   What is the most likely condition?   (1 mark)
6.2   List 4 steps in the immediate management.   (4 marks)
6.3   List 4 steps in the follow up of this patient.   (4 marks)
6.4   What is the best method of contraception?   (1 mark)

QUESTION 7

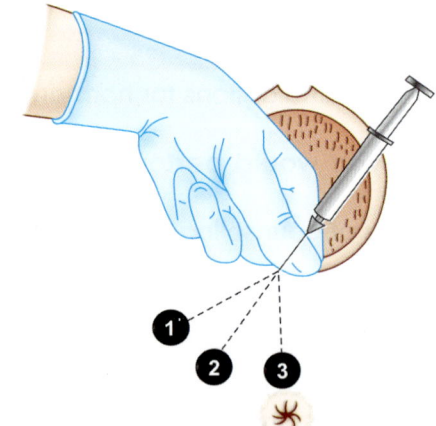

7.1   What is the disadvantage of performing an episiotomy along the line 3?
                                                                                                         (2 marks)

7.2   Select from the given samples the most appropriate material to suture an episiotomy.   (2 marks)
      a. No 1 polyglactin

  b. No 3/0 polyglactin
  c. Thick nylon
  d. 3/0 black silk
  e. No 0 polyglactin

7.3   What are the tissue planes which are cut while performing an episiotomy?
                                                                    (2 marks)
7.4   At which point will you commence suturing?   (2 marks)
7.5   What suturing technique would you use for (A) the vaginal mucosa and (B) the muscle layer?   (2 marks)

QUESTION 8

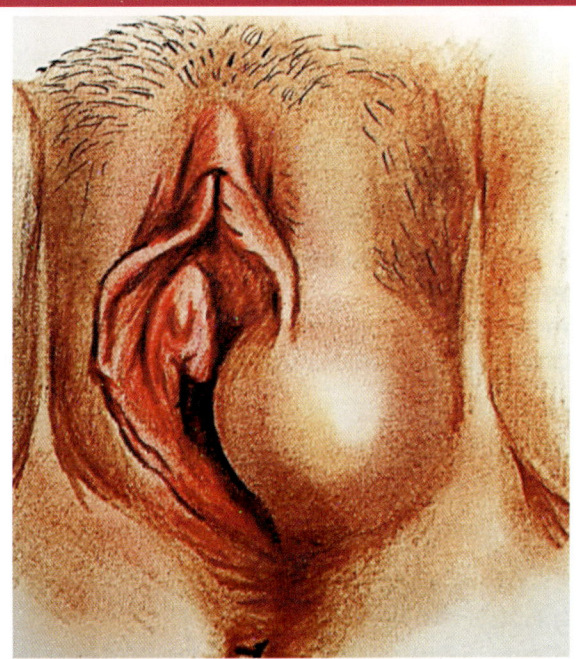

8.1   What is the condition shown in the picture?   (2 marks)
8.2   What is the cause?   (2 marks)
8.3   Mention a complication which can occur.   (2 marks)
8.4   Describe the surgical procedure which is used to treat this condition.
                                                                    (4 marks)

QUESTION 9

A woman is admitted with dribbling at a period of amenorrhoea of 32 weeks.
9.1   How would you confirm the diagnosis?   (1 mark)
9.2   List the investigations you would perform.   (2 marks)
9.3   List 3 drugs you would use in the management. Give reasons for the use of the drugs.   (3 marks)
9.4   Mention the POA at which you would deliver the baby.   (1 mark)
9.5   List 3 indications for early delivery.   (3 marks)

QUESTION 10

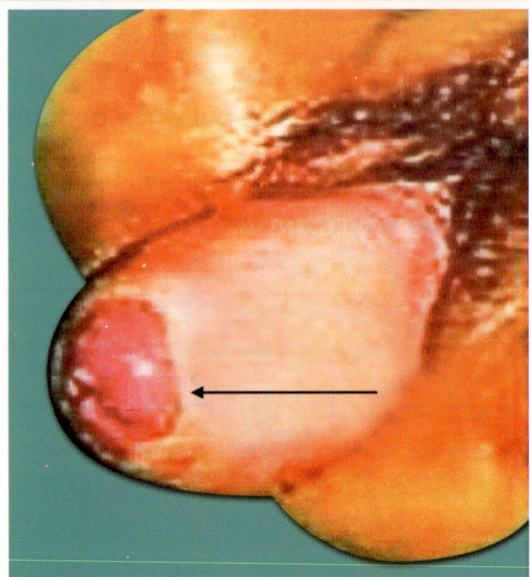

10.1 What is the abnormality shown by the arrow? (1 mark)

10.2 What is the cause for it? (2 marks)

10.3 How do you treat it? (4 marks)

10.4 List 3 complications which can occur if surgery is carried out without treating it. (3 marks)

ANSWERS FOR EXAMINATION PAPER 4

Answer 1.1

Occurrence of reduced baseline variability in the fetal heart tracing.

Answer 1.2

- Fetal hypoxia/acidosis
- Fetal sleep
- Use of narcotic analgesics
- Epidural analgesia
- Administration of dexamethasone

Answer 1.3

- The first step is to exclude fetal sleep by repeating the CTG after 1 hour.
- Do not give the next injection of pethidine or the top up dose of epidural analgesia.
- If the abnormality still persists perform fetal scalp blood sampling.
- Perform a caesarean section if there is fetal acidosis.

Answer 2.1

1. Engagement, flexion and descent.
2. Complete extension.
3. Further descent and internal rotation.
4. Restitution.

5. Depression of the head to deliver the anterior shoulder.
6. Elevation of the head to deliver the posterior shoulder.

Answer 2.2

1, 3, 2, 4, 5, 6.

Answer 3.1

- Webbing of the neck.
- Widely spaced nipples.
- Failure of development of secondary sexual characteristics.
- Increased carrying angle.

Answer 3.2

Turner syndrome.

Answer 3.3

Perform a karyotype to confirm the XO karyotype.

Answer 3.4

- Reassurance and explanation is essential.
- Give ethinyl estradiol at first to improve the secondary sexual characteristics and give life-long treatment with HRT. Calcium and vitamin D supplements and regular exercise is essential. Bone dinsitometry should be performed later.
- Refer to an endocrinologist for treatment with growth hormone before commencing estrogen.
- Refer to a cardiologist to exclude a structural lesion of the heart. Also refer to a ENT surgeon and an eye surgeon. Gonads should be removed if a Y chromosome is present.

Answer 3.5

- She should continue HRT during the entire life. A baseline dual energy X-ray absorptiometry scan should be done.
- Cyclical menstruation will occur due to HRT.
- Further development of secondary sexual characteristics will not occur.
- Normal sexual activity is possible.
- Fertility is possible only with ovum donation.

Answer 4.1

- Active thromboembolic disorder.
- Acute phase myocardial infarction.
- Previous stroke.
- Suspected or active breast or endometrial carcinoma.
- Active liver disease with abnormal liver function tests.

Answer 4.2

- ECG, lipid profile and fasting blood sugar

- Echocardiograph and assessment by a cardiologist if coronary heart disease is suspected.
- Liver function tests.
- Mammogram.
- Cervical smear.
- Transvaginal and abdominal ultrasound scan.

Answer 4.3

- She should take the pill regularly at the same time every day. Failure to do so may result in vaginal bleeding.
- She should attend the clinic immediately if she develops even mild bleeding.
- There is an increased risk of developing breast carcinoma, stroke and type 2 diabetes mellitus.
- There is an increased risk of developing DVT in women with other risk factors. If the woman is obese she should be advised to reduce weight.
- She should be reviewed at the clinic 3 months after commencing treatment and yearly thereafter.

Answer 5.1

Tetanus toxoid is given to ensure transplacental transfer of maternal antibodies to the fetus in order to prevent neonatal tetanus.

Answer 5.2

After 12 weeks.

Answer 5.3

0.5 ml is given by intramuscular injection. Two doses are given 6 weeks apart.

Answer 5.4

Only one booster injection is given between 20 and 28 weeks, if she has been immunized during the first pregnancy within 5 years.

Answer 6.1

Complete hydatidiform mole.

Answer 6.2

- Insert two 14 gauge cannulae and commence normal saline.
- Send blood for cross-matching. Observe for bleeding and transfuse, if necessary.
- Perform an USS to exclude retained products.
- Perform a suction evacuation if retained tissue is present.

Answer 6.3

- Perform serum beta hCG levels weekly until it becomes negative.
- If the hCG levels return to normal within 56 days after evacuation, hCG levels will be checked monthly for 6 months from the day of evacuation.
- If the hCG levels return to normal more than 56 days after evacuation, hCG levels will be checked monthly for 6 months after the values become normal.

- Women should be advised not to conceive till their follow up is complete. Women who need chemotherapy should not conceive for 1 year after the treatment is complete.

Answer 6.4

A reliable contraceptive method should be used for at least 6 months after the hCG level becomes normal.

If the hCG level is normal any method can be used. If hCG is elevated a barrier method should be used.

Answer 7.1

If the episiotomy undergoes extension during a difficult delivery the anal sphincters and the anal mucosa can get torn.

Answer 7.2

No. 0 polyglactin.

Answer 7.3

Vaginal mucosa, perineal muscles and the perineal skin.

Answer 7.4

At the apex of the vaginal mucosal cut.

Answer 7.5

Vaginal mucosa is sutured with continuous non-interlocking sutures and the perineal muscles are sutured with interrupted or continuous non-interlocking sutures.

Answer 8.1

A Bartholin's cyst.

Answer 8.2

It is a swelling caused by collection of the secretions of the Bartholin's gland due to blocking of the duct.

Answer 8.3

It can become infected forming a painful abscess.

Answer 8.4

Marsupialization is performed under general anaesthesia.

An incision is made on the inner aspect of the labium minus. The cyst cavity is opened and the fluid or pus is drained. The cyst wall is everted and sutured to the skin to maintain an opening to prevent re-collection of fluid.

Answer 9.1

Dribbling is diagnosed by performing a sterile speculum examination. Liquor is identified by the presence of flakes of vernix. The diagnosis can be confirmed if required by the alkaline pH or by performing the nitrazine blue test.

Answer 9.2

- Nitrazine blue test
- Full blood count
- C-reactive protein levels.
- High vaginal swab for culture and ABST
- USS for maturity, presentation, liquor volume and the position of the cord.
- CTG

Answer 9.3

- Nifidepine 20 mg twice daily is given as a tocolytic agent. It is the preferred tocolytic agent as it is effective, cheap and is given orally
- Betamethasone 12.5 mg intramuscularly; 2 injections are given 12 hours apart. This is given to bring about fetal lung maturity.
- Erythromycin 500 mg orally, 12 hourly, to prevent infection.

Answer 9.4

After 34 weeks.

Answer 9.5

Occurrence of:
- Chorioamnionitis
- Meconium staining of the liquor
- Fetal distress diagnosed by an abnormal CTG.

Answer 10.1

Decubitus ulcer.

Answer 10.2

It occurs in the most dependent part of the prolapse due to venous congestion and poor nutrition of the tissues.

Answer 10.3

The prolapse is kept reduced by insertion of a pessary till the ulcer heals. Application of estrogen cream is helpful in postmenopausal patients.

Answer 10.4

- Bleeding
- Infection
- Difficulty in dissecting the vaginal epithelium around the ulcer.

Examination Paper 5

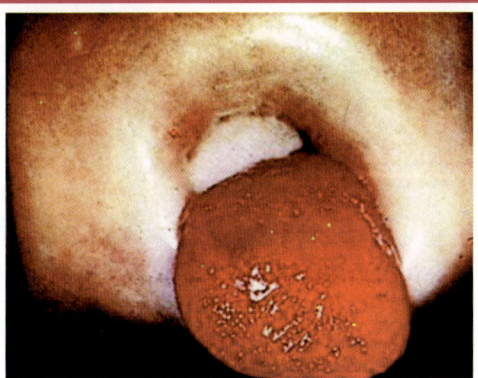

1.1 What is the condition shown in the picture of the cervix?   (1 mark)
1.2 List 3 symptoms.   (3 marks)
1.3 Name the surgical procedure used to treat this condition.   (1 mark)
1.4 Describe how the growth is removed at surgery.   (5 marks)

QUESTION 2

Using the principles of the mechanism of labour, list 5 steps in the management of a normal delivery commencing at the stage shown in the picture. (10 marks)

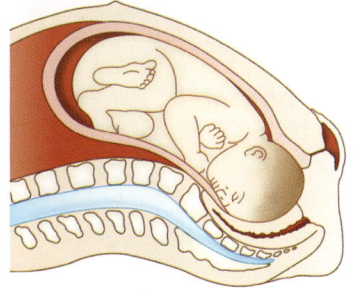
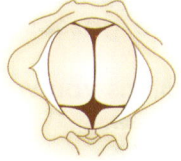

QUESTION 3

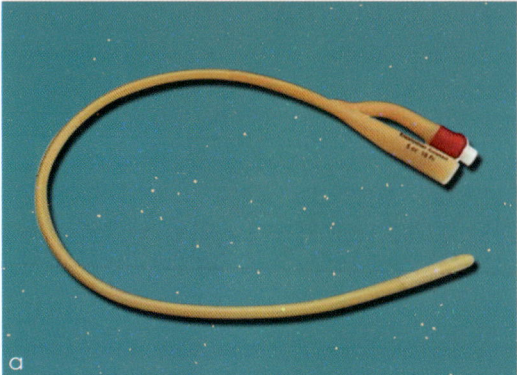

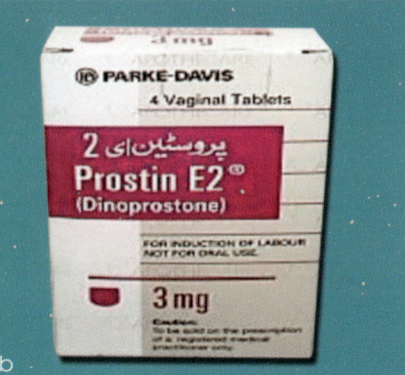

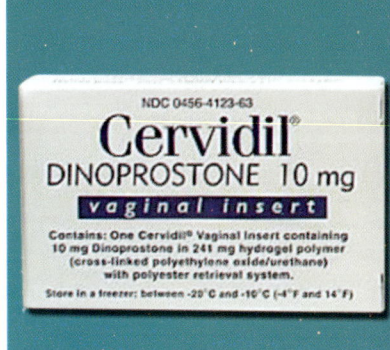

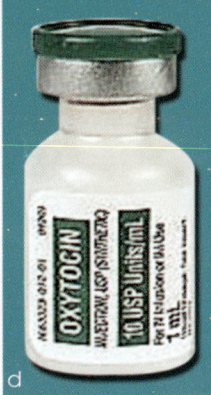

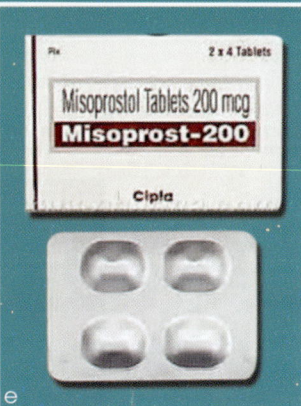

Which of the above are suitable for the following conditions? If a drug is used mention the dose and the frequency of administration.   (2 marks for each)

3.1   To ripen the cervix in a women with a previous caesarean section scar.

3.2   To induce labour in a stillbirth at 25 weeks.

3.3   To augment labour in a primipara with an occipito-posterior position at a cervical dilatation of 6 cm.

3.4   To induce labour in a third para with moderately severe PIH and a Bishop score of 2 at 38 weeks.

3.5   To induce labour in a primipara with a Bishop score of 7 at a POA of 41 weeks.

QUESTION 4

This is a device available for use in the labour room

4.1   Identify the equipment.   (1 mark)

4.2   What are the gasses delivered by this device?   (1 mark)

4.3   List 3 instructions you would give a patient regarding its use.   (6 marks)

4.4   List 2 side effects.   (2 marks)

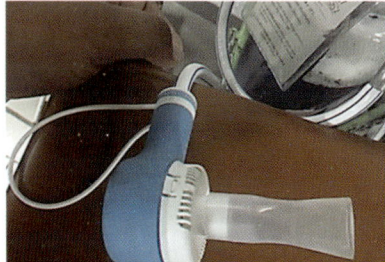

QUESTION 5

This is the report of a bone density scan (DEXA scan), which was performed on a 47-year-old patient, who had reached menopause 2 years ago. Her mother has had a hip fracture due to osteoporosis.

AP Spine: L1–L4 (BMD)

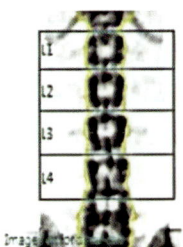

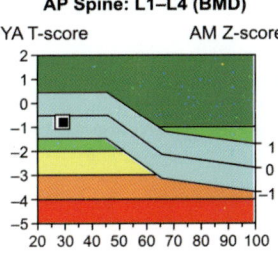

Region	BMD (g/cm^2)	YA T-score	AM Z-score
L1	0.990	−1.2	−0.6
L2	1.071	−1.1	−0.5
L3	1.137	−0.5	−0.0
L4	1.115	−0.7	−0.2
L1–L4	1.084	−0.8	−0.3

Age (years)
USA (Combined NHANES/Luner)

Left femur: Neck (BMD)

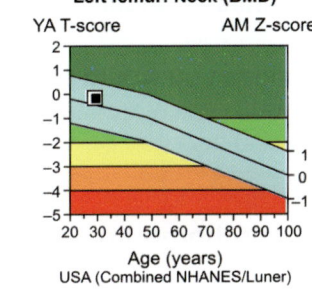

Region	BMD (g/cm^2)	YA T-score	AM Z-score
Neck, Left	1.014	−0.2	−0.3

Age (years)
USA (Combined NHANES/Luner)

Right femur: Neck (BMD)

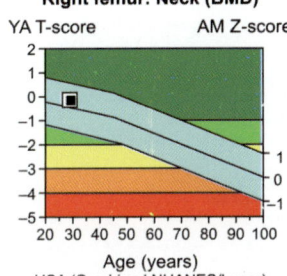

Region	BMD (g/cm^2)	YA T-score	AM Z-score
Neck, Right	1.006	−0.2	−0.2

Age (years)
USA (Combined NHANES/Luner)

5.1   Has this patient got osteoporosis? Give reasons for your answer. (2 marks)

5.2   List 4 first line treatment options. Give reasons for your selection. (4 marks)

5.3   Does she need HRT? Give reasons for your answer. (2 marks)

5.4   How will you follow up this patient? (2 marks)

QUESTION 6

6.1   Identify the instrument in the image. (1 mark)

6.2   List its uses in Gynaecological practice. (2 marks for any one use)

6.3   List three (3) common insertion points of this instrument into the **peritoneal cavity**. (3 marks)

6.4   What are the complications associated with the use of this instrument?
(2 marks)

6.5   How would you avoid these complications during its use?   (2 marks)

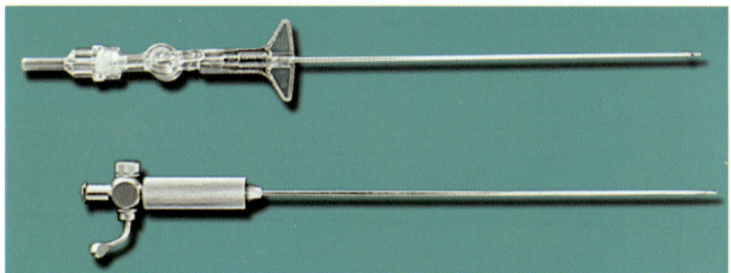

7.1   What are the types of urinary incontinence?   (0.5 × 4 = 2 marks)

7.2   How do you differentiate between these conditions from the history?
(4 marks)

7.3   What are the preliminary investigations you would perform in mixed urinary incontinence?   (4 marks)

This woman complained of pain and discharge from the caesarean section wound on the 4th postoperative day.

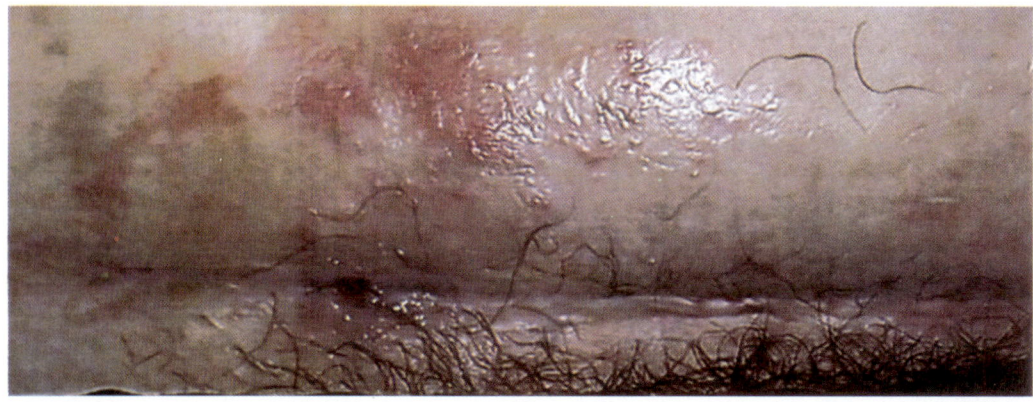

List 10 steps in the management of this patient in the appropriate order. (10 marks)

9.1   Identify the instrument.   (2 marks)

9.2   Mention the use of this instrument.   (2 marks)

9.3   Mention two possible advantages of use of this instrument compared to the traditional procedure.   (2 marks)

9.4   Mention one disadvantage of use of this instrument.   (2 marks)

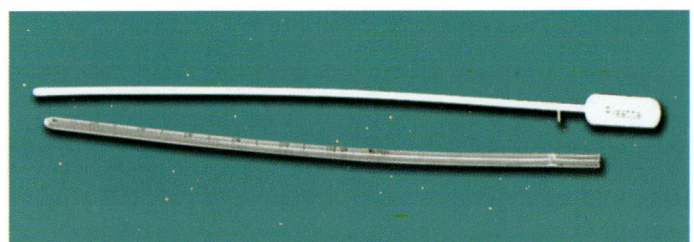

9.5 Pick out the other instruments required to use the above instrument and place them in the appropriate order of use.   (2 marks)

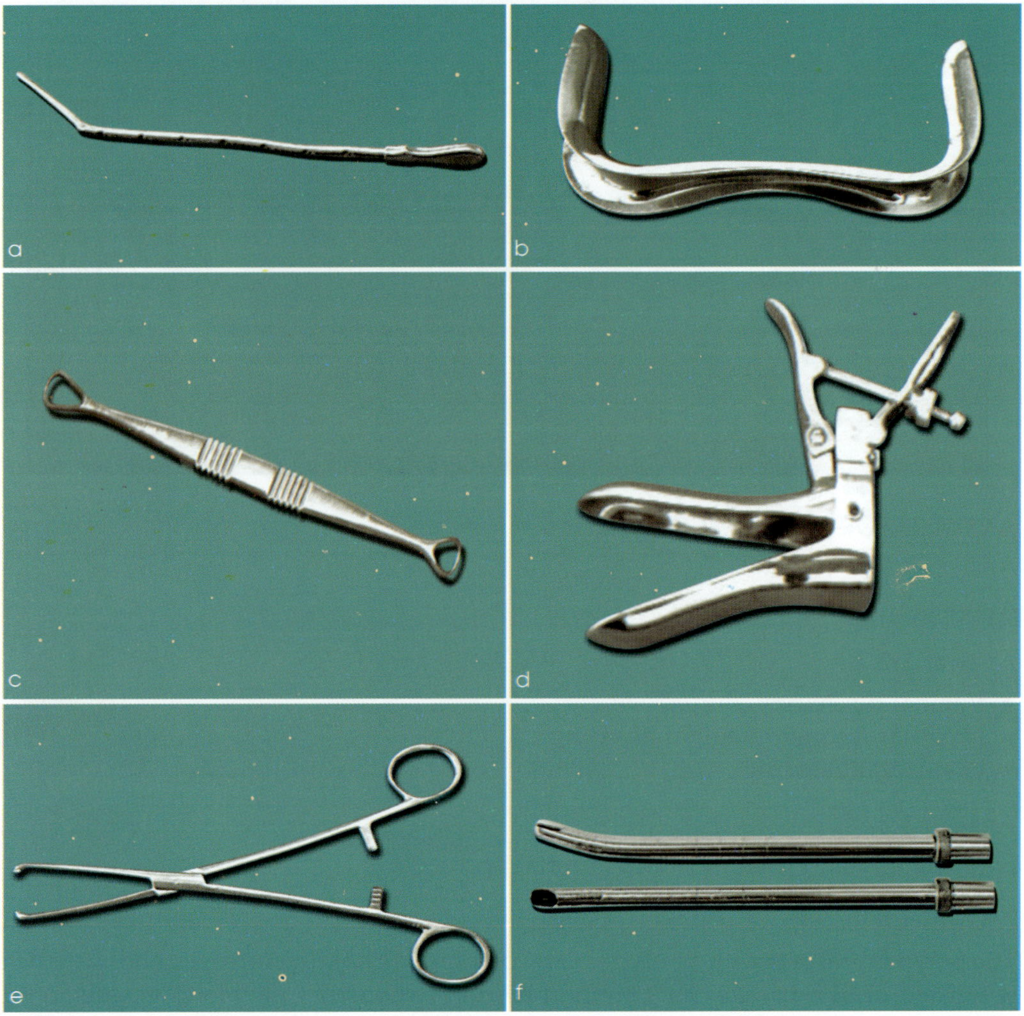

a

b

c

d

e

f

QUESTION 10

10.1 Name the pathological condition seen in the ultrasound image.   (1 mark)

10.2 List 3 abnormalities seen in the image.   (3 marks)

10.3 List 3 causes of this condition.   (3 marks)

10.4 Outline the management. (3 marks)

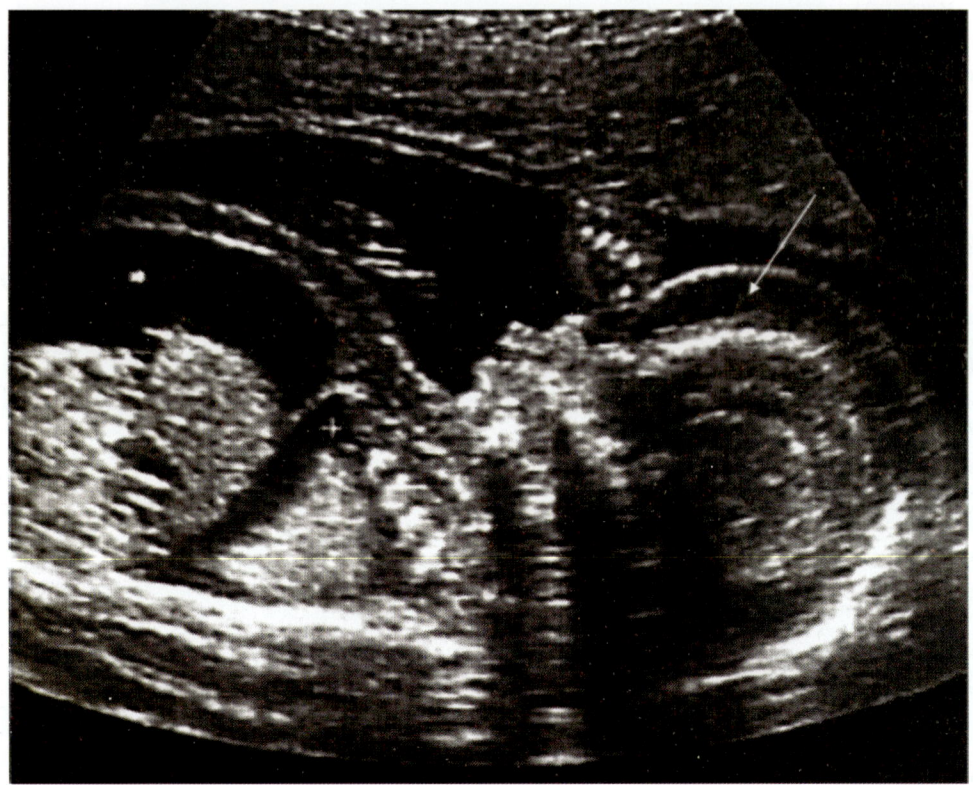

ANSWERS FOR EXAMINATION PAPER 5

Answer 1.1

A mucoid cervical polyp

Answer 1.2

- Vaginal discharge
- Irregular frequent vaginal bleeding
- Post-coital bleeding

Answer 1.3

Polypectomy and dilatation and curettage

Answer 1.4

The polyp is grasped with a polypectomy or a sponge holding forceps and the pedicle is twisted until it breaks. This method is used to constrict the blood vessels in the pedicle to prevent bleeding.

Answer 2

- At this point internal rotation of the head has commenced and the sagittal suture is in the mid-line. Place the patient in the dorsal position and advise her to bear down with the contractions.

- With further descent internal rotation will be complete, extension of the head will commence and crowning will occur. Keep the head flexed by applying gentle pressure on the occiput with two fingers till it passes under the sup-pubic arch.
- As the head passes beyond the sub-pubic arch it will extend fully. When the head is crowned perform an episiotomy and deliver the head. Support the perineum with a pad to prevent tears.
- External rotation and restitution will occur next and the anterior shoulder comes into view. It can be delivered by gentle downward traction of the fetal head. 5 units of oxytocin is given intravenously at this stage.
- Posterior shoulder will descend next and is delivered by elevating the body of the fetus. The rest of the body will follow completing the delivery.

Answer 3.1

a

Answer 3.2

e. Misoprostol 200 µg is inserted into the vagina, 6 hourly, up to a maximum of 4 doses.

Answer 3.3

d. Oxytocin 5 units in 500 ml of normal saline is used. The dose is commenced at 10 drops per minute and is adjusted at half hourly intervals until there are 4 contractions per 10 minutes, during the first stage. Amniotomy should be performed before commencing oxytocin.

Answer 3.4

b. Dinoprostone 3 mg is inserted into the posterior fornix. The dose is repeated after 6 hours if the patient is not in labour.

Answer 3.5

d. Oxytocin 5 units in 500 ml of normal saline is used. The dose is adjusted at half hourly intervals until there are 4 contractions per 10 minutes, during the first stage. Amniotomy should be performed before commencing oxytocin.

Answer 4.1

Self-controlled device to inhale entonox for pain relief in labour.

Answer 4.2

50% oxygen and nitrous oxide.

Answer 4.3

Offer the demand valve to the patient and advise to:
- Hold the mouthpiece between her teeth and breathe through her mouth only, sealing the mouthpiece with her lips.
- Commence inhalation when the pain starts.
- Continue to use the entonox throughout the pain and to breathe slowly and deeply.
- Discontinue the device in-between the contractions.

Answer 4.4

Nausea, vomiting, sedation, dizziness.

Answer 5.1

This patient has not got osteoporosis as the T-score is more than –2.5.

Answer 5.2

She has a family history of osteoporosis and is developing osteopenia as she has a T score of –1.2 in L1 and –1.1 in L2. A T score between –1.0 and –2.5 indicate low bone mineral density or osteopenia. Therefore, it is better to give calcium supplements.

First line treatment options include:
- Administration of bisphosphonates, calcium and vitamin D supplements,
- Advising exposure to morning sunlight.
- Improving her dietary intake of calcium by adding small fish, dried sprats and dairy products.
- Advising regarding non-weight bearing supervised exercises.

Answer 5.3

She does not need HRT for her bone health.

Answer 5.4

A DEXA scan should be repeated in 2–3 years for comparison.

Answer 6.1

Verres needle

Answer 6.2

- Insufflation of gas into the peritoneal cavity at laparoscopy.
- Drainage of pus from an abscess through the POD.

Answer 6.3

- Umbilicus
- Palmer's point
- Through the posterior fornix of the vagina.

Answer 6.4

Perforation of bowel and blood vessels.

Answer 6.5

- Lift the abdomen upon insertion.
- Check for two clicks.
- Perform Palmers test with a syringe.

Answer 7.1

- Stress urinary incontinence.
- Over active bladder (OAB)/urgency incontinence.
- Retention with overflow.
- True incontinence due to an urinary fistula.

Answer 7.2

- In stress incontinence, passage of urine occurs during activities which increase intra-abdominal pressure, such as coughing, laughing and even walking. The amount may be small and leaking will occur even if the bladder is not full.
- In over active bladder, the woman will be unable to hold the urine and she will leak a large volume of urine, if she is unable to reach the toilet immediately. There will be frequency as the woman will try to pass urine frequently, to avoid embarrassing situations.
- In true incontinence caused by a fistula, the woman will be constantly wet and the illness will commence after pelvic surgery or difficult childbirth.
- In the case of retention with overflow there will be difficulty in passing urine at first and this will be followed by leaking. This may be preceded by pelvic surgery, prolonged immobilization or a neurological illness.

Answer 7.3

- Maintain a bladder diary for three days to help to identify the type of incontinence.
- Perform urine full report and culture and ABST, to exclude urinary tract infection.
- Perform fasting blood sugar to exclude diabetes.
- Perform an USS to exclude urinary calculi and residual urine.

Answer 8

1. Obtain a swab from the wound for culture and ABST.
2. Clean the wound and the surrounding area with betadine solution.
3. Commence intravenous broad spectrum antibiotics.
4. Insert a sinus forceps into the raw area and explore the wound.
5. If an abscess cavity is found under the skin open the wound under local anaesthesia and drain the abscess. Remove any slough present.
6. Clean the wound with betadine, wash liberally with normal saline and place a dry dressing.
7. Continue daily cleaning with normal saline till the wound is clean. Change the antibiotics if necessary when the ABST report is available.
8. Oral antibiotics can be given once the acute phase subsides.
9. Carry out secondary suturing with silk/nylon under GA/LA once the wound is clean, free of slough and granulating.
10. Remove sutures after 10 days.

Answer 9.1

Pipelle endometrial biopsy curette.

Answer 9.2

It is used to obtain an endometrial sample for histology.

Answer 9.3

- It can be performed as an out-patient procedure.
- It is not necessary to anaesthetize the woman.

Answer 9.4

It is best avoided in women with focal thickening of the endometrium in the TVS. It is a blind procedure and an endometrial carcinoma can be missed.

Answer 9.5

d, e

Answer 10.1

Fetal hydrops

Answer 10.2

- Scalp oedema
- Fetal ascites
- Skin oedema

Answer 10.3

- Immune haemolysis due to presence of red cell antibodies
- Fetal cardiac abnormalities
- Fetal chromosomal/genetic abnormalities
- Fetal parvovirus infection

Answer 10.4

- If the POA is more than 34 weeks the best option is delivery by caesarean section.
- If the POA is less than 34 weeks and the cause is alloimmunisation perform exchange transfusion once in 2 weeks, to maintain the haemoglobin above 9 gr/dl. If the abnormality is due to any other cause aspiration of ascetic and pericardial fluid could be carried out.

Examination Paper 6

The appearance of a caesarean section wound on the 6th day after surgery is shown in the picture.

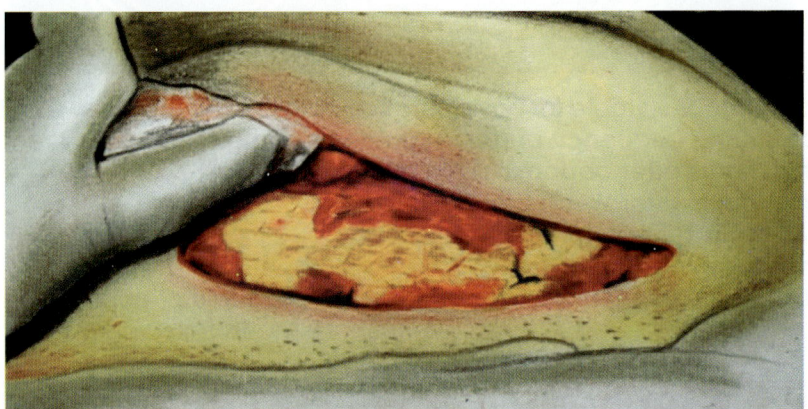

1.1 Describe the condition of the wound. (3 marks)
1.2 Outline your management in the appropriate order. (7 marks)

QUESTION 2

A 14-year-old girl attends the gynaecology clinic with a complaint of delay in menarche. Her current BMI is 24. Her secondary sexual characteristics are at Tanner stage 3.

Hormonal evaluation is given below:
- Serum estradiol: 50 pg/ml   (15–400 pg/ml)
- FSH: 2.8 IU/L   (less than 30 U/L)
- LH 2.3 IU/L   (less than 20 U/L)
- Prolactin: 95 mU/L   (83–357 mU/L)

2.1 What further information do you want to know from the patient? (2 marks)

2.2   What is the most likely diagnosis? Give your reasons.   (2 marks)
2.3   Mention 4 relevant investigations you would order.   (0.5 × 4 = 2 marks)
2.4   What is your immediate management?   (4 marks)

QUESTION 3

The following are used for relief of postoperative pain.

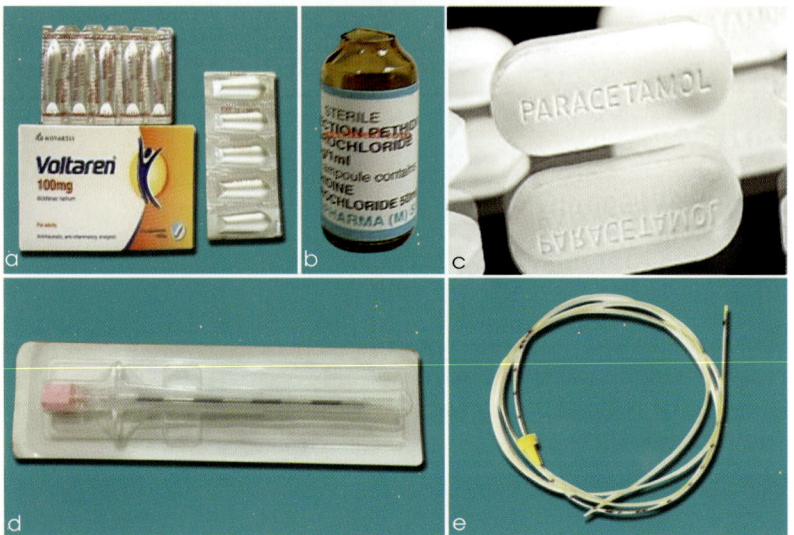

Mention 2 methods suitable for postoperative pain relief in the following situations. The dose and the frequency of administration of drugs should be mentioned.
3.1   First 24 hours after abdominal hysterectomy.
3.2   First 24 hours after Wertheims hysterectomy.
3.3   24–48 hours after vaginal hysterectomy.
3.4   72 hours after myomectomy.
3.5   First 24 hours after evacuation of retained products of conception.
                                          (2 marks for each correct answer)

QUESTION 4

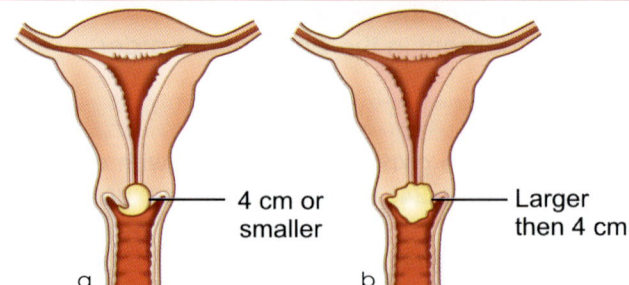

These 2 diagrams show two stages of cervical carcinoma.
4.1   Mention the stage of the disease in a and b.   (2 marks)
4.2   What further examinations and investigations should be performed to confirm the stage of the disease?   (4 marks)
4.3   What is your management of a and b?   (4 marks)

QUESTION 5

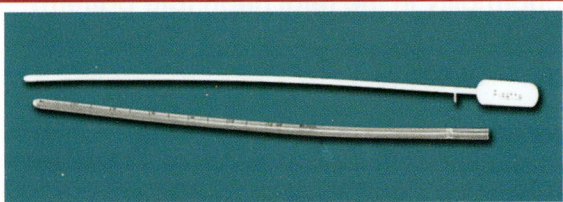

Demonstrate to the examiner how you would use the instrument. The method should be described in the proper order.   (10 marks)

QUESTION 6

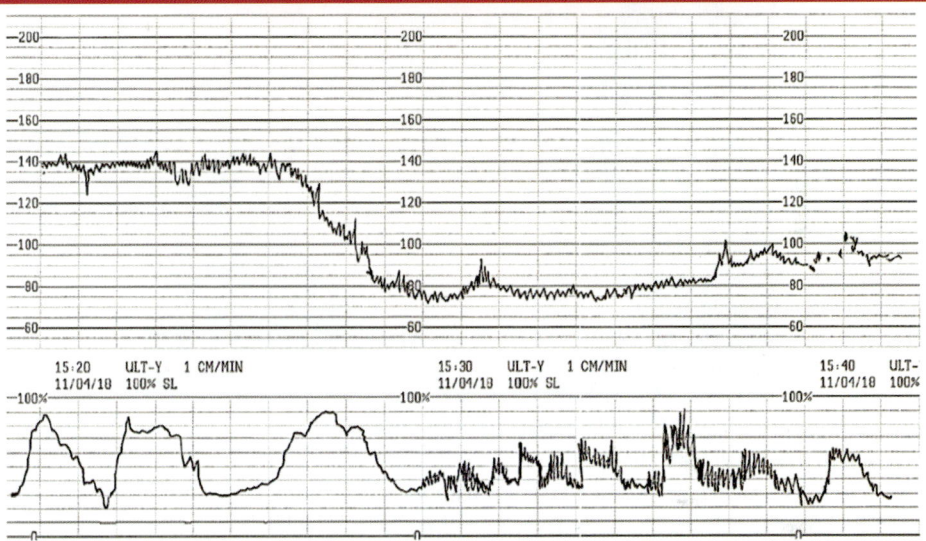

This CTG was performed in a fourth para at a cervical dilatation of 7 cm.

6.1   List 2 abnormalities seen in this CTG.   (0.5 × 2 = 1 mark)
6.2   What is the most likely cause in this case?   (1 mark)
6.3   List 3 steps in your management.   (3 marks)

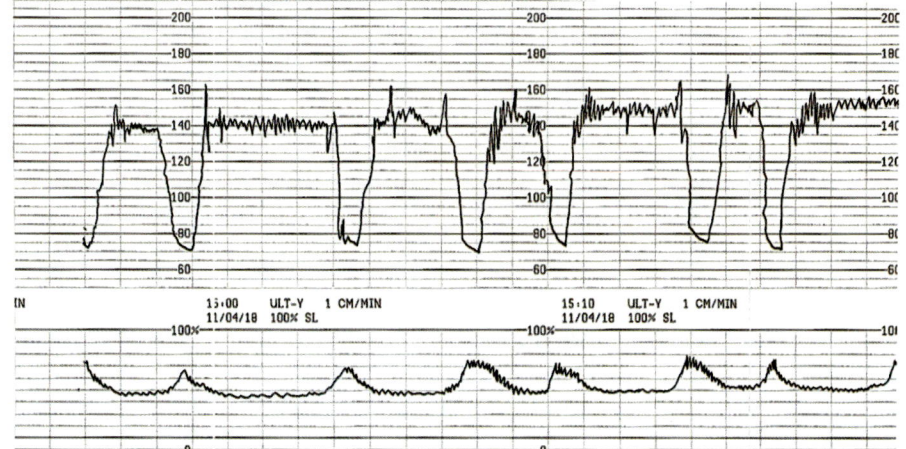

This CTG was performed on a fourth para at a cervical dilatation of 5 cm.

6.4   What is the abnormality in the fetal heart rate pattern?   (1 mark)
6.5   List 2 causes for it.   (2 marks)
6.6   What is your management?   (2 marks)

QUESTION 7

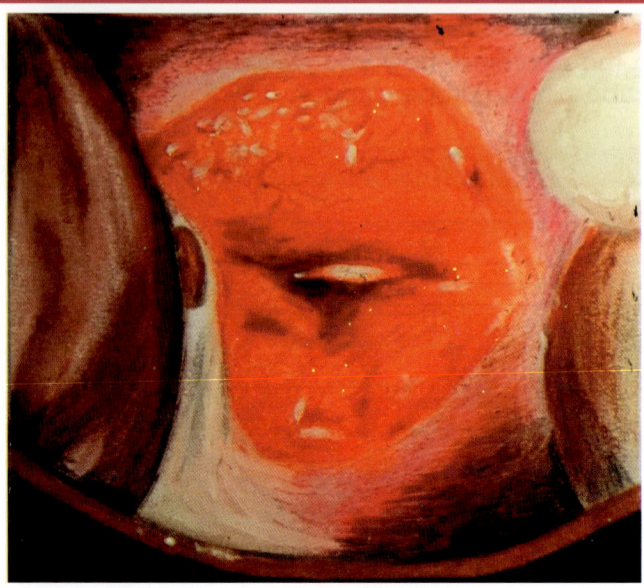

7.1   Describe the abnormality seen in this picture.   (2 marks)
7.2   What is your diagnosis?   (1 mark)
7.3   What is the pathological basis of this lesion?   (1 mark)
7.4   How do you clinically differentiate it from a malignant lesion?   (2 marks)
7.5   List the symptoms.   (0.5 × 2 = 1 mark)
7.6   How will you manage this patient?   (3 marks)

QUESTION 8

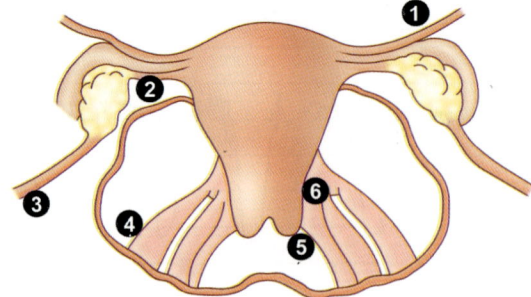

8.1   List the sites shown in the picture where the ureter can be damaged at hysterectomy.   (3 marks)
8.2   What are the other sites which are not shown in the picture where damage can occur?   (2 marks)

8.3   What are the clinical features of ureteric injury?   (2 marks)
8.4   How will you treat ureteric injuries?   (3 marks)

QUESTION 9

WBC	5.5%
NE	54.7
LY	34.1
MO	7.5
EO	3.0
BA	0.7
RBC	4.28
HGB	9.7
HCT	29.9
MCV	69.9
MCH	22.6
MCHC	32.4
RDW	18.4
PLT	331
MPV	8.8

This is the full blood count report of a primipara who attended the antenatal clinic at a POA of 20 weeks.

9.1   What is your diagnosis?   (1 mark)
9.2   Give reasons for your diagnosis.   (2 marks)
9.3   List 2 investigations you should do to confirm your diagnosis and mention the expected results.   (4 marks)
9.4   List 3 aspects in the management of this woman.   (3 marks)

QUESTION 10

A 40-year-old woman with two children complains of amenorrhoea for 6 months. Her last child is 5 years of age. She has previously had regular periods. Her BMI is 24 kg/m^2.

10.1 List 5 questions you would ask her.   (5 marks)
10.2 List 3 relevant investigations you would carry out.   (3 marks)
10.3 How will you diagnose premature menopause in this woman?   (2 marks)

ANSWER FOR EXAMINATION PAPER 6

Answer 1.1

This wound has been severely infected with collection of pus and has been opened in order to drain the pus. It has begun to heal with formation of granulation tissue at the periphery. However, there is some slough at the centre of the wound.

Answer 1.2

- Pus should be sent for culture and ABST. A broad spectrum antibiotic should be commenced and changed once the ABST report is available. The slough should be excised.
- Investigate and correct co-morbidities such as, diabetes, immune suppressive disorders and poor nutritional status.
- The wound should be cleaned with normal saline and a dry dressing should be applied twice daily at first and daily later.

- Secondary suturing should be done under local or spinal anaesthesia once the wound is clean, with no slough and granulation tissue has formed. Number 1 nylon is used for this purpose.
- Sutures are removed in 10 days.

Answer 2.1

- History of prolonged childhood illnesses such as renal diseases, meningitis, tuberculosis and malnutrition.
- Family history of delayed menarche.
- The increase in height during the previous year.

Answer 2.2

- Constitutional delay in menarche.
- The hormone levels are within the low normal range and breast development has reached Tanner stage 3. She is only 14 years of age and menstruation may occur within the next year.

Answer 2.3

- Ultrasound scan of the abdomen and pelvis.
- Renal function tests
- ESR
- Full blood count
- TSH levels
- X-ray bone age

Answer 2.4

If the investigations are normal observe for 1 year. However, reassurance and explanation is essential. Any intercurrent illness should be treated.

Answer 3.1

a. 75–100 mg per rectally 12 hourly
b. 75 mg by intramuscular injection 6 hourly.

Answer 3.2

b. 75 mg by intramuscular injection 6 hourly
d and e. Continuous epidural nalgesia can be given.

Answer 3.3

a. 75–100 mg per rectally 12 hourly
c. 500 mg 6 hourly.

Answer 3.4

a. 75–100 mg per rectally 12 hourly or when requested by the patient
c. 500 mg 6 hourly.

Answer 3.5

c. 500 mg 6 hourly.

Answer 4.1

a. Stage I B1
b. Stage I B2

Answer 4.2

Perform:
- A bi-digital examination with one finger in the vagina and one finger in the rectum to assess the spread to the parametrium and the lateral pelvic wall.
- CT scan to assess spread to the lymph nodes and the surrounding organs.
- Cystoscopy to assess spread to the bladder.
- Hysteroscopy and endometrial biopsy to assess spread to the uterus.
- Sigmoidoscopy to assess spread to the rectum.

Answer 4.3

- If the lesion is smaller than 4 cm (a—stage 1 B1) type 3 radical hysterectomy is performed. If the nodes contain cancer cells post-operative radiotherapy and chemotherapy with cisplatin is necessary.
- If the lesion is larger than 4 cm (b—stage 1 B2) the standard treatment is chemotherapy with cisplatin or cisplatin and 5 fluorouracil together with radiation therapy (chemoradiotherapy).
- 23 cycles of external beam therapy is given 5 days a week till the course is completed. 3 cycles of chemotherapy is given every Monday for 3 weeks. One week after completing external radio therapy 2–3 courses of brachytherapy are given weekly.

Answer 5

- Obtain consent.
- It is performed as an out-patient procedure without anaesthesia.
- Ask the patient to empty the bladder.
- Place in the lithotomy position. However, it can be performed in the dorsal position.
- Clean the vulva with an antiseptic solution.
- Perform a bimanual vaginal examination to determine the size and direction of the uterus.
- Insert a Cusco's speculum and expose the cervix. Hold the cervix with a vulsellum.
- Insert the Pipelle sampler gently into the uterine cavity. Attention should be paid to the size and the direction of the uterus to prevent perforation.
- Pull the plunger out to create a vacuum.
- Pull the external sheath in and out 3–5 times. Twist the external sheath during this step to obtain an adequate sample from all the walls of the uterus.
- Withdraw the instrument.
- Insert the sample into a bottle containing formalin.
- Inform the patient that she may have mild vaginal bleeding for 2–3 days.
- Give a date to attend the clinic after 3 weeks to obtain the histology report.

Answer 6.1

- Frequent irregular uterine contractions—hypertonic uterine activity.
- Deep deceleration in the fetal heart rate

Answer 6.2

It is due to hypertonic uterine activity most probably caused by improper use of oxytocin or due to precipitate labour as she is a fourth para.

Answer 6.3

- Stop the oxytocin drip or remove inserted prostaglandin.
- Give sublingual glyceryl trinitrate.
- Turn to the left lateral position and give oxygen.
- If the condition does not improve perform a caesarean section.

Answer 6.4

Recurrent deep atypical variable decelerations.

Answer 6.5

Acute fetal hypoxia due to:
- Cord prolapse
- Placental abruption
- Ruptured uterus

Answer 6.6

Deliver immediately by caesarean section.

Answer 7.1

A bright red clearly demarcated area is seen extending onto the ectocervix from the external os. The surface is intact.

Answer 7.2

Cervical ectropion

Answer 7.3

The columnar epithelium lining the endocervical canal grows over the squamous epithelium of the ectocervix. It appears red because the columnar epithelium is thin and the underlying blood vessels can be seen.

Answer 7.4

The surface is intact and there is no evidence of ulceration.

Answer 7.5

- Increase in the amount of the white vaginal discharge of leucorrhoea.
- Post-coital bleeding.

Answer 7.6

- A cervical smear should be performed.
- No treatment is required in most cases. The patient should be reassured after explaining the condition.
- If the discharge is troublesome cauterization can be performed. This procedure will destroy the columnar epithelium and healing will occur with the growth of

squamous epithelium. Cryotherapy is an option. Malignancy should be carefully excluded before performing the above procedures.

Answer 8.1

3, 4, 5, 6

Answer 8.2

The ureter can be damaged:
- In the ovarian fossa when attempts are made to remove an adherent ovary.
- When suturing the posterior flap of the vaginal vault.

Answer 8.3

A direct cut will manifest immediately. There will be leakage of urine through the vaginal vault even if a bladder catheter is *in situ*. There will be abdominal pain, abdominal distension and fever due to extravasation of urine into the peritoneal cavity. Haematuria may occur.

If the ureter is tied or if it is denuded of the blood supply necrosis will take 4–10 days and hence the above symptoms will occur later.

Answer 8.4

Surgery should be performed as soon as the diagnosis is made. Direct anastomosis of the cut ends or implantation into the bladder can be done. Surgery should be performed by an experienced consultant genitourinary surgeon.

Answer 9.1

Iron deficiency anaemia (IDA).

Answer 9.2

The diagnosis is most likely because the full blood count shows:
- Low haemoglobin percentage
- Low red cell count.
- Low MCV, MCHC and MCH

Answer 9.3

- Blood picture will show hypochromic microcytic anaemia.
- Serum ferritin below 15 ng/ml is diagnostic of IDA. Treatment is required if the level is below 30 ng/ml.

Answer 9.4

- 120 mg of iron should be given daily in the form of 2 ferrous gluconate (500 mg) or ferrous fumarate (180 mg) tablets which contain 60 mg of elemental iron. One tablet is given twice daily.
- The oral iron should not be taken with a main meal or with tea or coffee, as polyphenols found in these impair iron absorption. It should be taken at least one hour before a main meal with vitamin C or fruit juice. Antacids should not be taken at the same time. The calcium supplement should be taken at a different time as calcium inhibits iron absorption.

- Dietary advice should be given. She should be advised to eat food rich in iron such as green leaves, dried sprats, red meat and pulses.
- Worm treatment should be given and she should be advised regarding personal hygiene.
- The haemoglobin level is assessed after 2 weeks to assess the therapeutic response.
- If the diagnosis of IDA is correct the haemoglobin level should rise by 1 gm/dl (between 0.5 and 2 gm/dl).

Answer 10.1

Inquire regarding:
- Hot flashes.
- A history of recent uterine curettage.
- Taking anti-psychotic drugs or hormonal contraceptives.
- Surgery involving the cervix.
- Excessive hair growth.
- Headaches, visual disturbance, head injuries or meningitis.
- Symptoms of pregnancy.

Answer 10.2

- Urine hCG/serum beta hCG levels to exclude a pregnancy
- Hormone tests:
  - FSH and LH levels to exclude premature menopause.
  - Prolactin levels to exclude a pituitary tumour.
  - Testosterone levels to exclude hormone secreting ovarian or adrenal tumours.
  - Thyroxine levels to exclude thyroid dysfunction.
- Transvaginal USS to determine the endometrial thickness and to exclude cryptomenorrhoea or hormone secreting tumours.

Answer 10.3

Perform two FSH levels 6 weeks apart. The level should be more than 40 IU/ml.

Examination Paper 7

QUESTION 1

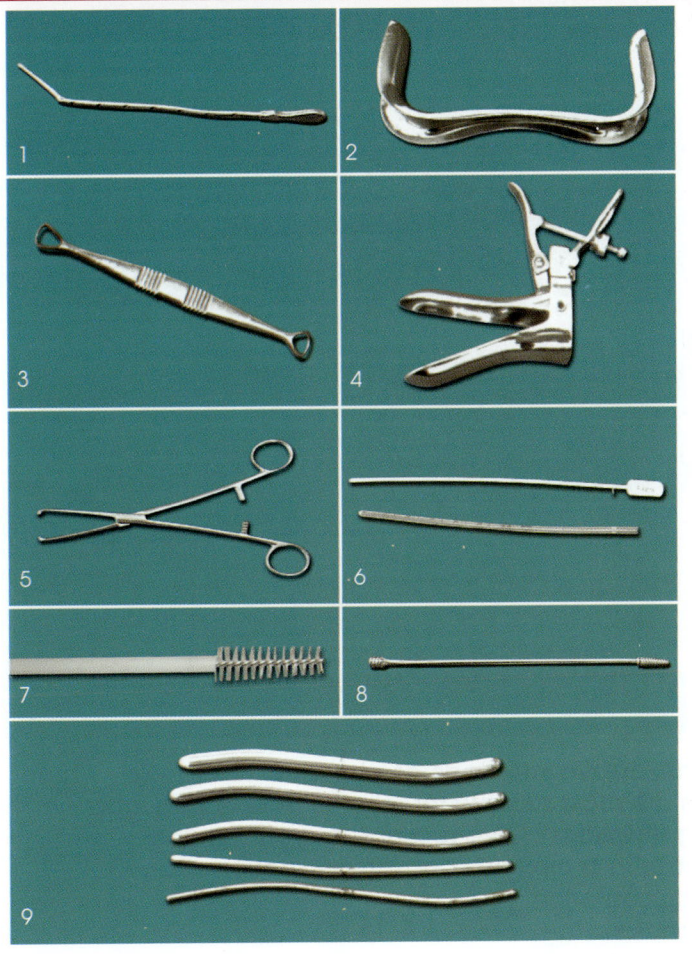

1.1   What is meant by ERPC, D&E and D&C?   (3 marks)
1.2   Pick the instruments required for the above procedures (from those given above) and place them in the appropriate order of use.   (3 marks)
1.3   Mention a complication which can occur during these procedures. (1 mark)
1.4   How do you identify the complication you have mentioned?   (1 mark)
1.5   How do you treat it?   (2 marks)

QUESTION 2

A 35-year-old woman complains of amenorrhoea for 18 months after birth of her second child. She has had a dilatation and curettage for secondary postpartum haemorrhage, 7 days after partus.

2.1   What is the most likely cause?   (2 marks)
2.2   List 2 other possible causes.   (2 marks)
2.3   How can you confirm the diagnosis?   (2 marks)
2.4   List 2 measures which could have been taken to prevent the occurrence of amenorrhoea.   (2 marks)
2.5   Mention the treatment of the cause you have mentioned in 2.1.   (2 marks)

QUESTION 3

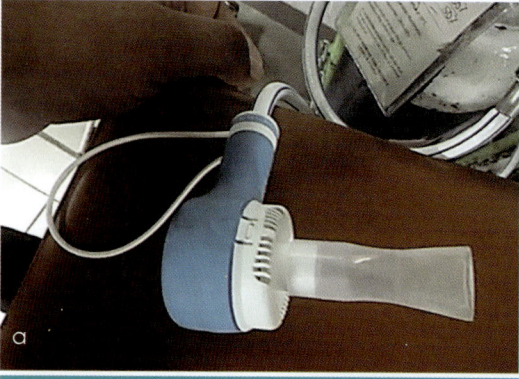
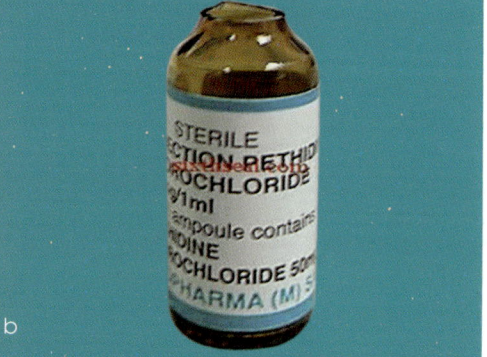
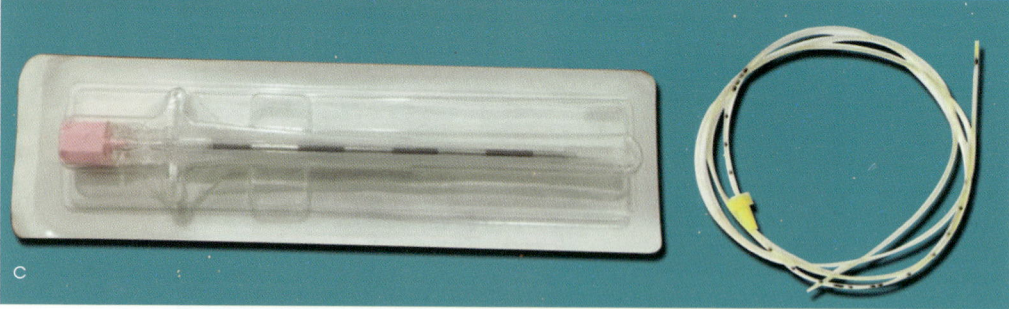

a   b

c

3.1   Name the above methods of obstetric analgesia. Which of the above methods are most suitable for relief of pain during labour in the each of the following situations? Give reasons for your choice.   (3 marks)
3.2. A woman with a previous caesarean section scar.
3.3. Breech presentation.
3.4. Mitral stenosis.

3.5   A woman who requests analgesia at a cervical dilatation of 9 cm.
3.6   Placental abruption.
3.7   Moderately severe pregnancy induced hypertension.
3.8   Twin pregnancy.   (1 mark for each correct answer from 3.2 to 3.6)

QUESTION 4

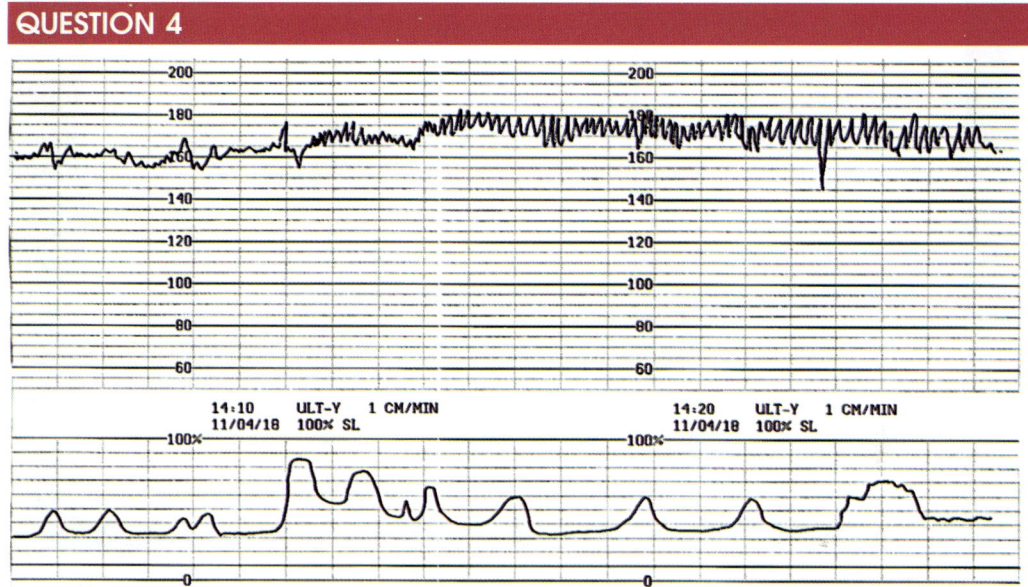

4.1   What is the abnormality seen in this CTG?   (1 mark)
4.2   Mention one criteria for identifying this abnormality.   (1 mark)
4.3   List 2 causes for this abnormality.   (2 marks)
4.4   What is your management?   (2 marks)
The CTG shown below was obtained from a woman in labour at a cervical dilatation of 5 cm.

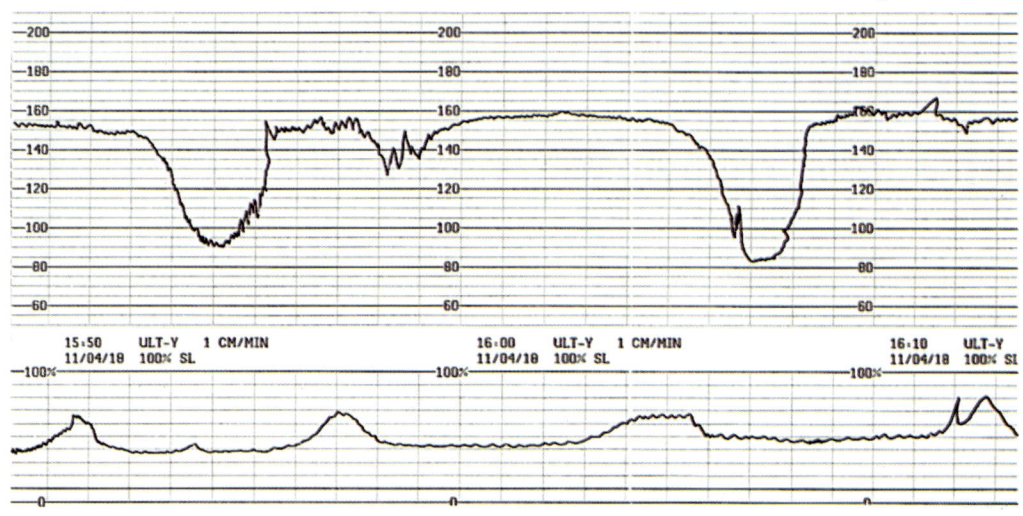

4.5   What is the abnormality seen in this CTG?   (2 marks)
4.6   What is your management?   (2 marks)

QUESTION 5

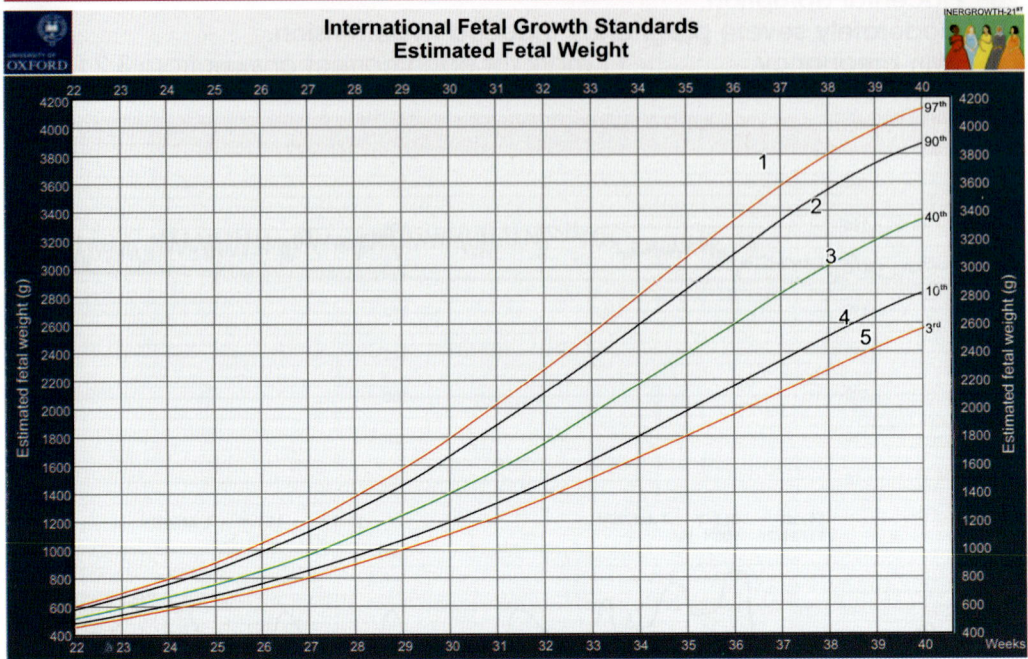

International Fetal Growth Standards
Estimated Fetal Weight

5.1   Mention the growth status of the babies in the graphs 1–5.   (5 marks)

5.2   Mention 2 methods of fetal surveillance you would carry out from **34 weeks**
        in the mother whose baby's growth falls into the graph 5.   (2 marks)

5.3   How and when will you deliver this woman? Give your reasons.   (3 marks)

QUESTION 6

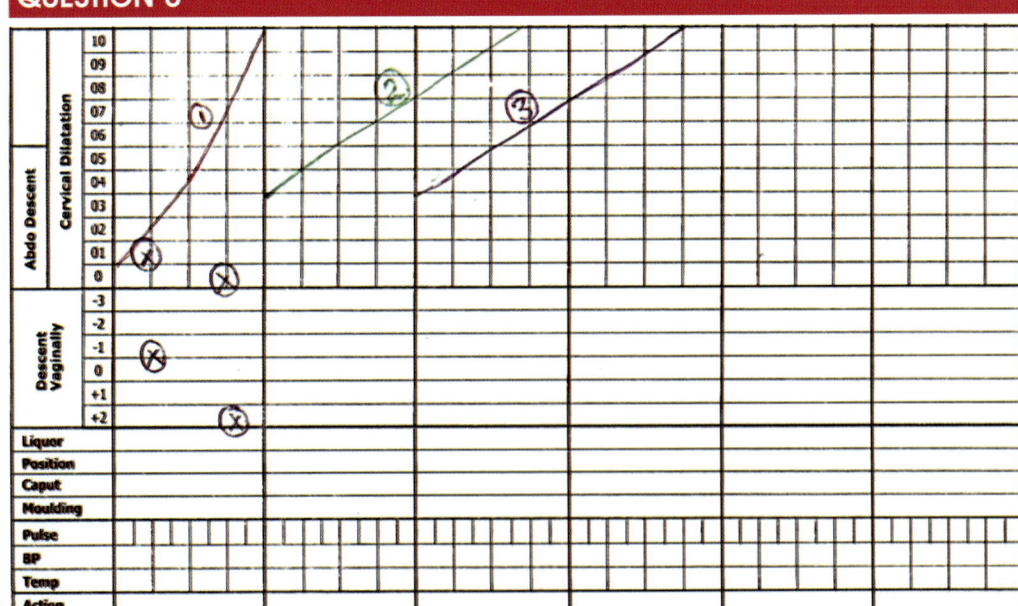

The graph 1 shows the rate of cervical dilatation in a multiparous woman who was admitted to the labour ward at a cervical dilatation of 1 cm.

6.1 What is shown by the 2nd graph?	(1 mark)
6.2 What is shown by the 3rd graph?	(1 mark)
6.3 What is the abnormality shown in the first graph?	(2 marks)
6.4 List 3 fetal and maternal risks of this condition.	(3 marks)
6.5 List 3 precautions you will take to minimize these risks.	(3 marks)

QUESTION 7

Test Report Status **Final**	Results	Biological Reference Interval	Units
	EIA-ENDOCRINOLOGY		

ANTI MULLERIAN HORMONE

ANTI-MULLERIAN HORMONE / MULLERIAN INHIBITING SUBSTANCE   <0.01   Low   ng/mL
                                                                                              0.672 -7.55

Comments

Comments for AMH

Clinical applications for serum AMH (anti-Müllerian hormone) measurement include the assessment of ovarian reserve, prediction of response to ovarian stimulation, prediction of time to menopause, surrogate biomarker for AFC in the diagnosis of PCOS and monitoring of granulosa cell tumours. Serum AMH level remains relatively stable throughout the menstrual cycle. Levels decrease significantly while using combined contraceptives.

Reference range:

	Median	5th – 95th centile
Healthy male	4.79	1.43 – 11.6

Healthy women by age (years)
[not on contraceptives]

20 – 24	3.97	1.66 – 9.49
25 – 29	3.34	1.18 – 9.16
30 – 34	2.76	0.67 – 7.55

		10th – 90th centile
35 – 39	2.05	0.77 – 5.24
40 – 44	1.06	0.09 – 2.96
45 – 50	0.22	0.05 – 2.06

		5th – 95th centile
Women with PCOS*	6.81	2.41 – 17.1

This report belongs to a 32-year-old woman.

7.1 List 2 possible causes	(2 marks)
7.2 List 2 presenting complaints.	(2 marks)
7.3 List 2 other investigations you would perform.	(2 marks)
7.4 How will you counsel this woman?	(4 marks)

QUESTION 8

What are the most suitable methods of hormone replacement therapy in the following circumstances? Give your reasons.   (2 marks each)

8.1 A 48-year-old woman who is under treatment for breast carcinoma and has reached menopause. She is complaining of vasomotor symptoms. She is on tamoxifen.

8.2 A 42-year-old woman who has infrequent periods and vasomotor symptoms. She needs contraception as well.

8.3 A 56-year-old obese woman who is a heavy smoker. She complains of vasomotor symptoms and loss of libido.

8.4 A 60-year-old woman with osteoporosis and hot flashes who has a history of VTE during her pregnancy 30 years ago. Her BMI is 24 kg/m^2.

8.5 A 40-year-old woman who has undergone hysterectomy and bilateral salpingo-oophorectomy for endometriosis.

QUESTION 9

An 18-year-old girl complains of failure to attain menarche. Her hormone profile is given below.

- Serum estradiol: 6 pg/ml (15–400 pg/ml)
- FSH: 60 IU/L (less than 30 U/L)
- LH 40 IU/L (less than 20 U/L)
- Prolactin: 200 mU/L (83–357 mU/L)

9.1 List 3 causes for her condition. (3 marks)

9.2 Which of the cause/s you have mentioned will result in short stature? (1 mark)

9.3 List 2 investigations you should perform to confirm your diagnosis. Give your reasons. (0.5 × 2 = 1 mark)

9.4 List 5 important steps in your management. (5 marks)

QUESTION 10

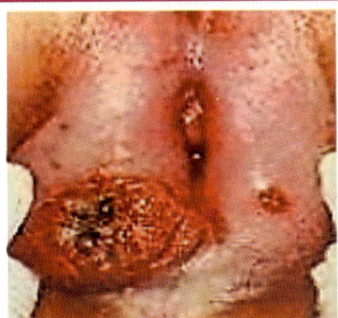

1

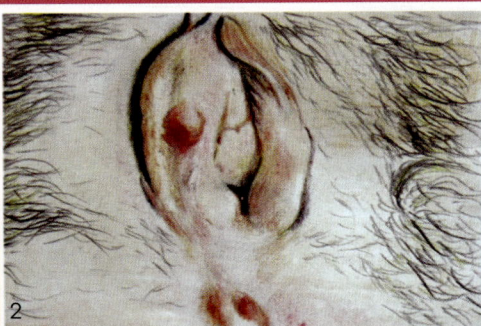

2

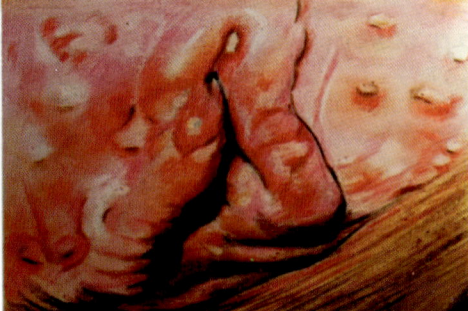

3

10.1 Mention a likely diagnosis in each of the above pictures of genital ulcers.

(3 marks)

10.2 How will you confirm the diagnosis in each of these conditions? (3 marks)

10.3 How will you treat each of these conditions? (3 marks)

10.4 Mention another condition which can be considered in the differential diagnosis of 2 and 3. (1 mark)

ANSWERS FOR EXAMINATION PAPER 7

Answer 1.1

ERPC Evacuation of retained products of conception. This is carried out to evacuate the uterus in cases of inevitable or incomplete miscarriage when the cervical os is open. Dilatation is not necessary.

D and E Dilatation and evacuation. This is carried out to evacuate a pregnant uterus in cases where the os is closed such as in a missed miscarriage. The os should be dilated to 10 Hegars.

D and C Dilatation and curettage. This is performed to obtain an endometrial sample for histology. The os should be dilated to 8 Hegars.

Answer 1.2

2, 5, 1, 9, 3

Answer 1.3

Perforation of the uterus.

Answer 1.4

The instrument by which the injury is caused will pass through the uterus without resistance. It will appear to pass beyond the measured length of the uterus.

Answer 1.5

If the perforation is caused by a small instrument such as an uterine sound or a small dilator repair is not necessary and the patient is kept under observation for 24 hours. If the perforation is caused by a large instrument such as a large dilator or a sponge holder, it is safer to close the perforation through a minilaparotomy or laparoscopy.

Answer 2.1

Asherman's syndrome.

Answer 2.2

• Lactation amenorrhoea
• Sheehan's syndrome.

Answer 2.3

Intrauterine adhesions can be seen on transvaginal scanning. Direct visualization can be done by hysteroscopy. FSH, LH, TSH and prolactin levels should be done to exclude a pituitary cause.

Answer 2.4

An IUCD should be kept *in situ* for 3 months or she should be given OCP for 3 cycles after postpartum curettage to prevent formation of adhesions.

Answer 2.5

The adhesions can be resected through the hysteroscope. An IUCD should be kept in the uterus for 3 months to prevent re-formation of adhesions.

Answer 3.1

a. Inhalation of entonox
b. Intramuscular pethidine
c. Continuous epidural analgesia.

Answer 3.2

Epidural analgesia is the best option. However, care should be taken if the patient requests increasing amounts of analgesia as it could be a warning sign of scar dehiscence.

Answer 3.3

Intramuscular pethidine 75 mg can be given 6 hourly till the cervical dilatation is about 8–9 cm. Entanox can be used thereafter. Nalorphine should be available to reverse neonatal respiratory depression whenever pethidine is used. Epidural analgesia is best avoided because it can impair the maternal expulsive efforts in the second stage.

Answer 3.4

Adequate pain relief is essential as pain can precipitate failure. Therefore, epidural analgesia is the best method of pain relief, except in cases with a gross reduction of the ejection fraction. Morphine can be given in the latter situation.

Answer 3.5

Inhalation of entonox is the best option. Pethidine is best avoided as delivery may occur within 4 hours, resulting in neonatal respiratory depression. It may be difficult to insert an epidural cannula to a patient in advanced labour.

Answer 3.6

Intramuscular pethidine 75 mg can be given 6 hourly till the cervical dilatation is about 8–9 cm. Entanox can be used thereafter. Nalorphine should be available to reverse neonatal respiratory depression, whenever pethidine is used. Epidural analgesia is contraindicated as coagulopathy may be present and the patient may be hypovolaemic.

Answer 3.7

Epidural anaesthesia will give adequate anaesthesia and will also reduce the blood pressure.

Answer 3.8

Epidural anaesthesia will give adequate pain relief during labour and will also provide adequate anaesthesia for procedures which may be required during delivery of the second twin.

Answer 4.1

Pseudo-sinusoidal pattern

Answer 4.2

The hallmark feature of a pseudo-sinusoidal trace is the prior (as in this case) or subsequent appearance of normal baseline variability and accelerations and the pattern will rarely exceed 30 minutes.

Answer 4.3

Fetal thumb sucking or administration of analgesia to the mother.

Answer 4.4

This CTG pattern does not indicate fetal hypoxia. Therefore, labour can be allowed to progress.

Answer 4.5

Prolonged type 2 decelerations

Answer 4.6

The baby should be delivered immediately by caesarean section as this pattern indicates acute fetal hypoxia.

Answer 5.1

1. Macrosomic baby most probably due to a pathological cause. However, a constitutionally large baby is a possibility.
2. Constitutionally large baby
3. Baby with a normal growth pattern
4. Constitutionally small baby who is continuing to grow at a slower rate.
5. Small for gestational age baby (SGA) who is continuing to grow at a slower rate. However, a constitutionally small baby is a possibility.

Answer 5.2

- Umbilical artery Doppler study is the best method to assess the well-being of a SGA fetus. If normal, the test is repeated every 14 days. Liquor volume can be assessed at the same time. If the umbilical artery Doppler flow indices are reduced, repeat measurements are carried out twice weekly. If end diastolic flow is reversed or absent, the fetus should be delivered as the POA is more than 34 weeks.
- The mother is advised to maintain a fetal movement chart.

Answer 5.3

As the growth seems to be continuing though at a slower rate delivery can be carried out at 38 weeks, if the umbilical artery Doppler flow studies are normal and the MCA Doppler studies are normal. Caesarean section is the safer method of delivery. Normal delivery can also be considered if the Doppler parameters are normal. If the umbilical artery blood flow is reduced early delivery by caesarean section is carried out at 37–38 weeks. However, MCA Doppler studies should be performed. Earlier delivery is indicated if the MCA Doppler is abnormal. If umbilical artery end diastolic flow is reversed or absent the fetus should be delivered, after a course of steroids, as the POA is more than 34 weeks.

Answer 6.1

The graph 2 shows the alert line or the normal rate of cervical dilatation in the active phase of the first stage of labour.

Answer 6.2

The 3rd graph is the action line. The rate of cervical dilatation is less than 2 cm for four hours.

Answer 6.3

The graph has moved to the left of the alert line. The progress of labour is very rapid resulting in precipitate labour. The cervix has dilated from 4 to 10 cm in 2 hours.

Answer 6.4

- Fetal distress causing fetal hypoxia
- Intracranial injuries due to changing pressures on the fetal head due to rapid expulsion.
- Uterine rupture can occur due to strong uterine contractions as this woman is a multipara.
- Perineal tears due to rapid delivery.

Answer 6.5

- If an oxytocin drip is running it should be stopped immediately. Intravenous tocolytics should be commenced.
- Continuous fetal heart rate monitoring should be commenced.
- Perineal tears should be prevented by controlling the delivery of the head by supporting the head with the left hand and the perineum with the right hand. An episiotomy may be given. Try to deliver the head in-between contractions.
- Patient should be kept under observation for vaginal bleeding and haemodynamic compromise during and after labour, to detect uterine rupture.

Answer 7.1

- Premature ovarian failure
- Prolonged use of oral contraceptives.

Answer 7.2

- Secondary amenorrhoea/oligomenorrhoea
- Infertility
- Climacteric symptoms such as hot flushes.

Answer 7.3

Perform
- Two serum FSH levels at an interval of 6 weeks to confirm premature menopause.
- TSH and anti-thyroid antibody levels
- Anti-nuclear antibody tests

Answer 7.4

She should be informed that:
- Her ovarian function is reduced due to a low reserve of eggs
- Further tests should be done to exclude/confirm premature menopause and the presence of any other chronic disease condition.
- She will need hormone replacement therapy if premature menopause is confirmed.
- She will respond poorly to attempts to induce ovulation with drugs and therefore IVF may not be successful with her own eggs.
- The only option for fertility is to undergo IVF with ovum donation.

Answer 8.1

Selective noradrenaline reuptake inhibitor (SNRI) venlafaxine 37.5 mg twice daily, can be used. This is a non-hormonal preparation which does not interfere with the action of tamoxifen and will relieve vasomotor symptoms. Other non-hormonal preparations such as fluoxetine and paroxetine which are selective serotonin re-uptake inhibitors (SSRIs) cannot be used as they interfere with the action of tamoxifen.

Answer 8.2

A combined oral contraceptive pill containing 30 μg of estradiol can be used. This will give relief from vasomotor symptoms and provide contraception as well. Also conjugated equine estrogen 0.625–1.25 mg can be given and a LNG-IUS can be inserted to provide contraception and protection for the endometrium.

Answer 8.3

Tibalone 1.25–2.5 mg daily is suitable for this woman. Tibalone is a synthetic preparation with estrogen, progesterone and testosterone effects. It is suitable for this woman as she has a higher risk of VTE and is complaining of loss of libido. Tibalone carries a lower risk of VTE and will improve libido as it has a testosterone action as well.

Answer 8.4

A transdermal estrogen patch releasing between 25 and 100 μg daily can be used to avoid first pass effect through the liver, thereby reducing the risk of VTE. A LNG-IUS can be inserted to provide protection for the endometrium. The patch should be changed twice or thrice a week.

Answer 8.5

Conjugated equine estrogen 0.625–1.25 mg can be commenced 1 year after surgery to prevent recurrence of endometriosis due to estrogens. Estrogen only HRT carries a lower risk of breast carcinoma and is the preferred method for hysterectomised women as they do not need endometrial protection.

Answer 9.1

- Tuner syndrome
- Gonadal agenesis
- Premature ovarian failure/resistant ovary syndrome

Answer 9.2
Tuner syndrome

Answer 9.3
- Perform a karyotype to confirm Tuner syndrome and XY gonadal agenesis.
- Perform an USS to assess the condition of the ovaries and the presence of the uterus and the vagina. The ovaries are normal but small in resistant ovary syndrome, streaky in Turner syndrome and absent in gonadal agenesis. The uterus and the vagina will be present in all the above patients, including in XY gonadal agenesis as müllerian inhibiting factor is absent.

Answer 9.4
- Reassurance and explanation regarding the treatment and the expected results is the first step in the management.
- Estrogen is given for about a year for the development of the breasts.
- She should be referred to an endocrinologist for treatment with growth hormone to improve the height.
- This is followed by hormone replacement therapy for life with combined estrogen and progesterone to restore monthly menstruation and to prevent osteoporosis.
- Fertility can be achieved only by IVF with ovum donation.
- She should be referred to a cardiologist to exclude a structural lesion of the heart.
- Sexual function is possible because a patent vagina is present.

Answer 10.1
1. Carcinoma of the vulva
2. Primary syphilis
3. Genital herpes

Answer 10.2
1. Biopsy and histological examination
2. VDRL reaction is a screening test for syphilis. Diagnosis can be confirmed by demonstrating treponema pallidum by dark field microscopy of scrapings from the ulcer or by FTA or TPHA.
3. Electron microscopy and culture or PCR test of scrapings from the ulcer.

Answer 10.3
1. Radical vulvectomy is performed once the diagnosis is confirmed.
2. Benzathene penicillin is given as a single intramuscular dose of 2.4 mega units.
3. Oral acyclovir 800 mg given 5 times a day for 5 days will relieve symptoms and duration of viral shedding.

Answer 10.4
- Lymphogranuloma venereum
- Granuloma inguinale

Examination Paper 8

AP Spine: L1–L4 (BMD)

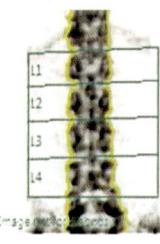

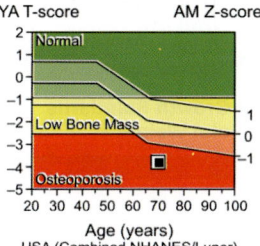

YA T-score   AM Z-score

Normal

Low Bone Mass

Osteoporosis

20 30 40 50 60 70 80 90 100
Age (years)
USA (Combined NHANES/Luner)

Region	BMD (g/cm²)	YA T-score	AM Z-score
L1	0.673	–3.8	–1.8
L2	1.713	–4.1	–2.1
L3	1.775	–3.5	–1.6
L4	1.728	–3.9	–1.9
L1–L4	0.725	–3.8	–1.8

Left femur: Total (BMD)

YA T-score   AM Z-score

Normal

Low Bone Mass

Osteoporosis

20 30 40 50 60 70 80 90 100
Age (years)
USA (Combined NHANES/Luner)

Region	BMD (g/cm²)	YA T-score	AM Z-score
Neck, Left	0.739	–2.2	–0.3
Total, Left	0.778	–1.8	–0.1

Right femur: Total (BMD)

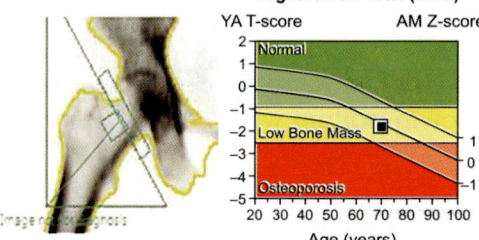

YA T-score   AM Z-score

Normal

Low Bone Mass

Osteoporosis

20 30 40 50 60 70 80 90 100
Age (years)
USA (Combined NHANES/Luner)

Region	BMD (g/cm²)	YA T-score	AM Z-score
Neck, Right	0.730	–2.2	–0.3
Total, Right	0.774	–1.9	–0.2

329

These images were obtained during a radiological examination which was performed on a 55-year-old woman.

1.1   What is seen in the above images?   (1 mark)

1.2   What is the clinical significance of this abnormality?   (1 mark)

1.3   What are the diagnostic criteria for the severity of loss of bone mineral density in the above investigation?   (2 marks)

1.4   List 4 risk factors for the above condition.   (0.5 × 4 = 2 marks)

1.5   List 3 first line non-hormonal methods of treating this condition.   (3 marks)

1.6   What is the definitive treatment?   (1 mark)

QUESTION 2

List 2 drugs which are used in each of these clinical conditions in a pregnant woman. Mention the dose and the reason for use.

2.1   Type 2 diabetes mellitus

2.2   Eclampsia

2.3   Intrapartum antibiotic prophylaxis in Group B streptococcal infection

2.4   Preterm labour

2.5   Heart failure   (2 marks for each correct answer)

QUESTION 3

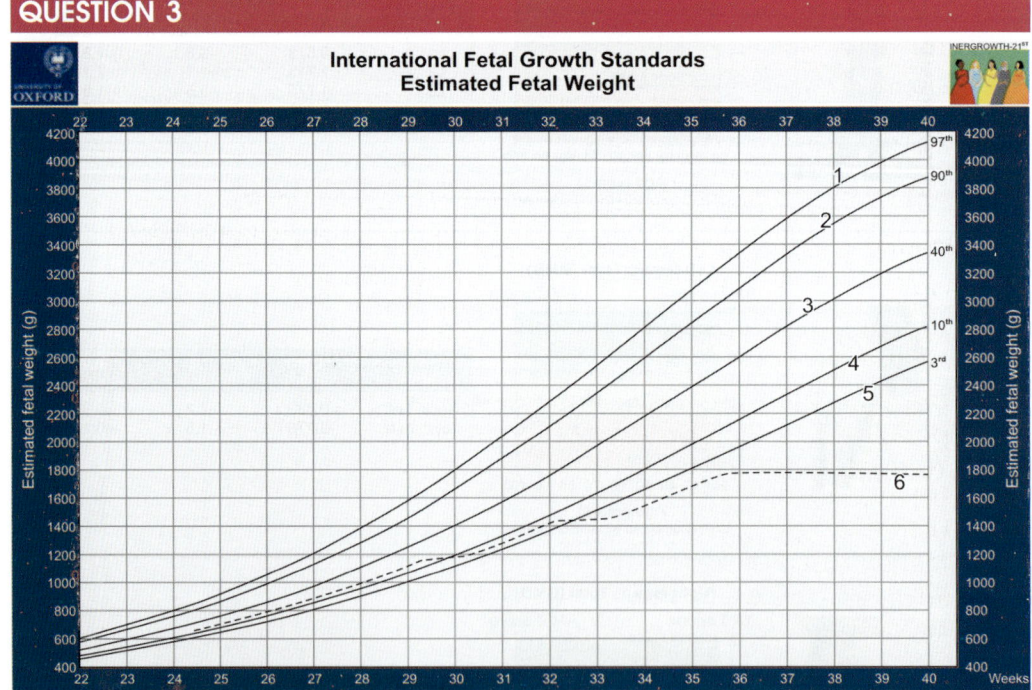

3.1   Describe the abnormality in the growth pattern which has occurred in the fetus in the 6th graph.   (2 marks)

3.2   List 4 causes for this abnormality.   (2 marks)

3.3   How does the growth pattern of the fetus in the fifth graph differ from that in the 6th graph?   (0.5 × 4 = 2 marks)

3.4 What is the best method of surveillance for the fetus in the 6th graph?
(2 marks)

3.5 When will you deliver the fetus in the 6th graph? Give your reasons. (2 marks)

QUESTION 4

4.1 List the important criteria you would check in a woman listed for major surgery during the preoperative ward round in the previous afternoon.
(1 mark each for any five points)

4.2 Mention your check list before sending the patient to the theatre in the morning.
(One mark each will be given for the first 4 points which are essential. One mark will be given for any one of the other points = 5 marks)

QUESTION 5

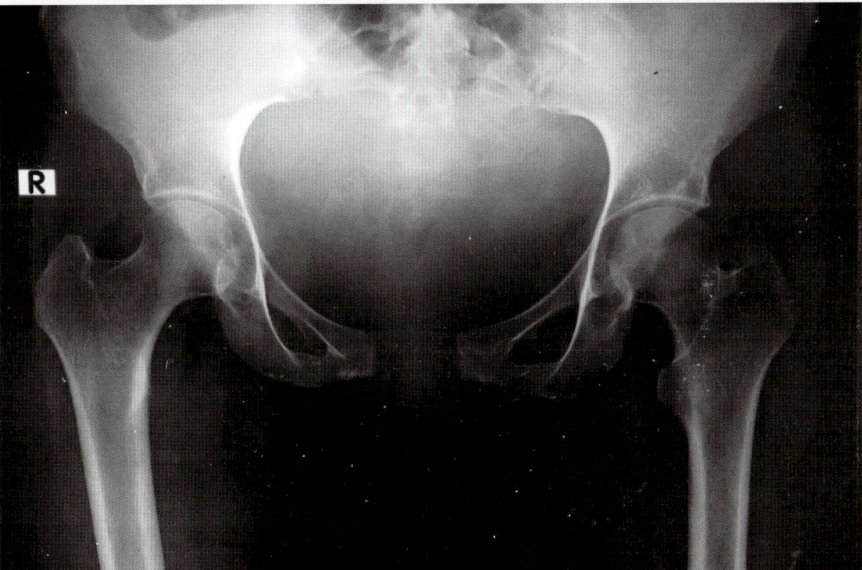

5.1 Describe the abnormality/abnormalities seen in this X-ray, which was performed in a woman on the third day after normal delivery.   (1 mark)

5.2 What is your diagnosis?   (1 mark)

5.3 List 3 presenting symptoms.   (3 marks)

5.4 List 2 predisposing factors.   (2 marks)

5.5 Mention the first line management.   (2 marks)

5.6 What is the next step in the management if the first line management is not successful?   (1 mark)

QUESTION 6

6.1 How do you diagnose stress incontinence?   (2 marks)

6.2 What are the preliminary investigations you would perform in stress incontinence?   (3 marks)

6.3 What is your initial management of stress incontinence?   (3 marks)

6.4 What is the next step in the management if the symptoms persist after preliminary treatment? (2 marks)

QUESTION 7

A 14-year-old girl attends the gynaecology clinic with a complaint of delay in menarche. Her current BMI is 24. Her secondary sexual characteristics are at Tanner stage 2. Her height is 148 cm.

Hormonal evaluation is given below:

- Serum estradiol: 6 pg/ml (15–400 pg/ml)
- FSH: 1 IU/L (less than 30 U/L)
- LH 0.8 IU/L (less than 20 U/L)
- Prolactin: 95 mU/L (83–357 mU/L)

7.1 What further information do you want to know from the patient? (2 marks)
7.2 What is the most likely diagnosis? (2 marks)
7.3 Mention the investigations you would order. (2 marks)
7.4 What is your immediate management? (4 marks)

QUESTION 8

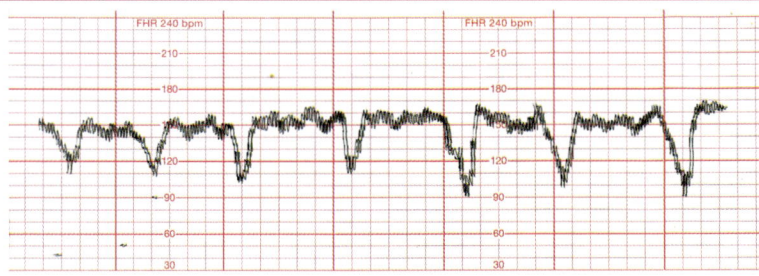
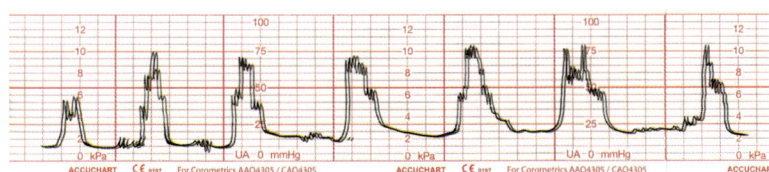

This is the CTG of a multipara whose cervical dilatation is 8 cm.

8.1 Name the decelerations seen in this CTG. (2 marks)
8.2 What is the cause for these decelerations? (2 marks)
8.3 Mention 3 normal features seen in this CTG. (3 marks)
8.4 How will you manage this woman? (3 marks)

QUESTION 9

a. No 1 polyglactin
b. No 3/0 polyglactin
c. No 2 nylon
d. No 2 black silk

e. No 2 polyglactin
f. No 2/0 polyglactin
g. No 0 polyglactin
h. No 1 nylon

Select 2 most appropriate suture materials from the samples given above to suture the following. (2 marks for each)

9.1   An episiotomy
9.2   A vestibular tear
9.3   The uterus at caesarean section

9.4 To perform a cervical circlage
9.5 A cervical tear

QUESTION 10

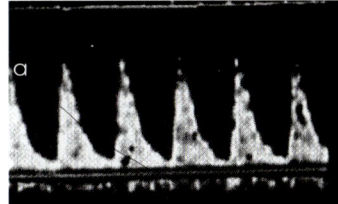 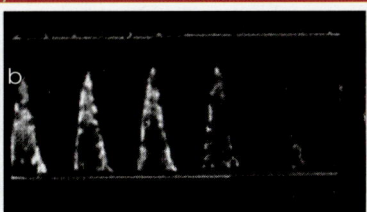 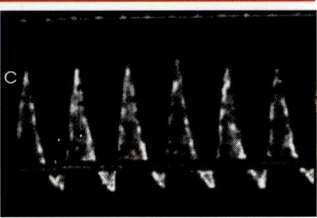

10.1 Mention the abnormalities seen in the umbilical artery Doppler flow in each
      of the above images.   (6 marks)
10.2 What is your management for b, if the POA is 34 weeks?   (2 marks)
10.3 What is your management for c, if the POA is 31 weeks?   (2 marks)

ANSWERS FOR EXAMINATION PAPER 8

Answer 1.1

It is an image of a DEXA scan (dual-energy X-ray absorptiometry) showing
osteoporosis from L1 to L4. and loss of bone mineral density (osteopenia) in both
femur and hip joints.

Answer 1.2

She is at risk of fracturing her spine with minimal trauma especially in the region
from L1 to L4.

Answer 1.3

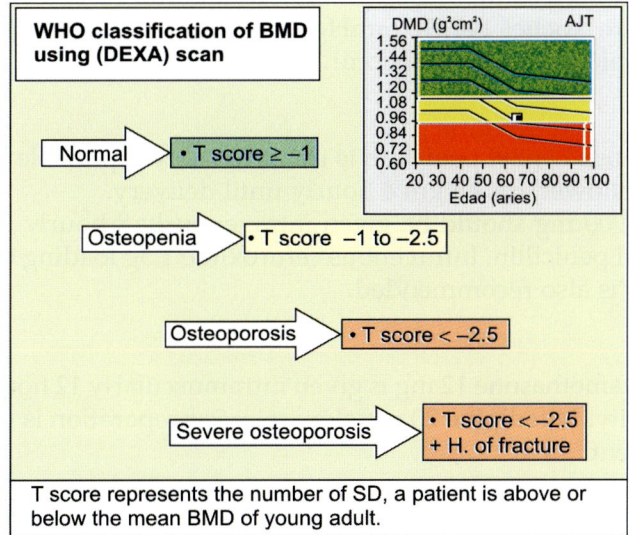

Answer 1.4

• Early menopause or oophorectomy before the age of 45 years.

- Heavy smoking and drinking.
- BMI of less than 21 kg/m².
- Use of corticosteroids.

Answer 1.5

- Give alendronate, calcium and vitamin D supplements.
- Exposure to morning sunlight daily for about half an hour.
- Supervised weight training and exercise. Care should be taken to prevent falling.
- Stop smoking.
- Consume a balanced diet containing calcium, vitamins and proteins. This should include, small fish, milk, grains, dried sprats, green leaves and fruits.

Answer 1.6

Commence on continuous combined HRT.

Answer 2.1

Metformin 500 mg twice or thrice daily is given for the control of mild uncomplicated cases with a FBS of less than 7. Soluble insulin is indicated if the fasting blood sugar is more than 7 mmol/L or in women with macrosomia or polyhydramnios. Three premeal doses are given.

Answer 2.2

Magnesium sulphate 4 gr loading dose is given by slow IV injection followed by 1 g IV infusion hourly. This is given to control fits and the drug is continued till the fits are under control.

Intravenous hydralazine 10 mg bolus is given by slow IV injection to rapidly reduce the blood pressure, if it is higher than 160/110 mmHg. This is followed by an infusion containing 20 mg in 500 ml of normal saline. The drip is continued till the blood pressure reaches 140/90 mmHg. Blood pressure should be checked every 10 minutes as rapid reduction can occur.

Answer 2.3

3 gm of intravenous benzyl penicillin is given as soon as possible after the rupture of membranes followed by 1.5 gm 4 hourly until delivery.

Clindamycin 900 mg should be given intravenously 8 hourly to those who are allergic to benzyl penicillin. Intravenous cefuroxime 1.5g loading dose followed by 750 mg 8 hourly is also recommended.

Answer 2.4

Two doses of betamethasone 12 mg is given intramuscularly 12 hours apart to cause fetal lung maturity. Nifedipine 20 mg slow release preparation is given twice daily as a tocolytic agent.

Answer 2.5

Furosemide 20–40 mg is given intravenously twice or thrice daily to reduce the lung congestion.

Oral digoxin 0.125 mg is given daily to improve cardiac function.

Answer 3.1

The growth has been slow from the beginning but it has been within the 10th centile till the 29th week. Pathological growth restriction has commenced at about 29 weeks and 5 days.

Growth has stopped after 35 weeks. This could be due to severe placental insufficiency from early pregnancy or due to a serious fetal abnormality and hence there is a risk of sudden fetal death.

Answer 3.2

- Chronic renal disease
- Chronic hypertension
- Anti-phospholipid syndrome
- Chromosomal abnormalities in the fetus.

Answer 3.3

The fetus in the 5th graph is continuing to grow steadily though at a slower rate and could be a constitutionally small baby. There is a lower risk of sudden fetal death as the growth is continuous.

Answer 3.4

Perform umbilical artery Doppler and middle cerebral artery Doppler studies

Answer 3.5

Delivery is best carried out at 36 weeks after a course of corticosteroids, because the fetal growth has stopped, indicating the occurrence of severe placental insufficiency and risk of sudden intrauterine death.

Answer 4.1

Confirm whether
- The patient has been listed for the correct procedure and whether the indication is justified.
- The results of the investigations are available and they are normal. If further investigations are needed arrange for them to be done immediately.
- Any medical problems have been treated and whether she has any allergies.
- Four copies of the operation list has been sent to the relevant individuals.
- Blood has been reserved.
- Informed consent has been obtained and whether the patient has any further questions.
- Prophylactic treatment such as thromboprophylaxis has been arranged, if required.
- She is on any medication and whether anticoagulants have been omitted.
- She has been advised to fast for 6 hours.

Answer 4.2

Check whether
1. The patient has been prepared and listed for the correct surgical procedure.
2. The patient is fasting.
3. The blood is ready.

4. Consent has been obtained.
5. Reports of all the investigations are available.
6. The blood pressure is normal.
7. She has taken the morning dose of any medications she is on at present.
8. The area has been shaved.
9. Jewelry and dentures have been removed.

Answer 5.1

There is significant separation of the pubic symphysis. The other bony structures appear normal.

Answer 5.2

Postpartum pubic symphysis diastasis

Answer 5.3

- Severe pain over the pubic symphysis.
- Difficulty in walking due to the pain.
- Midline lower abdominal pain.
- Difficulty in passing urine.

Answer 5.4

- Prolonged pushing during the second stage.
- Delivery of a large baby.

Answer 5.5

- Apply a pelvic binder.
- Give analgesics.
- Allow weight bearing when the pain subsides.

Answer 5.6

Carry out surgical correction.

Answer 6.1

In stress incontinence, passage of urine occurs during activities which increase intra-abdominal pressure, such as coughing, laughing and even walking. The amount may be small and leaking will occur even if the bladder is not full.

Answer 6.2

- Urine full report and culture and ABST, to exclude urinary tract infection
- Fasting blood sugar to exclude diabetes

Answer 6.3

- Maintain a bladder diary for 3 days to exclude mixed incontinence
- Treat urinary tract infection if present.
- Reduce weight.
- Treat chronic cough.
- Stop smoking.
- Commence pelvic floor exercises as the first line treatment.

Answer 6.4

- Surgery can be considered after review by a multidisciplinary team
- A transobturator tape is the procedure of choice because it is performed outside the pelvic cavity and the risk of bladder injury is minimal.
- Colposuspension can be performed through the abdominal route or by laparoscopy. It is the procedure of choice when an abdominal hysterectomy is needed or when mid-urethral tape procedures have failed.

Answer 7.1

Inquire regarding:
- Stress, excessive exercise
- Head injuries, meningitis, headaches and visual disturbance
- Symptoms of impaired thyroid and adrenal function.
- Impaired sense of smell
- Use of anti-psychotic, performance enhancing or addictive drugs.

Answer 7.2

Hypogonadotropic hypogonadism due to a hypothalamic or pituitary cause.

Answer 7.3

- Estimate GnRH, TSH, ACTH and growth hormone levels.
- Test the visual fields.
- Perform CT/MRI scan of the brain.
- Perform X-ray wrist for bone age.

Answer 7.4

- Management depends on the cause.
- Advice should be sought from an endocrinologist.
- Stress and excessive exercise should be prevented.
- Any drugs should be discontinued.
- Surgery or laser treatment should be performed if a tumour is present.
- All the hormones which are deficient should be replaced. If pituitary hormones are deficient replacement should commence with ACTH and TSH. Gonadotropins are given later to bring about ovulation, sexual maturation and menstruation.

Answer 8.1

Type 1 decelerations.

Answer 8.2

They occur due to head compression during the late first stage and the second stage of labour and are not pathological.

Answer 8.3

- The fetal heart rate is within the normal range.
- The beat-to-beat variability is normal.
- There are regular uterine contractions in the tocogram.

Answer 8.4

Labour should be allowed to progress anticipating normal vaginal delivery.

Answer 9.1

a or g

Answer 9.2

b or f

Answer 9.3

a or e

Answer 9.4

d or h

Answer 9.5

f or b

Answer 10.1

a. Reduced end diastolic flow
b. Absent end diastolic flow
c. Reversed end diastolic flow.

Answer 10.2

- Admit to hospital.
- Give a course of corticosteroids
- Perform middle cerebral artery Doppler flow studies.
- Perform CTG twice daily for 48 hours.
- Deliver in 48 hours by caesarean section after completing the course of corticosteroids if MCV Doppler studies are abnormal.

Answer 10.3

- Admit to hospital.
- Give a course of corticosteroids.
- Perform ductus venosus Doppler studies.
- Deliver by caesarean section if the ductus venosus Doppler flow is abnormal. Even if the ductus venosus Doppler flow is normal deliver at 32–33 weeks.

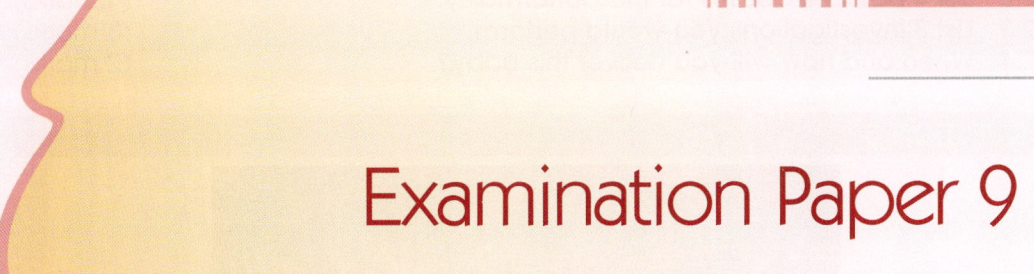

Examination Paper 9

Select 2 most appropriate suture materials from the samples given below to suture the following.

(2 marks for each)

a. No 1 polyglactin
b. No 3/0 polyglactin
c. No 2 nylon
d. No 2 Black silk
e. No 2 polyglactin
f. No 2/0 polyglactin
g. No 0 polyglactin
h. No 1 nylon

1.1 To ligate the uterine and the ovarian pedicle at hysterectomy.
1.2 To suture the abdominal wall in a wound which has undergone dehiscence.
1.3 To repair the ovary after cystectomy.
1.4 To repair a bladder injury.
1.5 To suture the anal mucosa during repair of a 4th degree perineal tear.

QUESTION 2

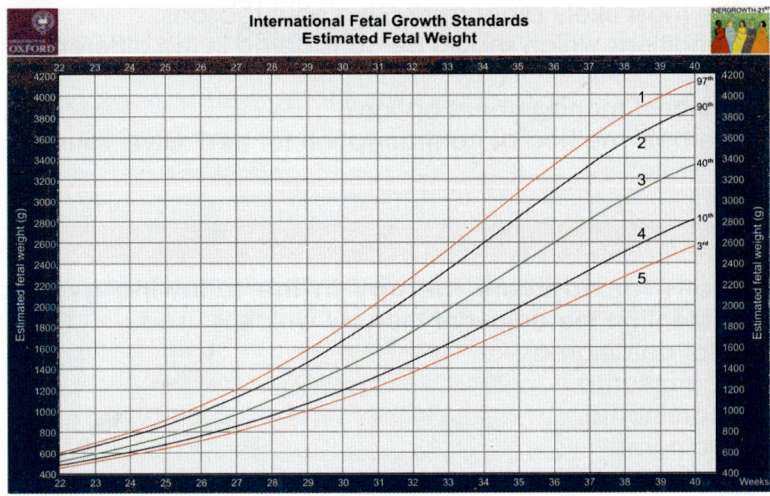

2.1   Explain the abnormality in the growth pattern of the baby in the 1st graph.

(1 mark)

2.2   List 4 possible causes for this abnormality.   (4 marks)

2.3   List 3 investigations you would perform.   (3 marks)

2.4   When and how will you deliver this baby?   (2 marks)

QUESTION.3

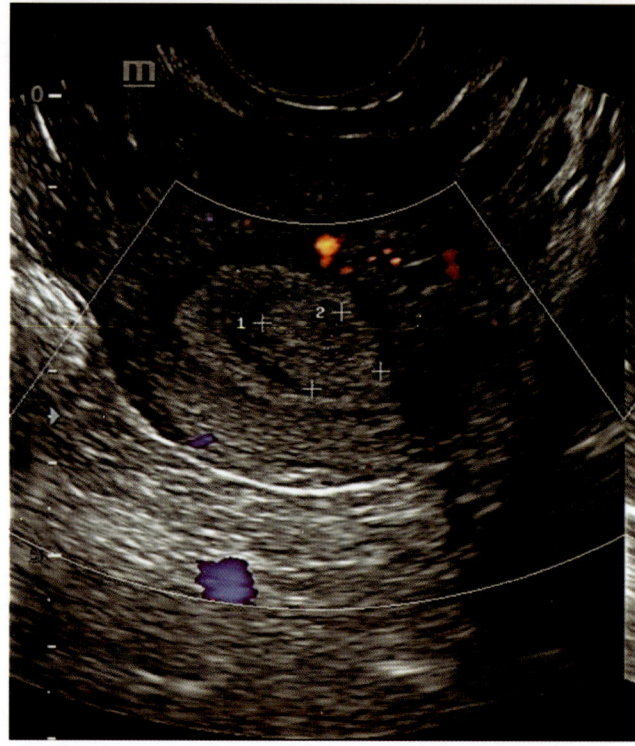

This ultrasound image was obtained when a TVS was performed on a 44-year-old woman who complained of heavy menstrual bleeding.

3.1   What is the most likely diagnosis? Give your reasons.   (4 marks)

3.2   List two conditions which should be considered in the differential diagnosis.

(1 mark)

3.3   What is the best management option?   (3 marks)

3.4   What is the best method of contraception for her? Give your reasons.

(2 marks)

QUESTION 4

List 2 indications for adjuvant therapy in the following gynaecological malignancies. Mention the adjuvant therapy which is used.   (2 marks each)

4.1   Endometrial carcinoma

4.2   Cervical carcinoma

4.3   Ovarian carcinoma

4.4   Vulval carcinoma

4.5   Vaginal carcinoma

QUESTION 5

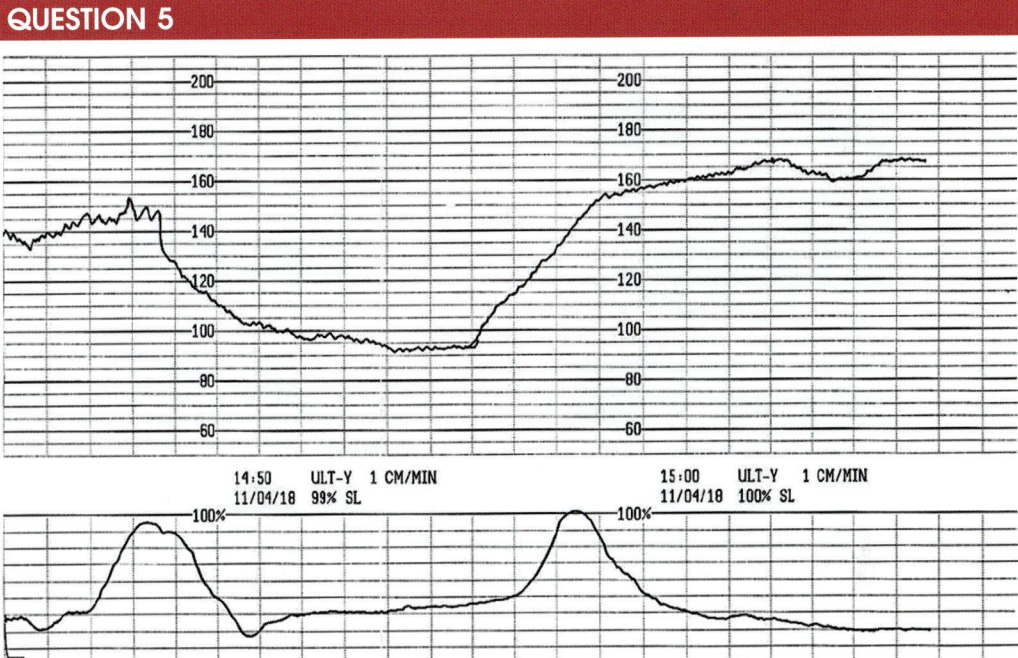

This CTG was obtained from a woman in the active phase of the first stage of labour.

5.1   List 3 abnormalities seen in the fetal heart rate pattern.   (2 marks)

5.2   List 2 causes for this abnormality.   (0.5 × 2 = 1 mark)

5.3   What is your management?   (2 marks)

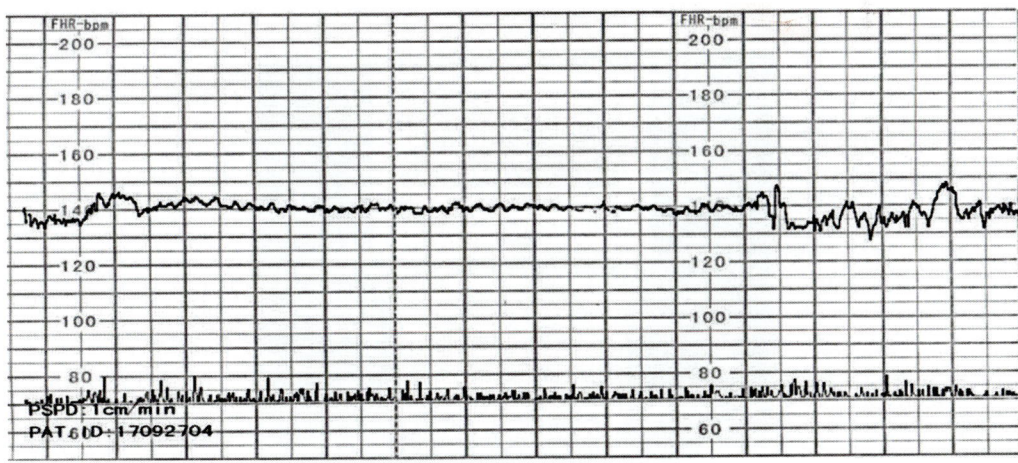

5.4   Describe the fetal heart rate pattern seen in this CTG.   (2 marks)

5.5   What is the reason for it?   (2 marks)

5.6   What is the next step in the management?   (1 mark)

QUESTION 6

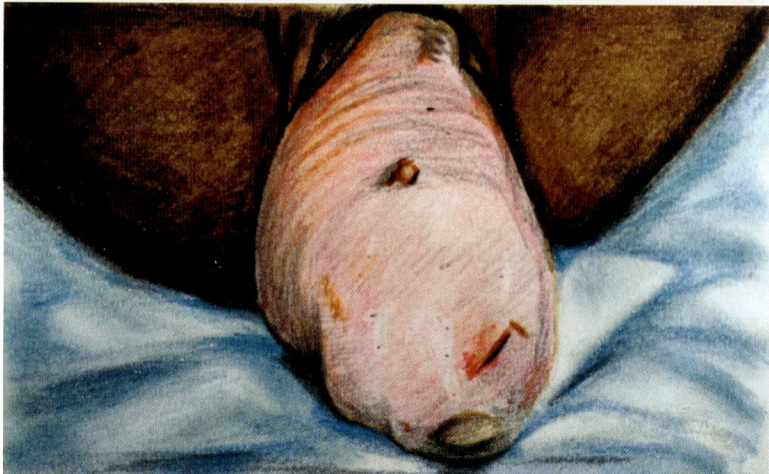

The following image was obtained from a woman who complained of a lump at the vulva. What is the best option of treatment in each of the following clinical situations?

6.1   If the woman is 38 years of age and has no fertility wishes.   (2 marks)
6.2   If the woman is 30 years of age with one child and wishes to conceive soon.
                                                                           (2 marks)
6.3   If the woman is 35 years of age and wishes to preserve her uterus, but does not wish to conceive soon.   (2 marks)
6.4   If the woman is 80 years of age with a history of recent myocardial infarction. A ring pessary which was inserted had fallen off after 2 days.   (2 marks)
6.5   If the woman is 6 weeks pregnant.   (2 marks)

QUESTION 7

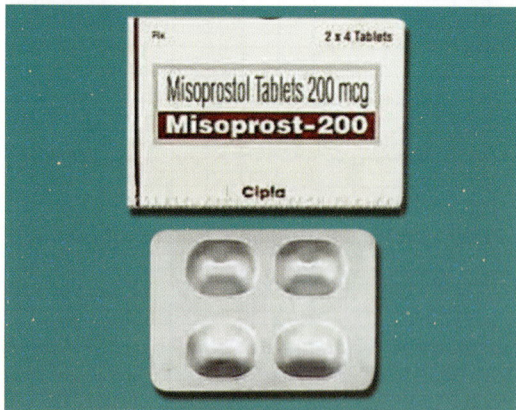

Mention the dose and mode of administration of the tablets shown above in the following conditions.   (2 marks for each correct answer)
7.1   Termination of pregnancy in the first trimester.
7.2   Incomplete miscarriage in the first trimester.
7.3   Intrauterine death at 32 weeks.

7.4   Missed miscarriage in the first trimester.
7.5   Intrauterine death between 18 and 26 weeks.

QUESTION 8

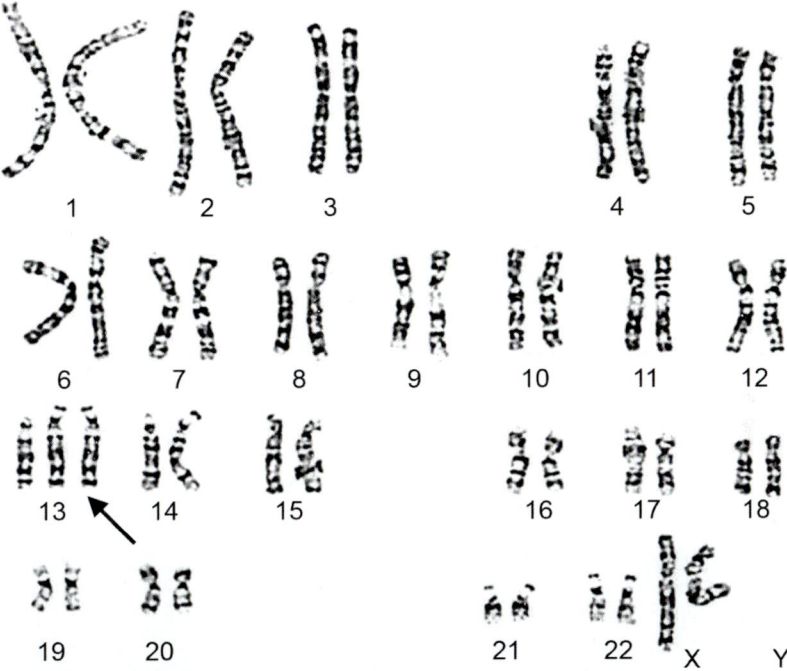

This is a Karyotype report of a baby who showed dysmorphic features at delivery.
Parents are planning another pregnancy and are seeing you for advice.

8.1   Describe the abnormality seen in the report.   (2 marks)
8.2   What tests would you perform on the parents?   (2 marks)
8.3   What is the risk to the future offspring of this couple?   (4 marks)
8.4   List the advices you can give these parents if they wish to have another baby.
                                                                       (2 marks)

QUESTION 9

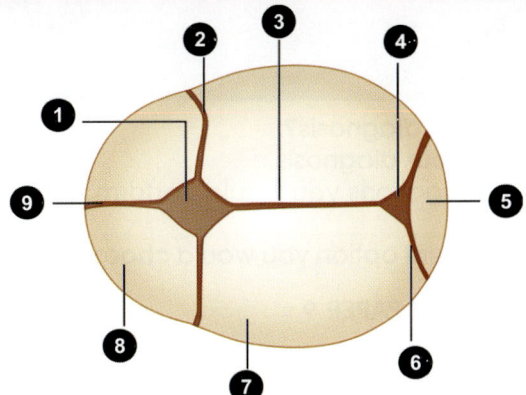

9.1   Name the parts of the fetal skull.   (0.5 × 8 = 4 marks)
9.2   Name 2 presentations in which the anterior fontanelle can be palpated by
           vaginal examination during labour.   (0.5 x 2 = 1 mark)
9.3   Name the diameters of the fetal skull and the corresponding fetal presenta-
           tions.   (5 marks)

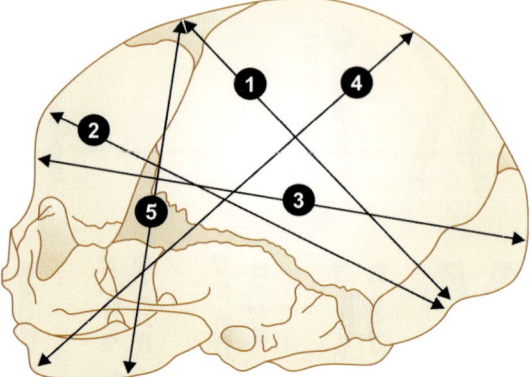

QUESTION 10

This is a transvaginal ultrasound image of a 30 year-old woman with one child
who attended the clinic with a complaint of abdominal discomfort and distension.

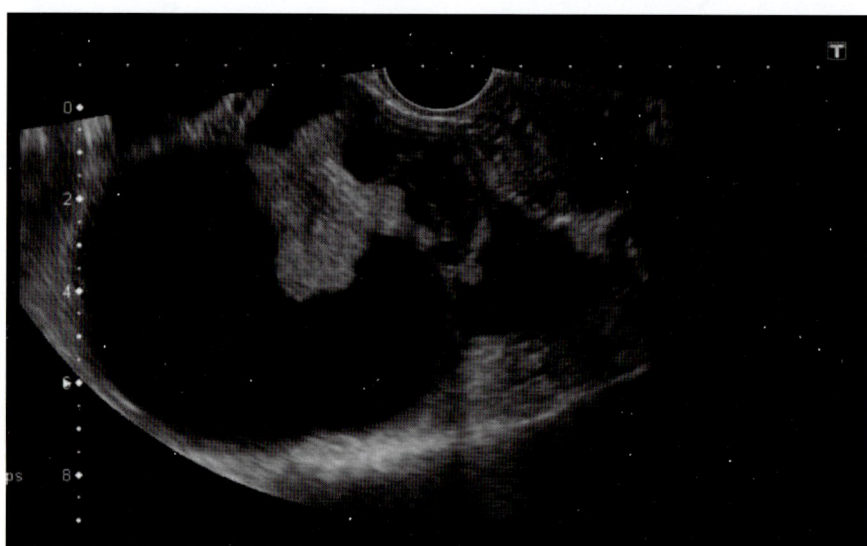

10.1 What is the most likely diagnosis?   (1 mark)
10.2 List four reasons for your diagnosis.   (4 marks)
10.3 List three other investigations you would perform to confirm your diagnosis.
                                                                         (3 marks)

10.4 What is the management option you would choose for this patient? (2 marks)

ANSWERS FOR EXAMINATION PAPER 9

Answer 1.1

a or e

Answer 1.2
c or h

Answer 1.3
b or f

Answer 1.4
f or b

Answer 1.5
b or f

Answer 2.1
This baby's weight has been above the 10th centile from the beginning. Therefore it could be constitutional or due to a pathological cause that has been present from the beginning.

Answer 2.2
- Type 1 or type 2 diabetes in the mother
- Fetal tumour/fetal hydrops
- Constitutionally large baby
- Chromosomal abnormalities.

Answer 2.3
Perform
- HbA1c to exclude maternal diabetes mellitus.
- Ultrasound scanning to exclude fetal abnormalities, fetal tumours and fetal hydrops. Cell free fetal DNA studies to exclude fetal chromosomal abnormalities.
- Umbilical artery Doppler studies to assess fetal well-being.

Answer 2.4
It is best delivered by caesarean section at 37–38 weeks or earlier if the umbilical artery Doppler studies are abnormal.

Answer 3.1
- Endometrial polyp
- There is a well circumscribed focal thickening of the endometrium. There is no evidence of myometrial infiltration.

Answer 3.2
- Endometrial carcinoma
- Endometrial hyperplasia

Answer 3.3
Perform hyteroscopic polypectomy followed by histological examination.

Answer 3.4
LNG IUS as it provides protection for the endometrium.

Answer 4.1

- Stage IB onwards
- Histological grade 3 at any stage
  Pelvic radiotherapy and brachytherapy are given.

Answer 4.2

- Stage IB2 onwards
- Positive lymph nodes following surgery at any stage.
  25 cycles of pelvic radiotherapy is given 5 days a week till the course is completed. Chemotherapy with cisplatin is given on every Monday for 3–6 cycles. 2–3 courses of brachytherapy is given weekly after completing pelvic radiotherapy.

Answer 4.3

- Stage 2 onwards
- Clear cell carcinoma at any stage
  Chemotherapy with cisplatin and pacitaxel is used. 6 cycles are given at 3 weekly intervals.

Answer 4.4

Pelvic radiotherapy is given if nodes are found to be positive after surgery or for histological grade 3 tumours.

Answer 4.5

Brachytherapy is used to treat all stages of the disease. Pelvic radiotherapy is given if the tumour volume is large.

Answer 5.1

- Prolonged deceleration followed by fetal tachycardia
- Loss of beat to beat variability.

Answer 5.2

Loss of baseline variability indicates fetal CNS depression due to hypoxia and the deceleration could be due to cord compression.

Answer 5.3

The baby should be delivered by caesarean section.

Answer 5.4

It shows a period of good fetal heart rate variability and accelerations followed by a period of reduced baseline variability in the middle. The variability shows recovery towards the end.

Answer 5.5

Fetal sleep.

Answer 5.6

No action is needed and the patient is kept under observation.

Answer 6.1

Perform a vaginal hysterectomy and repair as it appears to be a large third or fourth degree prolapse.

Answer 6.2

A ring pessary can be inserted as a temporary measure if she wishes to conceive soon.

Answer 6.3

Sacro hysteropexy is the best option. Manchester repair may not be successful as it appears to be a large third or fourth degree prolapse.

Answer 6.4

Insert a ring pessary with support or a Behring pessary. If the above methods fail perform a colpocleisis under local anaesthesia.

Answer 6.5

Insert a ring pessary.

Answer 7.1

Give 800 µg vaginally or sublingually 3 hourly × maximum of 3 doses within 12 hours.

Answer 7.2

Give 600 µg sublingually as a single dose or 400 µg orally as a single dose or 400–800 µg vaginally as a single dose and leave to work for 1–2 weeks.

Answer 7.3

Give 25 µg vaginally every 6 hours. If bleeding or infection is present give 25 µg orally every 2 hours.

Answer 7.4

Give 800 µg vaginally 3 hourly × 2 doses or sublingually 600 µg 3 hourly × 3 doses and leave to work for 1–2 weeks.

Answer 7.5

Give 200 µg vaginally or sublingually 6 hourly × maximum of 4 doses.

Answer 8.1

There is an unbalanced translocation of chromosomes 20 to 13.

Answer 8.2

Karyotyping should be carried out on both parents.

Answer 8.3

This is a case of Patau syndrome caused by a translocation between chromosomes 13 and 20 which can run in the family.

If mother is a carrier of a balanced translocation, there is a 10–12% risk of another abnormal baby. If father is a carrier of a balanced translocation, there is a 3% risk of a baby with Patau's syndrome.

Answer 8.4

The abnormality may be coming from one of the parents or may have arisen *de novo* in the child. To identify that we need to do karyotyping of both parents.

If one of the parents has the translocation and they decide to embark on a pregnancy chorionic villous sampling should be done at 11–13 weeks to exclude an unbalanced translocation in the fetus. Adoption may be an option especially if the mother is carrying the translocation.

Answer 9.1

1. Anterior fontanelle
2. Coronal suture
3. Sagittal suture
4. Posterior fontanelle
5. Occipital bone
6. Lamboid suture
7. Parietal bone
8. Frontal bone
9. Frontal suture

Answer 9.2

Occipitoposterior position and brow presentation.

Answer 9.3

1. Suboccipito-bregmatic diameter (9.5 cm) occurs in vertex presentation with occipitoanterior position
3. Occipitofrontal diameter (11.5 cm) occurs in occipito-posterior position
4. Mentovertical diameter (13.5 cm) occurs in brow presentation
5. Submento-bregmatic diameter (9.5 cm) occurs in face presentation with mento-anterior position

Answer 10.1

A malignant ovarian tumour.

Answer 10.2

It is most probably a malignant tumour because:
• It is a multilocular large cyst with thick septa and a thick wall.
• There is a solid area.

Answer 10.3

• CA 125
• CT/MRI scan of the abdomen and pelvis
• Lactate dehydrogenase and AFP levels

Answer 10.4

Exploratory laparotomy is performed. If the presence of ascites is confirmed, the tumour stage is above stage I. Therefore, TAH, BSO, infracolic omentectomy and full surgical staging is performed even though this woman is young and has only one child. If the tumour is stage IA unilateral salpingo-oophorectomy, infracolic omentectomy and biopsy of the other ovary can be done.

Examination Paper 10

This is the cardiotocogram of a woman in labour. The cervical dilatation is 5 cm.

1.1   Mention 2 abnormalities.   (2 marks)

1.2   What is the cause of this abnormality?   (1 mark)

1.3   What is your management?   (2 marks)

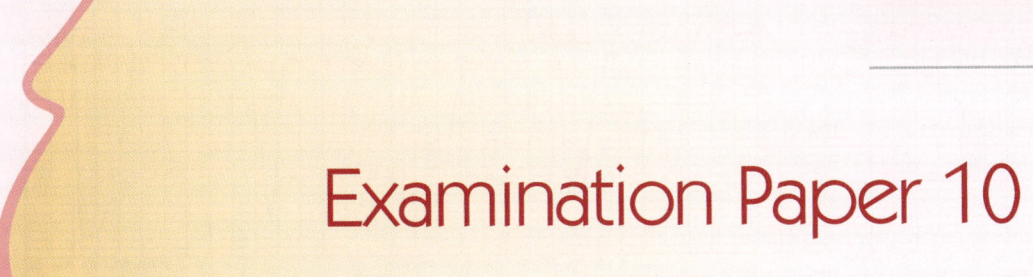

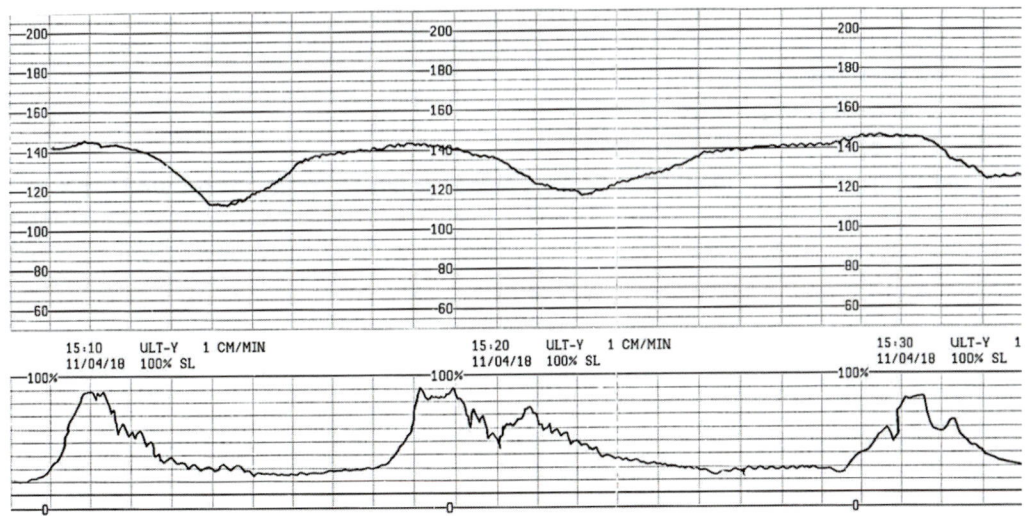

This is the cardiotocogram of a woman in labour. The cervical dilatation is 7 cm.

1.4   Mention 2 abnormalities.   (2 marks)

1.5   List 2 possible causes.   (2 marks)

1.6 What is your management? (1 mark)

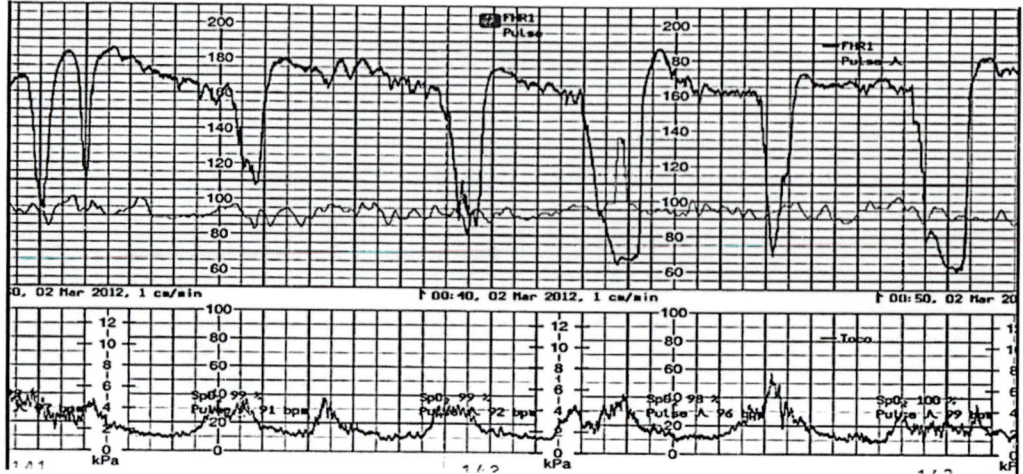

QUESTION 2

2.1 List the criteria which are used in the biophysical profile. (5 marks)

2.2 Calculate the biophysical profile from the data given below and mention the next step in the management. (3 marks)

- CTG reactive
- Largest amniotic fluid pool more than 2 cm
- Fetal breathing movements—less than 30 seconds of fetal breathing in 30 minutes
- One gross body movement
- One episode of limb flexion

2.3 List 2 difficulties in using the biophysical profile to assess fetal well-being (2 marks)

QUESTION 3

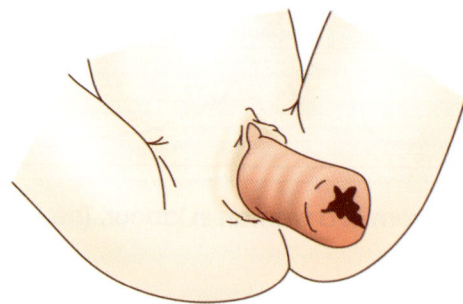

3.1 What is the condition shown in the picture? (2 marks)

3.2 List 3 methods of treating this woman if she wishes to preserve her fertility. (3 marks)

3.3 List the disadvantages of two of the methods you have mentioned. (5 marks)

QUESTION 4

Mention a drug which is one of the first line drugs, but is best avoided in a pregnant woman, for the clinical conditions mentioned below. (2 marks for each correct answer)

4.1 Typhoid fever
4.2 Chlamydial infection
4.3 Heart burn
4.4 Vomiting
4.5 Urinary tract infection

QUESTION 5

5.1 Calculate the Bishop score from the findings of vaginal examinations in the 3 clinical situations given below.   (6 marks)
     A. Cervix is 2 cm long soft and in mid position.
        The os is dilated to 2 cm.
        The station of the head is –2
     B. Cervix is 1 cm long, soft and anterior
        The os is dilated to 2 cm
        The station of the head is –2
     C. Cervix is not effaced, firm and posterior
        The os is dilated to 1 cm
        The station of the head is –2
5.2 Mention the Bishop score which is necessary to induce labour successfully.
                                                                          (2 marks)
5.3 Mention 2 methods which can be used to improve the Bishop score in a woman with a previous lower segment caesarean section scar.   (2 marks)

QUESTION 6

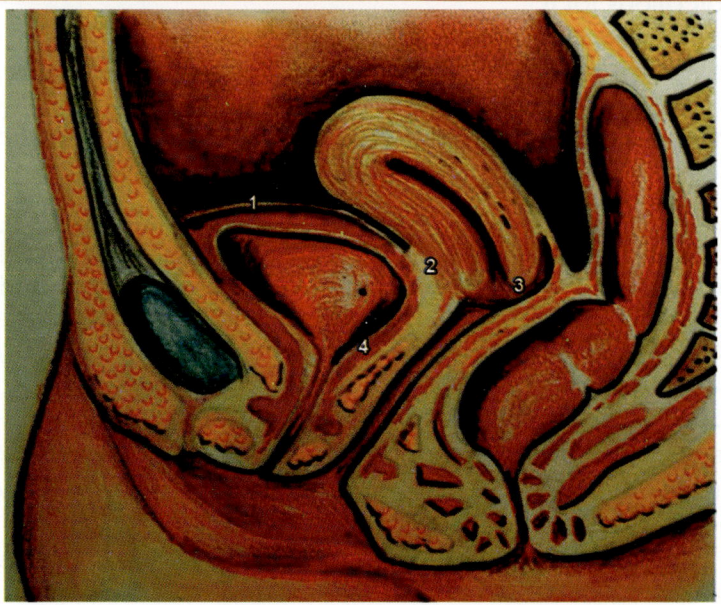

6.1 Indicate the places shown in the picture where the bladder can be damaged at abdominal hysterectomy and mention how the damage can occur.

(2 marks)

6.2 Mention another site where the bladder can be damaged. (1 mark)

6.3 List 3 precautions you can take to prevent bladder injury. (3 marks)

6.4 How can you diagnose bladder injury? (2 marks)

6.5 How can you treat bladder injury? (2 marks)

QUESTION 7

A 20-year-old nulliparous woman complains of amenorrhoea and galactorrhoea for 5 months.

7.1 List 3 questions you would ask her. (3 marks)

7.2 What is the first investigation you would perform? (2 marks)

7.3 List 3 steps in your management if the results of the above investigation is elevated. (3 marks)

7.4 List 4 drugs which could cause the above condition. (0.5 × 4 = 2 marks)

QUESTION 8

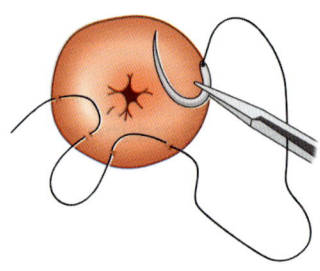 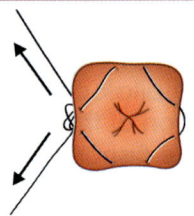

8.1 Name this procedure. (1 mark)

8.2 List 3 indications for it. (3 marks)

8.3 List 3 contraindications for it. (3 marks)

8.4 What advise will you give the patient regarding removal of the stitch?

(2 marks)

8.5 Mention why this procedure is not carried out during the first trimester.

(1 mark)

QUESTION 9

A 50-year-old woman complains of sudden onset of dyspnoea and chest pain 4 days after hysterectomy. Her BMI is 35 kg/m². She has diabetes mellitus which is well controlled. Her blood pressure is 90/60 mmHg, the respiratory rate is 28/minute and the temperature is 37.6°C.

9.1 List 3 possible causes for her condition. (3 marks)

9.2 List 4 steps in your immediate management. (0.5 × 4 = 2 marks)

9.3 List the investigations you would perform immediately to arrive at a diagnosis. Give reasons for performing the tests. (2 marks)

9.4 What is your immediate management if deep vein thrombosis is found in the left calf.

QUESTION 10

National Partogram

H. 1255

Name: Age: BHT. No:

Gravida: Parity: Blood Group: Date and Time:

Special Problems: Special Instructions:

Time of V/E																										
Hours		1	2	3	4	5	6	7	8	9	10	11	12	13	14	15	16	17	18	19	20	21	22	23	24
Fetal Heart Record in 1st Stage	≥180																								
	170																								
	160																								
	150																								
	140																								
	130																								
	120																								
	110																								
	100																								
	<100																								
CTG																										
Contraction free interval + duration of contraction	1																								
	2																								
	3																								
	4																								
	5																								
Oxy dose ml-h/ dpm																										
Abdo Descent / Cervical Dilatation	10																								
	09																								
	08																								
	07																								
	06																								
	05																								
	04																								
	03																								
	02																								
	01																								
	0																								
Descent Vaginally	-3																								
	-2																								
	-1																								
	0																								
	+1																								
	+2																								
Liquor																										
Position																										
Caput																										
Moulding																										
Pulse																										
BP																										
Temp																										
Action																										

The cervical dilatation of a multiparous patient is shown in the above partogram. She has one low intensity uterine contraction once in 10–15 minutes. Her POA is 40 weeks. Her fetal heart tracing is shown below.

10.1 Name the abnormality seen in the partogram.   (2 marks)

10.2 List 2 possible causes for this abnormality.   (2 marks)

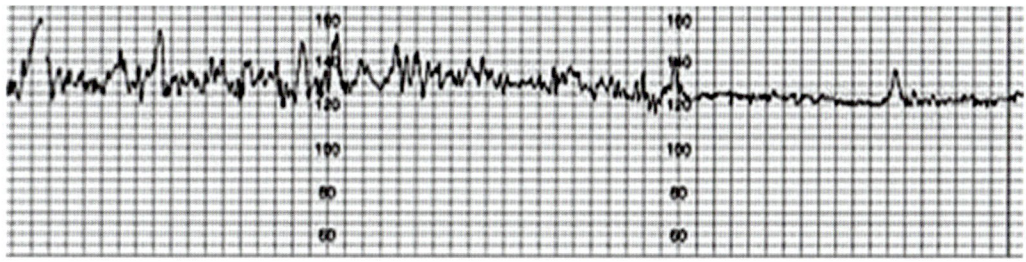

10.3 Mention your observations regarding the fetal heart rate tracing of this woman. (3 marks)

10.4 What is the best management option? (3 marks)

ANSWERS FOR EXAMINATION PAPER 10

Answer 1.1

- Late decelerations which are taking a long time to reach the baseline
- Reduced fetal heart rate variability—silent pattern

Answer 1.2

It occurs due to prolonged fetal hypoxia caused by chronic uteroplacental insufficiency, which may have been present from the antenatal period.

Answer 1.3

Immediate delivery should be carried out by caesarean section.

Answer 1.4

- Recurrent atypical variable decelerations with a deep amplitude and post-deceleration overshoots.
- Increased baseline heart rate.

Answer 1.5

Fetal hypoxia due to cord compression or cord prolapse.

Answer 1.6

Immediate delivery is indicated as the decelerations are recurrent and deep indicating acute fetal hypoxia.

Answer 2.1

- CTG
- Amniotic fluid volume
- Fetal breathing movements
- Fetal body movements
- Fetal tone

Answer 2.2

6 : It is low as the normal score should be more than 8 and repeat scanning should be performed in about 8 hours to exclude fetal sleep.

Answer 2.3

It requires ultrasound observation for 30 minutes. A low sore may be obtained during fetal sleep.

Answer 3.1

A second degree uterovaginal prolapse with hypertrophic elongation of the cervix and a small decubitus ulcer.

Answer 3.2

- Insert a pessary if she wishes to conceive soon.
- Perform sacrohysteropexy.
- Perform a Manchester repair.

Answer 3.3

Insertion of a pessary can cause pressure necrosis with vaginal discharge and bleeding. The pessary has to be replaced once in 6 months to avoid these complications. The pessary may fall off.

Manchester repair may cause cervical incompetence resulting in second trimester miscarriages and preterm labour. It can also cause cervical stenosis and cervical dystocia during labour.

Answer 4.1

Chloramphenicol

Answer 4.2

Doxycycline

Answer 4.3

Omeprazole

Answer 4.4

Ondansetron

Answer 4.5

Norfloxacin

Answer 5.1

a = 6, b = 7, c = 2

Answer 5.2

7

Answer 5.3

- Insertion of a Foley catheter with a 30 cc bulb into the internal os.
- Artificial separation of the membranes.

Answer 6.1

2 and 3

At 2 the bladder can be damaged when it is being pushed down to expose the cervix.

At 3 the bladder can be damaged while the cervix is being removed, if the bladder has not been pushed down below the cervix. A stitch can pass through the bladder at the same point when the anterior flap of the vaginal vault is being sutured.

Answer 6.2

The bladder can also be damaged while opening into the peritoneal cavity.

Answer 6.3

- Insert an indwelling urinary catheter before commencing pelvic surgery.
- Enter into the peritoneal cavity at the highest point in the abdominal incision.
- Push the bladder down gently to expose the cervix only after finding the plane between the uterus and the bladder.
- Push the bladder well below the cervix at total hysterectomy.

Answer 6.4

- A direct injury can be diagnosed at surgery or there will be leaking of urine through the vagina when the catheter is removed.
- It can be confirmed by filling the bladder with methylene blue and demonstrating leaking of the dye through the vagina.

Answer 6.5

- If the injury is detected at the time of surgery, it should be repaired immediately.
- If detected later catheter drainage is carried out for 3–4 weeks. Most of the small injuries will heal.
- Injuries which fail to heal should be repaired when infection and induration subside.

Answer 7.1

- Has she got headaches or visual disturbances?
- Has she had even a first trimester miscarriage?
- Is she taking any drugs?

Answer 7.2

Serum prolactin levels

Answer 7.3

If the prolactin levels are high:
- Perform MRI scan of the pituitary fossa.
- Examine the visual fields.
- Refer to a surgeon if a pituitary macroadenoma is found.
- Treat with bromocriptine or cabergoline if a microadenoma is present.

Answer 7.4

Drugs causing hyperprolactinaemia include phenothiazine, trifluoperazine (Stelazine), haloperidol (Haldol), chlorpromazine, benzodiazepines, risperidone, tricyclic antidepressants, metoclopramide, domperidone, ranitidine, famotidine, methyldopa, oral contraceptive pills, DMPA and many others.

Answer 8.1

Application of McDonald's cervical circlage.

Answer 8.2

- History of 3 or more recurrent mid-trimester miscarriages.
- History of 3 or more recurrent preterm deliveries.
- Cervical length of less than 2.5 cm on the TVS during the second and third trimesters.

Answer 8.3

Presence of:
- Uterine contractions.
- Ruptured membranes.
- An abnormal fetus

Answer 8.4

The stitch should be removed at 38 weeks or earlier, if she goes into labour.

Answer 8.5

First trimester miscarriages are usually caused by fetal abnormalities and not due to cervical incompetence.

Answer 9.1

- Myocardial infarction
- Pulmonary embolism
- Severe sepsis

Answer 9.2

- Insert a 14 gauge cannula and start a slow infusion of normal saline.
- Give oxygen by face mask.
- Arrange for immediate review by the medical team.
- Admit to the ICU.

Answer 9.3

- ECG and troponin T to exclude/diagnose myocardial infarction.
- Serum lactate levels. Severe sepsis is diagnosed if it is more than 2 mmol/L.
- Chest X-ray to exclude lung pathology.
- USS of the abdomen and pelvis to exclude the presence of a collection of pus.
- Duplex scan of the lower limbs to exclude DVT.
- Full blood count, serum bilirubin and serum creatinine levels. Severe sepsis with multi-organ involvement is diagnosed if the platelet count is less than 100×10^9, bilirubin is more than 2 mmol/L and creatinine is more than 2 mmol/L.

Answer 9.4

- Commence intravenous unfractionated heparin for 48 hours.
- Perform CTPA to confirm pulmonary embolism.
- Give streptokinase if there is massive pulmonary embolism.
- Perform APTT daily during treatment with intravenous unfractionated heparin
- Follow up with subcutaneous LMWH 60 mg twice daily.

Answer 10.1

Prolonged latent phase.

Answer 10.2

Inadequate uterine contractions
  The patient may not be in labour. As she is a multiparous woman, the cervix may be dilated up to 2–3 cm before onset of labour.

Answer 10.3

The fetal heart rate is within the normal range.

There is fetal cycling activity with a period of good baseline variability followed by a period of low baseline variability. This pattern is regarded as normal.

Answer 10.4

This patient is most probably not in labour. Therefore, she should be kept under observation in the ward and a vaginal examination should be performed after 4 hours.

Examination Paper 11

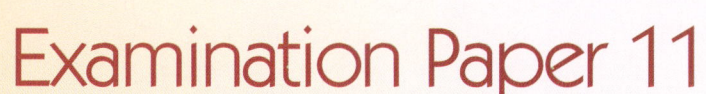

QUESTION 1

1.1 List 4 clinical observations which will allow early diagnosis of a blood transfusion reaction. (4 marks)
1.2 How will you manage a transfusion reaction? (6 marks)

QUESTION 2

A woman is admitted with a history of purulent vaginal discharge and high fever (39°F) 5 days after vaginal hysterectomy.
2.1 How will you clinically identify severe sepsis in the ward? (3 marks)
2.2 List 4 investigations which are necessary to diagnose severe sepsis according to the Sepsis Related Organ Failure Assessment Criteria. Mention the values which would indicate severe sepsis. ($0.5 \times 4 = 2$ marks)
2.3 What is your immediate lifesaving management? (5 marks)

QUESTION 3

3.1 List 3 criteria required to diagnose hyperemesis gravidarum. (3 marks)
3.2 List 4 investigations which should be performed in a woman who is admitted for the management of vomiting during pregnancy. ($0.5 \times 4 = 2$ marks)
3.3 List: (a) Two first line antiemetic drugs, (b) two second line antiemetic drugs used in the treatment of hyperemesis gravidarum. ($0.5 \times 4 = 2$ marks)
3.4 Mention 2 supportive treatment methods. (2 marks)
3.5 List 2 serious complications. ($0.5 \times 2 = 1$ mark)

QUESTION 4

A couple attend the preconception clinic. The male partner is found to be positive for HIV infection.

List the important steps in your management. (10 marks)

QUESTION 5

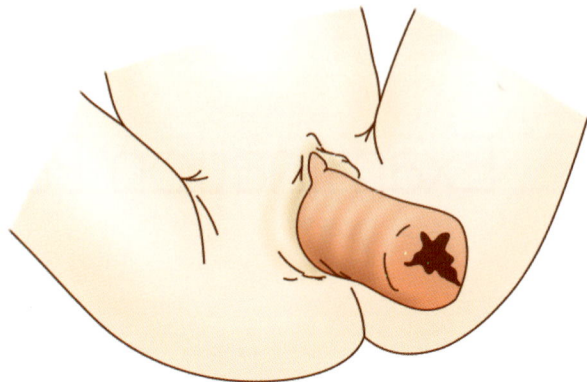

This image was obtained from a 30-year-old woman who attended the gynaecology clinic. She wishes to conceive soon and requests insertion of a pessary to relieve her symptoms.

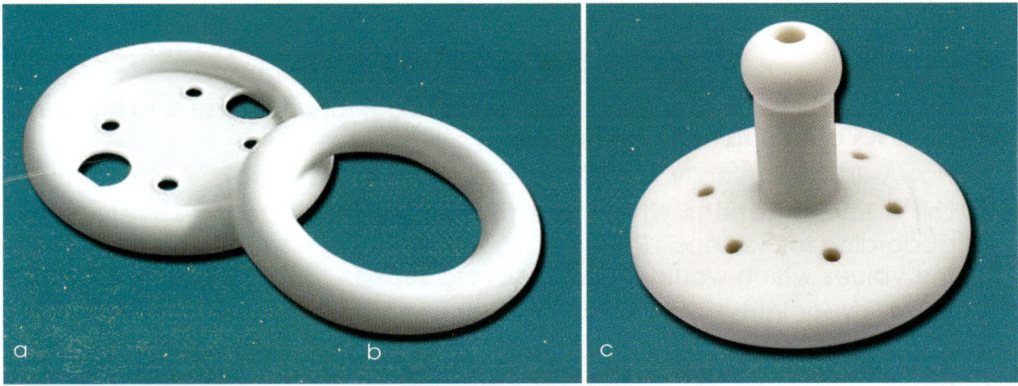

5.1   Which one of the above are most suitable for her? Give your reasons.
(2 marks)

5.2   How can you select a pessary with the appropriate diameter?   (2 marks)

5.3   List the steps you would follow during insertion of the pessary.   (3 marks)

5.4   List 2 advises you would give the woman regarding after care of the pessary.
(3 marks)

QUESTION 6

Describe in detail how you would instruct a junior registrar to repair a burst abdomen, which has occurred on the fifth postoperative day, in a woman who had undergone surgery for ovarian carcinoma.   (10 marks)

   (This question is intended for postgraduate students.)

QUESTION 7

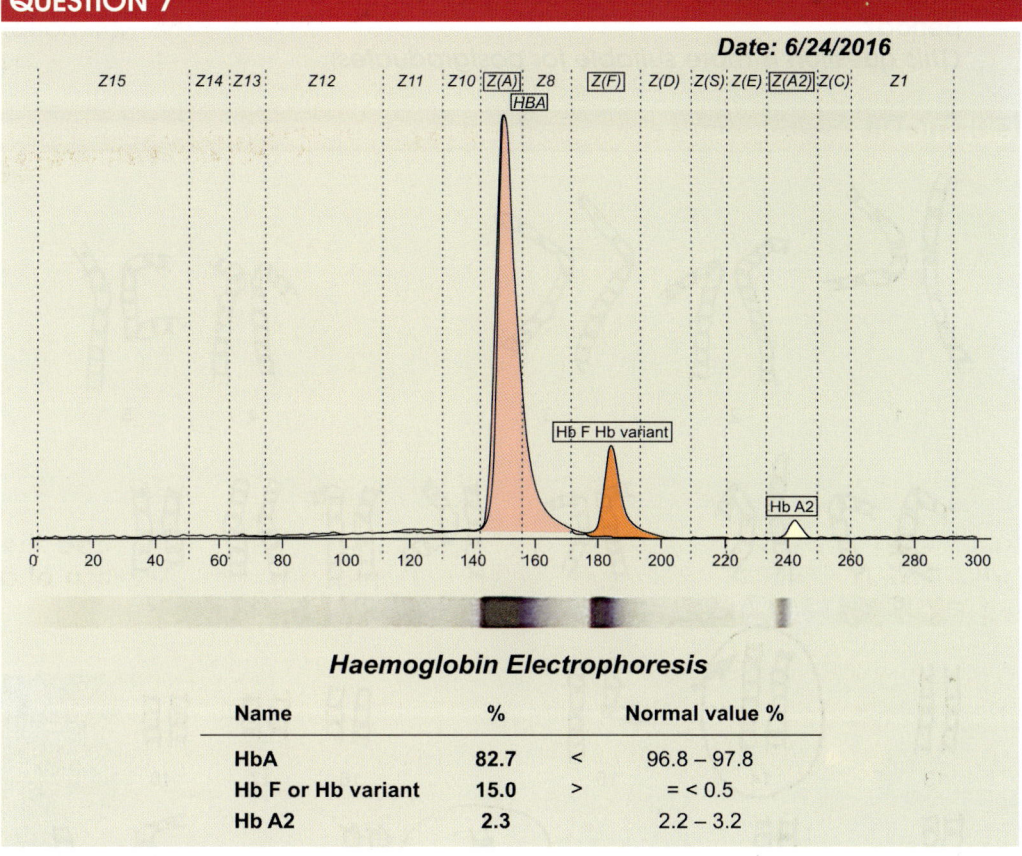

Date: 6/24/2016

Haemoglobin Electrophoresis

Name	%		Normal value %
HbA	82.7	<	96.8 – 97.8
Hb F or Hb variant	15.0	>	= < 0.5
Hb A2	2.3		2.2 – 3.2

This investigation was performed in a woman who had a haemoglobin level of 10 gm/dl at a POA of 16 weeks.

7.1   What is the probable diagnosis? Give your reasons.   (02 marks)

7.2   How will you assess the risk to her fetus?   (02 marks)

7.3   Mention an investigation which should be performed before commencing treatment.   (02 marks)

7.4   How will you treat her?   (04 marks)

QUESTION 8

A primipara is admitted at a POA of 38 weeks with fever and myalgia of three days duration. The NS 1 antigen is positive. She is tachypnoeic with a pulse rate of 130/min and BP of 90/50 mmHg.

The full blood count revealed the following: white cell count $1.5 \times 10^9/L$, haemoglobin 14 g/dl with a PCV of 45% and platelet count of $88 \times 10^9/L$.

SGPT 1000 U/L

SGOT 1650 U/L.

She complains of reduced fetal movements and the CTG showed reduced baseline variability.

8.1   What is her clinical condition?   (2 marks)

8.2   What is your immediate management?   (4 marks)

8.3 What would be your management plan for the delivery and postpartum period? (4 marks)
(*This question is more suitable for postgraduates*)

QUESTION 9

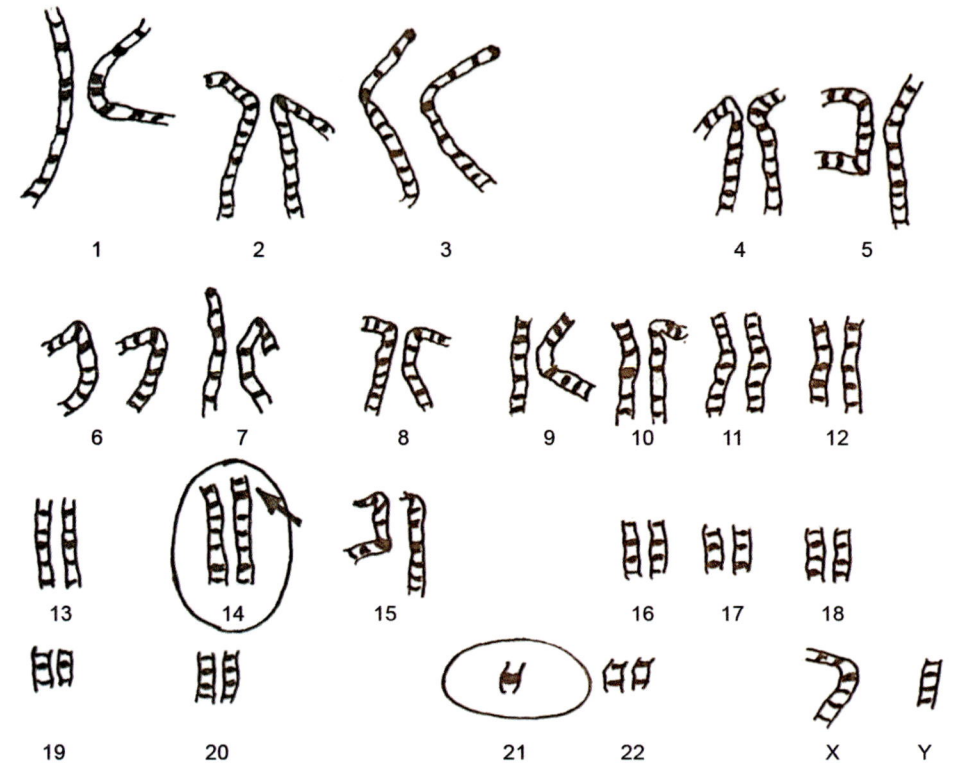

This karyotype was performed on a newborn baby with dysmorphic features.

9.1 What is the abnormality seen in this karyotype? (2 marks)
9.2 What is your diagnosis? (2 marks)
9.3 What is the investigation/s which should be performed in the parents to determine the prognosis for a future pregnancy? (2 marks)
9.4 What is the genetic abnormality which may be present in the parents? (2 marks)
9.5 If the mother has the abnormality how will you counsel the parents regarding a future pregnancy? (2 marks)

QUESTION 10

10.1 What methods would you adopt to prevent the occurrence of congenital rubella? (3 marks)
10.2 How can you diagnose fetal rubella infection? (5 marks)
10.3 Is there any method to prevent the occurrence of maternal rubella infection and fetal rubella infection if a non-immune woman is exposed to rubella at a POA of 6 weeks? (2 marks)

ANSWERS FOR EXAMINATION PAPAER 11

Answer 1.1

- Generalized itching
- Generalized skin rash
- Fever and chills
- Difficulty in breathing

Answer 1.2

If a reaction develops:

- Stop the blood transfusion and remove the blood pack immediately
- Administer 0.5 cc of 1:1000 adrenaline solution by intramuscular injection
- Raise the foot end of the bed. Give oxygen by face mask.
- Start a normal saline infusion.
- Nebulize with salbutamol.
- Administer hydrocortisone 100 mg intravenously .
- Administer chlorpheniramine 25 mg intravenously.
- Send the blood pack for reporting to the blood bank.
- Send the patient's blood and urine samples and the blood pack for investigation for transfusion reaction.

Answer 2.1

Presence of 2 or more of the quick sepsis related organ failure assessment criteria indicate severe sepsis.

- Respiratory rate greater than 22
- Altered mental status with GCS less than 12
- Systolic blood pressure less than 100 mm Hg.

Answer 2.2

- Serum lactate levels more than 2
- Full blood count—platelet count less than 100×10^9
- Serum bilirubin more than 2 mmol/L
- Serum creatinine more than 2 mmol/L

Answer 2.3

- Insert two 14-gauge cannulae.
- Commence IV crystalloid solution 30 ml/kg for hypotension.
- Send blood and a high vaginal swab for culture and ABST and commence intravenous broad spectrum antibiotics.
- Admit to the ICU.
- Give intravenous vasopressors (norepinephrine or epinephrine), if the systolic blood pressure drops to less than 65 mmHg after fluid resuscitation.

Answer 3.1

- Protracted nausea and vomiting in the first trimester of pregnancy.
- Dehydration and electrolyte imbalance.
- More than 5% pre-pregnancy weight loss.

Answer 3.2

- Serum electrolytes
- Urine full report and urine for ketone bodies
- USS to exclude hydatidiform mole and multiple pregnancy
- Liver function tests
- Full blood count.

Answer 3.3

A
- Prochlorperazine 5–10 mg 6–8 hourly orally; 12.5 mg 8 hourly IM/IV
- Promethazine 12.5–25 mg 4–8 hourly orally, IM or IV
- Chlorpromazine 10–25 mg 4–6 hourly orally, IV or IM

B
- Metoclopramide 5–10 mg 8 hourly orally, IV or IM (maximum 5 days duration)
- Domperidone 10 mg 8 hourly orally; 30–60 mg 8 hourly per rectally
- Ondansetron 4–8 mg 6–8 hourly orally; 8 mg over 15 minutes 12 hourly IV.

Answer 3.4

Supportive treatment includes:
- Normal saline infusion with added potassium chloride. The infusion should be guided by the serum electrolytes and the level of hydration.
- Oral or intravenous thiamine supplements.
- Thromboprophylaxis with LMWH during the period of hospitalization.

Answer 3.5

- Wernicke's encephalopathy
- Electrolyte imbalance.

Answer 4

- The woman should be informed only after obtaining consent from the male partner.
- Both partners should be tested for other sexually transmitted infections.
- The male partner should be counselled regarding the drug treatment of the condition. He should be referred to the STD clinic.
- Other sexual contacts of the man should be traced and tested.
- Both partners should be advised on safe sex with the use of condoms.
- Conception is possible by timed natural intercourse at the time of ovulation if the man is on cART and has had a zero viral load for 6 months. In other cases IUI can be performed with washed sperms. Donor insemination is another option.
- The woman should be tested for HIV during the pregnancy.
- Vertical transmission does not occur if the woman is negative for HIV.

Answer 5.1

'b' is the most suitable pessary as she has a second degree prolapse and she is actively engaged in sex.

Answer 5.2

Two fingers are inserted into the posterior fornix and the distance from the posterior fornix to the under surface of the symphysis pubis is measured in centimeters on the fingers. This distance is taken as the diameter of the pessary.

Answer 5.3

- The pessary is lubricated and squeezed to reduce the diameter.
- It is inserted into the vagina and is placed in the correct position.
- The patient is asked to cough and strain to exclude descent of the pessary.

Answer 5.4

- She should change the pessary once in 6 months.
- She should seek treatment if there is offensive discharge or bleeding. However, mild discharge may be present.
- Estrogen cream may be necessary if there is vaginal dryness or pressure wounds in the vaginal mucosa.

Answer 6

- Reassure the patent.
- Explain regarding her condition and the nature of the surgery and obtain informed consent.
- Help should be obtained from the surgical team.
- The surgery is performed under general anaesthesia.
- Send blood and a swab from the wound for culture and ABST.
- Commence intraoperative, intravenous, broad spectrum antibiotics.
- Ensure adequate hydration.
- Clean the area with a mild antiseptic solution taking care not to contaminate the bowel.
- Remove any existing sutures and enter into the peritoneal cavity.
- Resect any gangrenous portions of the bowel. A defunctioning colostomy may be necessary in some cases.
- Use liberal amounts of warm saline to wash out the peritoneal cavity.
- Apply a few deep tension sutures for additional support and close the abdominal wall with interrupted polypropylene or nylon no.1 sutures.
- Close the skin with interrupted nylon or silk mattress sutures if the wound is clean, leave it open if the wound is grossly contaminated.
- Continue broad spectrum antibiotics.
- Debrief the patient on the next day.

Answer 7.1

- She is a thalassemic trait.
- The HbA level is reduced and there is a small amount of HbF. A small amount of HbA2 is also seen.

Answer 7.2

- Haemoglobin electrophoresis should be carried out in her husband. If he is not a thalassemic trait there is no risk of the fetus having thalassemia major.
- If the husband is also a thalassemic trait amniocentesis should be done to exclude the occurrence of thalassemia major in the fetus.

Answer 7.3

Serum ferritin levels.

Answer 7.4

- She should be commenced on folic acid 5 mg daily.
- Dietary advice should be given. If the serum ferritin levels are low she should be advised to eat food rich in iron such as green leaves, red meat and pulses.
- She should be commenced on oral iron tablets (120 mg of elemental iron daily) if the serum ferritin level is below 30 ng/ml.
- Treatment should be monitored by performing haemoglobin levels monthly

Answer 8.1

Dengue haemorrhagic fever.

Answer 8.2

- Call the medical team immediately
- Admit to the ICU
- Multidisciplinary approach should be carried out with a physician, intensivist, anaesthetist, paediatrician/neonatologist, radiologist and a haematologist.
- Monitor according to dengue monitoring red chart for patients with fluid leakage. Monitor BP, pulse rate and respiratory rate continuously. Insert a catheter and monitor urine output hourly and assess fluid balance 3 hourly. Urine output should be maintained at 0.5–1 ml/kg/hour. Assess the haematocrit 3 hourly. Perform FBC twice a day, SGPT/SGOT and serum electrolytes daily. Assess capillary refilling time hourly.
- Give 2500 ml of fluid daily. Intravenous fluids should include normal saline or Hartman solution. Since the patient has a high PCV a bolus of colloid (dextran 40 or Tetrastarch) should be given as 10 ml/kg (500 ml total for an average adult) over an hour. In the midway of the bolus, furosemide 10–20 mg should be given. Furosemide can be repeated, if necessary.
- Perform serum albumin, serum calcium and creatinine, blood glucose levels, blood gases and PT/INR daily.
- Perform USS daily to assess liver damage, ascites and pleural effusion as well as fetal well-being.
- Send blood for cross matching and reserve blood and platelets.
- Inform relations regarding the patient's condition.

Answer 8.3

- Unless to save the mother's life, lower segment caesarean section (LSCS) or induction of labour should be avoided during the critical (plasma leakage) phase.
- Even though there is evidence of fetal compromise this should be disregarded till the patient recovers from the critical phase. Priority should be given to the mother's life and decision making should involve the multi-disciplinary team.
- If patient goes into spontaneous labour during the critical phase take steps to:
  - Maintain the platelet count above 50×10^9
  - Give single donor platelet transfusion, if platelet transfusion is necessary
  - Prevent vaginal tears by performing an episiotomy.
  - Anticipate and manage postpartum haemorrhage. Cross-match five pints of blood. Manage the third stage actively.
- Continue the same management in the ICU during the postpartum period.

Answer 9.1

There is an unbalanced translocation between chromosomes 21 and 14.

Answer 9.2

Translocation Down's syndrome.

Answer 9.3

Karyotyping should be performed on both parents.

Answer 9.4

A balanced translocation may be present in one of the parents.

Answer 9.5

If the mother has a balanced translocation the chance of recurrence is 12%. They can embark on a pregnancy, but chorionic villous sampling should be done at 11–13 weeks. Adoption or IVF with donor eggs are options.

Answer 10.1

- Vaccinate all girls at school or in the immediate postpartum period.
- At preconception counseling all women should be screened for rubella specific IgG antibodies. Non immune women should be offered vaccination and contraception for 2 months.
- All women should be screened for rubella specific IgG antibodies at the booking visit and non-immune women should be advised to avoid exposure.

Answer 10.2

The occurrence of rubella infection is diagnosed by:
- Four fold rise in rubella specific IgG antibody titer between acute and convalescent serum specimens, or
- Positive serologic test for rubella-specific IgM antibody.
- If a non-immune woman is exposed to rubella the first step in the management is to test the maternal serum for rubella specific IgG and IgM antibodies immediately and after 3 weeks.
- Presence of IgM antibodies in the first or second samples indicate acute infection with a high risk of congenital rubella.
- If IgM is negative and there is a significant increase in IgG in the second sample infection may have occurred but there is a reduced risk of congenital rubella.
- If IgM is negative and there is no rise in IgG antibodies there is no possibility of acute infection and the patient can be reassured.
- The risk of congenital rubella is 90% when maternal infection occurs before 11 weeks of gestation, 33% at 11–12 weeks, 24% at 15–16 weeks, < than 1% between 16 and 20 weeks and 0% after 20 weeks
- Fetal infection can be directly diagnosed by testing for rubella specific DNA by PCR on chorionic villous sampling at 12 weeks and on amniotic fluid at 14–16 weeks. However, serological testing for rubella infection in the mother is regarded as confirmatory of congenital rubella infection.

• USS is less useful to diagnose fetal infection as rubella causes mainly auditory, neurological and ocular lesions which cannot be detected by US scanning.

Answer 10.3

There is no method to prevent maternal infection as the immunoglobulin is not effective and the vaccine is contraindicated as it is a live attenuated vaccine.

Birth of an affected baby can only be prevented by termination of the pregnancy if maternal infection is confirmed by the presence of IgM antibodies or a 4-fold rise in IgG antibodies before 16 weeks.

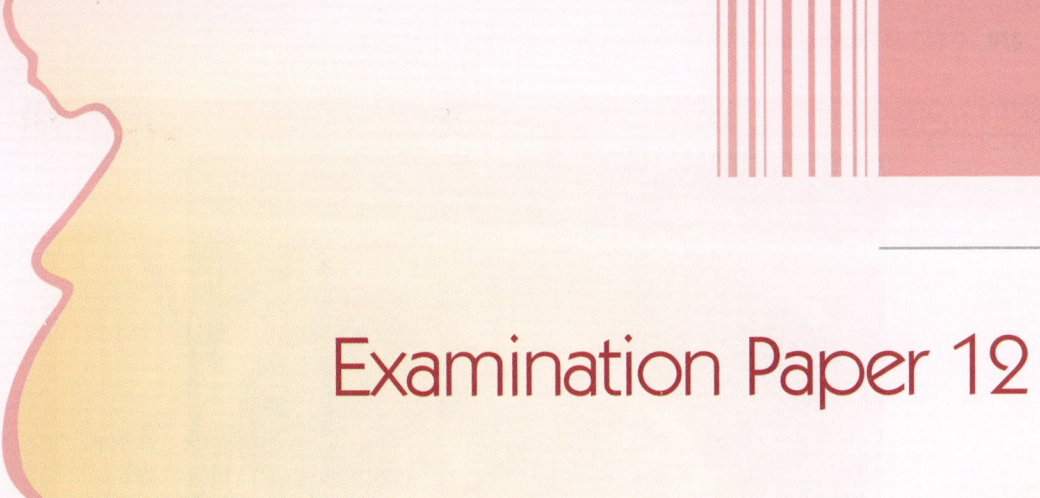

Examination Paper 12

QUESTION 1

List two methods of contraception which are most suitable in the following situations.   (2 marks for each correct answer)

1.1 A 42-year-old woman
1.2 A breastfeeding woman 3 weeks after partus.
1.3 A breastfeeding woman 6 weeks after partus.
1.4 For emergency contraception within 72 hours
1.5 For emergency contraception up to 5 days.

QUESTION 2

What advise will you give a couple regarding future pregnancies if the male partner is suffering from

2.1 Huntington's disease?   (2 marks)
2.2 Haemophilia?   (2 marks)

What advise will you give a couple regarding future pregnancies if one partner is suffering from:

2.3 Cystic fibrosis?   (2 marks)
2.4 Phenyl ketonuria?   (2 marks)
2.5 What advise will you give a couple regarding future pregnancies if they have one child with Edward syndrome?   (2 marks)

QUESTION 3

3.1 How do you diagnose an infralevator haematoma?   (4 marks)

How do you treat:

3.2 A small infralevator haematoma?   (3 marks)
3.3 A large infralevator haematoma with haemodynamic compromise?
                                                                         (3 marks)

QUESTION 4

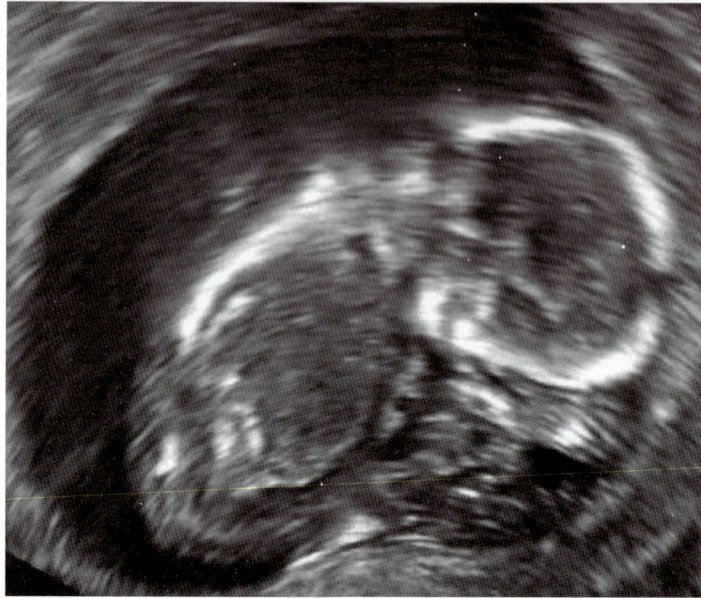

From Wikipedia commons

4.1 This ultrasound scan image belongs to a woman who attends the antenatal clinic at a POA of 13 weeks. The fetal heart beat is absent. What is the best management option?   (2 marks)

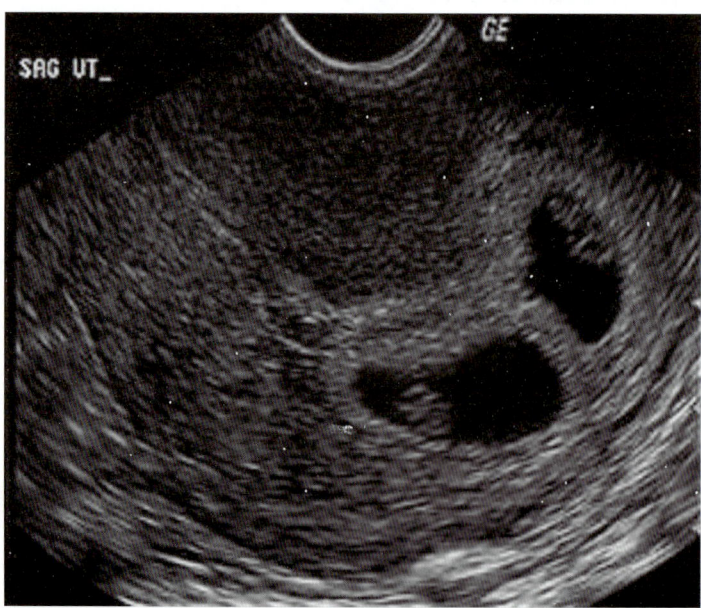

4.2 This ultrasound scan image belongs to a woman who attends the antenatal clinic at a POA of 6 weeks. The fetal heart beat is absent in the smaller sac. What is the best management option?   (3 marks)

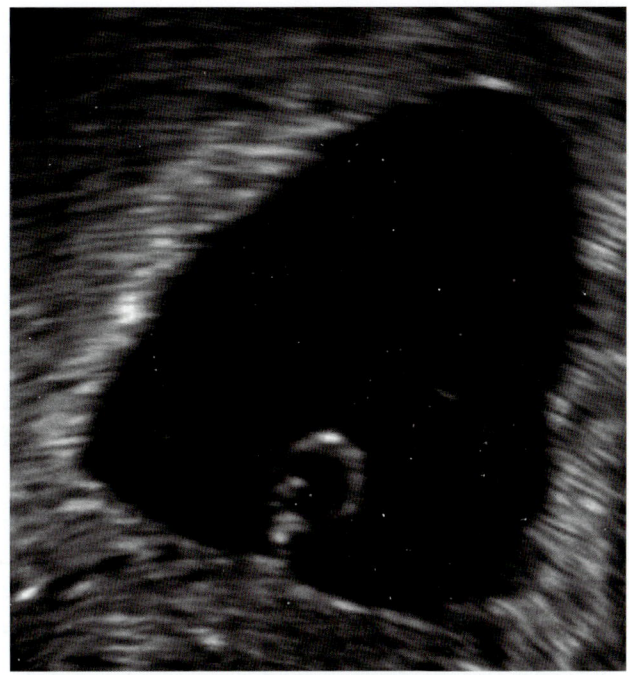

From Wikipedia commons

This ultrasound scan image belongs to a woman who attends the antenatal clinic at a POA 8 weeks.

4.3   What is your diagnosis? Give your reasons.   (2 marks)
4.4   How will you manage this woman if the fetal heart beat is not found after one week?   (3 marks)

QUESTION 5

5.1   List the steps involved in ovarian stimulation for IVF.   (5 marks)
5.2   How do you diagnose ovarian hyperstimulation?   (2 marks)
5.3   What is your management if ovarian hyperstimulation is suspected during an IVF cycle?   (3 marks)

QUESTION 6

List the precautions you would take to prevent ureteric damage at hysterectomy.
                                                                                  (10 marks)

QUESTION 7

A woman develops moderately severe vaginal bleeding 7 days after normal vaginal delivery. This was preceded by fever and purulent vaginal discharge.

7.1   Name this condition.   (1 mark)
7.2   List 2 causative factors.   (2 marks)
7.3   List 4 investigations you would perform.   (4 marks)
7.4   List the steps in your immediate management in the appropriate order.
                                                                                  (3 marks)

QUESTION 8

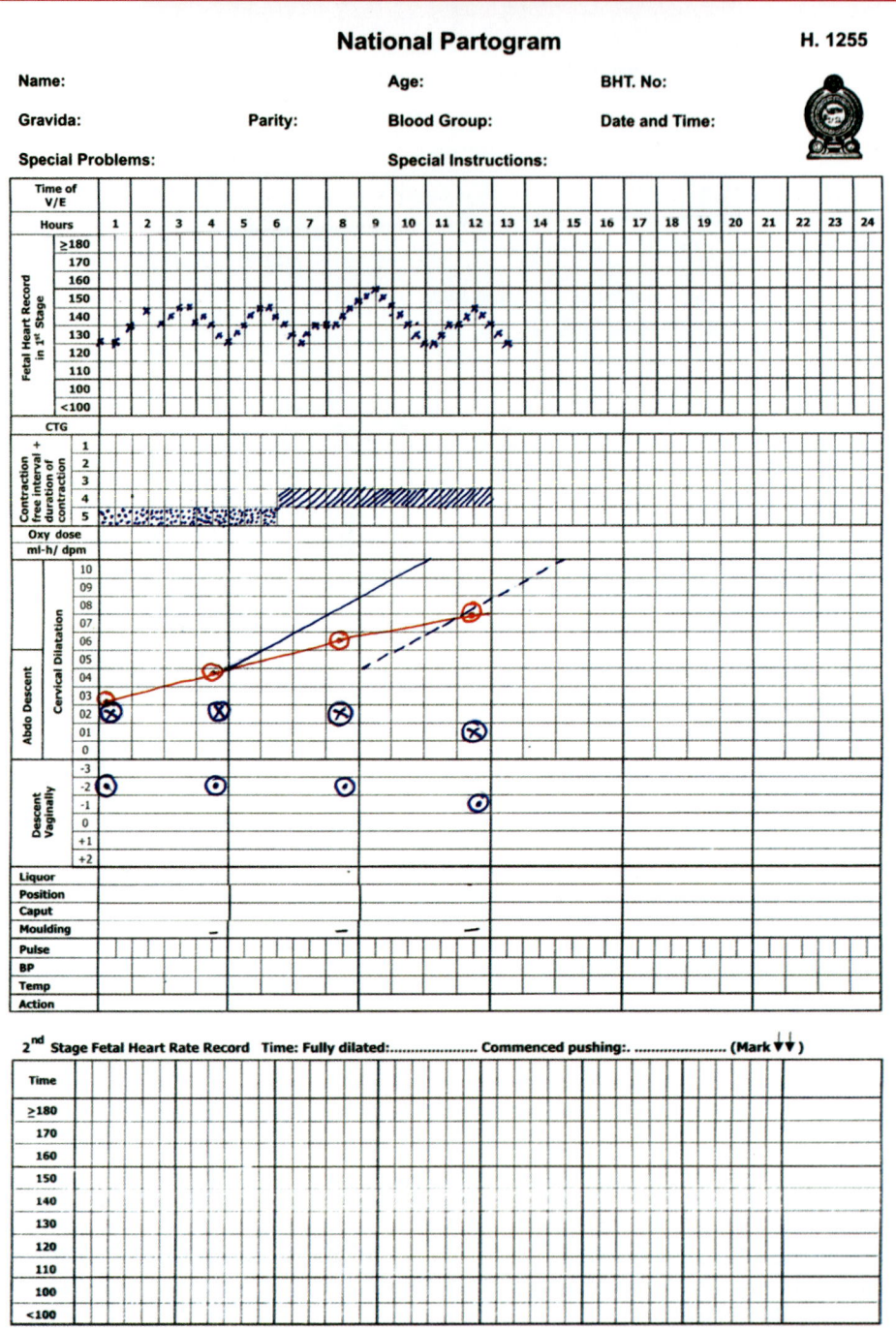

What is the best management option if the above partogram was obtained on a:

8.1 Woman in labour with a breech presentation? (2 marks)

8.2 Woman in labour with a previous caesarean section scar? (2 marks)

8.3   Woman in labour with a Dichorionic and diamniotic twin pregnancy? (2 marks)

8.4   Woman in labour with an occipitoposterior position and an android pelvis? (2 marks)

8.5   Woman in labour with a mentoanterior face presentation? (2 marks)

QUESTION 9

9.1   Mention the chorionicity and amnionicity of twins shown in each of the scan images. (3 marks)

9.2   Describe how you would determine the chorionicity and amnionicity of twins. (7 marks)

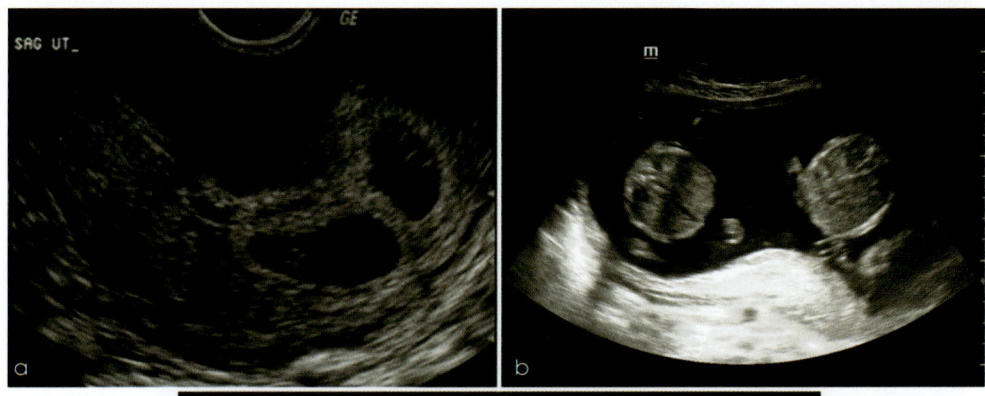

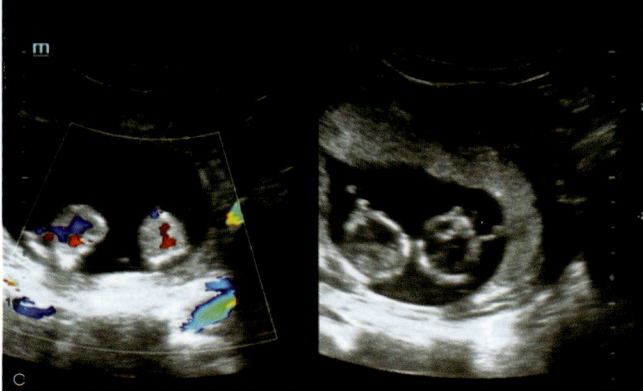

QUESTION 10

List the steps in the procedure you would follow when discharging a patient from hospital after normal delivery. (10 marks)

ANSWERS FOR EMAINATION PAPER 12

Answer 1.1

Copper IUCD, LNG-IUS, progesterone implant

Answer 1.2

DMPA, progesterone implant.

Answer 1.3

Copper IUCD, LNG-IUS, progesterone implant.

Answer 1.4

Give:
- 1 dose of levonorgestrel 1.5 mg (postinor 1) or two 0 .75 mg tablets (postinor 2) 12 hours apart
- 1 dose of ulipristal 30 mg
- 2 doses of 2 tablets of combined oral contraceptive pills taken 12 hours apart
- Insert a copper IUCD

Answer 1.5

Give 1 dose of ulipristal 30 mg or insert a copper IUCD.

Answer 2.1

The parents should be told that there is a 50% chance of the child being affected as it is an autosomal dominant disease. Therefore, chorionic villous sampling should be performed at 12–13 weeks.

Answer 2.2

A male with haemophilia will not produce affected children, if he is married to a normal female. However, all the female children will be carriers and they can produce affected male children, if they get married to a normal male.

Answer 2.3

Since cystic fibrosis is an autosomal recessive disease they will not have an affected child as the other partner is normal. Therefore, they can embark on a pregnancy. 50% of the children will be carriers. They have a 25% chance of having an affected child if the other partner is a carrier.

Answer 2.4

Since phenyl ketonuria is an autosomal recessive disease they will not have an affected child as the other partner is normal. Therefore, they can embark on a pregnancy. 50% of children will be carriers. They have a 25% chance of having an affected child if the other partner is a carrier.

Answer 2.5

Both parents should be tested for the presence of a balanced translocation. If the mother has a balanced translocation the risk of transmission is 12%. If the father has a balanced translocation the risk of transmission is 3%. They can embark on a pregnancy, but chorionic villous sampling should be done at 12–13 weeks. If neither parents have a balanced translocation and the previous baby is affected due to a mutation and there is no risk for future pregnancies if the mother is under 40 years of age.

Answer 3.1

- The patient may complain of pain in the vagina or in the rectum after delivery.
- She may develop retention of urine.

- There may be unexplained tachycardia and low blood pressure in the absence of vaginal bleeding.
- Examination may reveal a soft boggy mass in the lateral vaginal wall.

Answer 3.2

A small infralevator haematoma does not need drainage and the patient can be kept under observation.

Answer 3.3

Since this patient has haemodynamic compromise she should be having a moderate collection of blood. The best management option is to drain the haematoma and to control further bleeding, by applying figure of eight sutures. It is not possible to find the individual bleeding vessels in this situation. A vaginal pack can be inserted to control further bleeding. Insertion of a vaginal pack alone may not be sufficient as the haematoma is large. She will need resuscitation with intravenous fluids and blood transfusion.

Answer 4.1

Expectant management can be carried out for 3 weeks, if the patient is willing and there is no infection or excessive bleeding. A coagulation profile should be performed. If expectant management fails, or if the patient is not willing for expectant management, insert 200 µg of misoprostol 6 hourly for a maximum of 4 doses.

Answer 4.2

Reassurance and explanation is essential. She should be told that mild bleeding may occur, but most probably the live fetus may continue to grow. Expectant management is carried out. Serial scans are performed weekly.

Answer 4.3

A diagnosis of wrong dates or failing pregnancy can be made as there is only a yolk sac and a fetus is not seen. A repeat scan should be performed in 1 week to confirm the diagnosis.

Answer 4.4

If the repeat scan confirms a missed miscarriage expectant management may be carried out for three weeks if the patient is willing and there is no infection or excessive bleeding. A coagulation profile should be performed. If expectant management fails insert 800 µg of misoprostol vaginally. Insert 2 doses 3 hourly and observe for 1–2 weeks in the absence of infection or bleeding.

Answer 5.1

- Commence GnRH at the midluteal phase of the previous cycle.
- Commence FSH 75 IU daily from the 3rd day of the treatment cycle.
- TVS is performed daily to assess the follicular size and to detect hyperstimulation.
- If the follicular size is smaller than 0.8 cm by the 7th day step up the dose to 150 IU.

- FSH is administered until the 9th–16th day of cycle till follicles with dimensions equal to or more than 17 mm are found. Serum estradiol levels should be over 150 pg/mL per follicle which is equal to or greater than 17 mm in diameter.
- 5000 IU recombinant human chorionic gonadotropin is injected at this stage.

Answer 5.2

The woman will complain of abdominal pain, dyspnea, vomiting, fever and abdominal distension. PCV will reveal haemoconcentration. Serum proteins may be low. Ultrasound scan will reveal enlarged ovaries (up to 12 cm) and ascites.

Answer 5.3

- Cancel the cycle.
- Freeze any mature ova.
- Treat with intravenous fluids, analgesics and antiemetics. Avoid NSAIDs.
- Surgery should be avoided.

Answer 6

- Ureteric stenting is performed before commencing surgery in Piver type 2 and type 3 hysterectomies and in cases where adhesions are anticipated as in cases of endometriosis and PID.
- If a broad ligament fibroid or a cervical fibroid is present, it is better to reduce the size of the tumour by giving 3.75 mg of GnRH once a month for 3 months. The tumour should be enucleated before commencing the hysterectomy.
- The infundiblopelvic ligament should be clamped as medially as possible.
- Care should be taken to identify the ureter while removing adherent ovarian remnants from the ovarian fossa.
- Push the bladder well below the cervix as the ureter will move downwards with the bladder.
- The first transversely applied clamp for the uterine artery should be placed high. The tissues should be dissected to expose the uterine artery, to allow the clamp to include the artery only.
- The vertical clamp which is applied next for the transverse cervical ligament and the uterine artery should be placed medially "hugging" the uterus, as the ureter is closest to the uterus at this point.
- Avoid applying another transverse clamp to remove the cervix.
- Do not take deep needle bites when suturing the posterior flap of the vaginal vault.
- Though it is not mandatory to trace the ureter when performing a straight forward hysterectomy for a non-malignant condition, it may be safer to palpate the ureter at the end of the procedure.
- During a vaginal hysterectomy the bladder should be moved well above the fundus and laterally. The ureter will then move away with the bladder.

Answer 7.1

Secondary postpartum haemorrhage.

Answer 7.2

- Retained placental tissue
- Infection.

Answer 7.3
- Blood and high vaginal swab for culture and ABST
- Full blood count
- C-reactive protein levels.
- Ultrasound scanning.

Answer 7.4
- Insert two 14 gauge cannulae and commence an intravenous infusion of crystalloids.
- Send blood for cross-matching and reserve 3 pints.
- Commence intravenous broad spectrum antibiotics after sending blood and vaginal discharge for culture and ABST.
- Commence blood transfusion if there is haemodynamic compromise.
- Perform evacuation under general anaesthesia if retained products are found on the ultrasound scan.
- ICU admission may be required if there is haemodynamic compromise or severe sepsis.

Answer 8.1
Perform a caesarean section.

Answer 8.2
Perform a caesarean section.

Answer 8.3
Perform an amniotomy and commence an oxytocin infusion.

Answer 8.4
Perform a caesarean section.

Answer 8.5
Perform an amniotomy and commence an oxytocin infusion.

Answer 9.1
a. Dichorionic and diamniotic twins.
b. Monochorionic and diamniotic twins.
c. Monochorionic and monoamniotic twins.

Answer 9.2
- This is done by ultrasound scanning in late first trimester between 11 and 13 weeks.
- The following are assessed to determine the chorionicity.
  - The number of placental masses.
  - The lambda or T sign—ultrasound diagnosis of chorionicity is mainly based on the presence of the 'lambda' or 'twin peak' sign in dichorionic twins or 'T sign' in monochorionic twins at the membrane placenta interface.
  - Membrane thickness.
  - Discordant fetal sex.

- Monochorionic twins will have a thin separating membrane, the T sign and a single placental mass. They will be of the same sex.
- Dichorionic twins will have a thick dividing membrane, the lambda sign and two placental masses. They can be of the same or different sexes.
- Monoamniotic twins will have all the characteristics of monochorionic twins and will lie within one amniotic sac.

Answer 10

- The woman is discharged 24 hours after an uncomplicated normal vaginal delivery.
- The birth should be registered.
- The baby should be given the BCG vaccination and should be discharged by the paediatric house officer.
- Examine the woman for:
  - Excessive bleeding
  - Height of the fundus which should be below the umbilicus
  - The consistency of the uterus
  - Distension of the bladder
  - Temperature
- Advise the woman:
  - Regarding the proper technique of breastfeeding.
  - Regarding contraception.
  - To take a well-balanced diet with adequate amount of fruits and vegetables.
  - To drink plenty of water.
  - Regarding care of the episiotomy.
  - That she can have a bath daily.
  - Regarding the need to attend the postnatal clinic in 6 weeks.
- Give the BCG vaccination card.
- Mild analgesics such as paracetamol should be given for 5 days. In some units antibiotics may be given in cases where an episiotomy has been performed.

Examination Paper 13

Fetal Kick Count Chart

Hours	M	T	W	Th	F	S	Su
.00							
.30							
.00							
.30							
.00							
.30							
.00							
.30							
.00							
.30							
.00							
.30							

(Week)

1.1 How do you instruct a woman to maintain the above kick count chart?
(2 marks)

1.2 List 2 tests you would perform in your first line management if a woman complains of reduced fetal movements at a POA of 38 weeks.
(2 marks)

1.3 What is the next investigation you would perform if the above tests are normal but the woman complains of persistent reduction of fetal movements?
(1 mark)

1.4 List 3 risk factors which should be excluded in this woman. (3 marks)

1.5 What is the best management option, if this woman is readmitted 3 days later with the same complaint? She has no other risk factors. (2 marks)

QUESTION 2

A woman is admitted with a complaint of lower abdominal pain at a POA of 34 weeks.

2.1 How will you diagnose preterm labour?   (2 marks)
2.2 List three tocolytic drugs which are used to treat preterm labour. (3 marks)
2.3 Which of the above drugs will you use? Give your reasons.   (1 mark)
2.4 The CTG of this woman is given below. What is your management option?
                                                                      (2 marks)

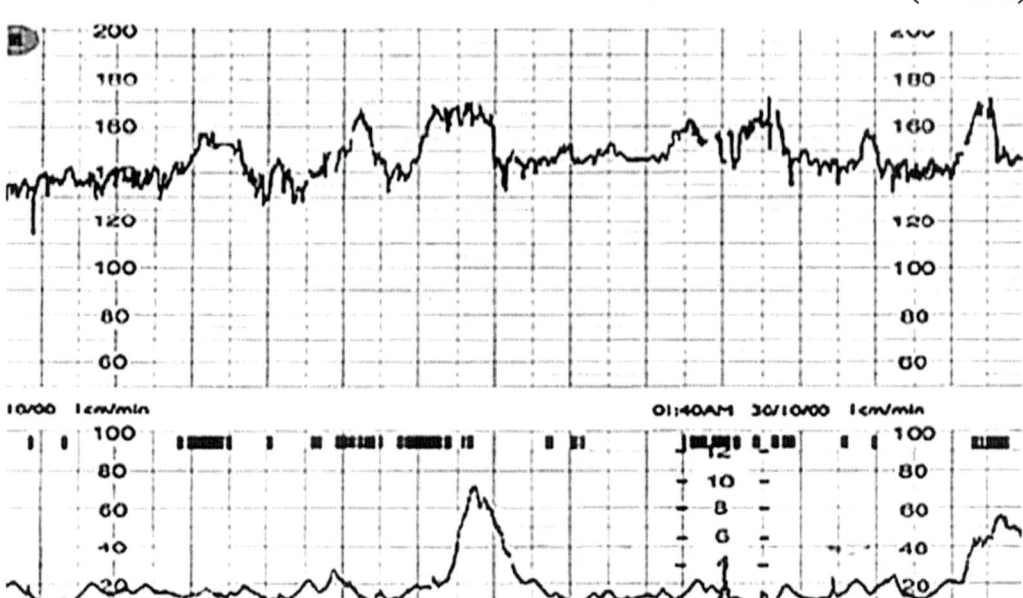

2.5 The CTG of a multiparous woman in preterm labour at a POA of 34 weeks is given below. What is the best management option? Give your reasons.
                                                                      (2 marks)

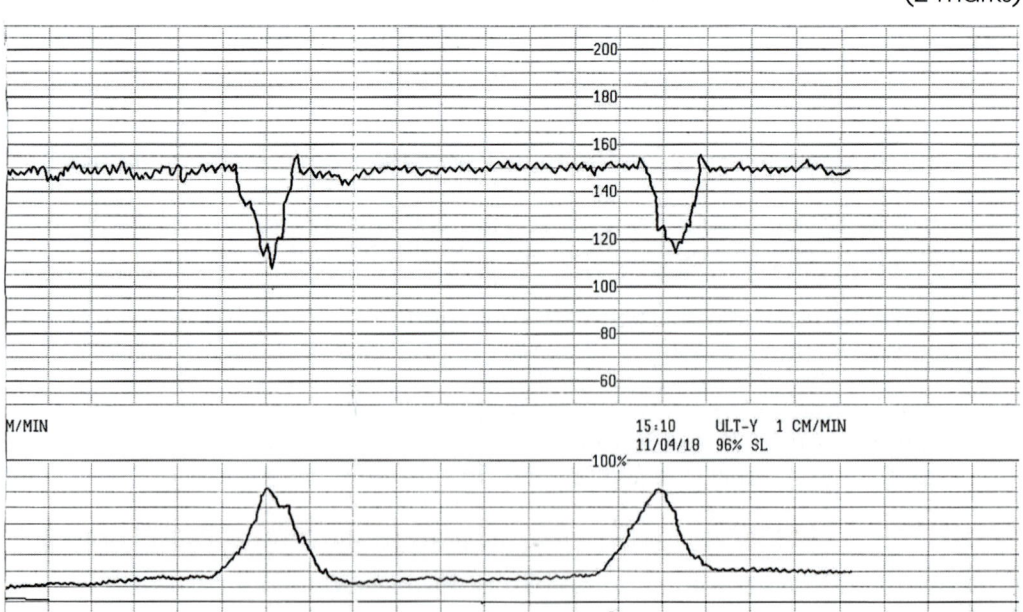

QUESTION 3

A primipara complains of dyspnoea on severe exertion at a POA of 20 weeks. On examination a cardiac murmur is found.

3.1   List 2 pathological cardiac murmurs which occur in a pregnant woman. (2 marks)

3.2   List 3 investigations which should be performed. (3 marks)

3.3   What is the NYHA cardiac grade of this woman? (1 mark)

3.4   List 4 steps in the antenatal care. (2 marks)

3.5   What is the best method of delivery, if her cardiac grade remains the same at term? (2 marks)

QUESTION 4

Select 2 methods of contraception which are most suitable for a woman:

4.1   With frequent irregular bleeding without a structural lesion, 6 months after the third pregnancy at the age of 35 years.

4.2   With venous thromboembolism.

4.3   With prolonged immobilization.

4.4   Who has delivered her sixth child 24 hours ago and is not consenting for sterilization.

4.5   Who is 39 years of age and is undergoing the third caesarean section.

(2 marks for each correct answer)

QUESTION 5

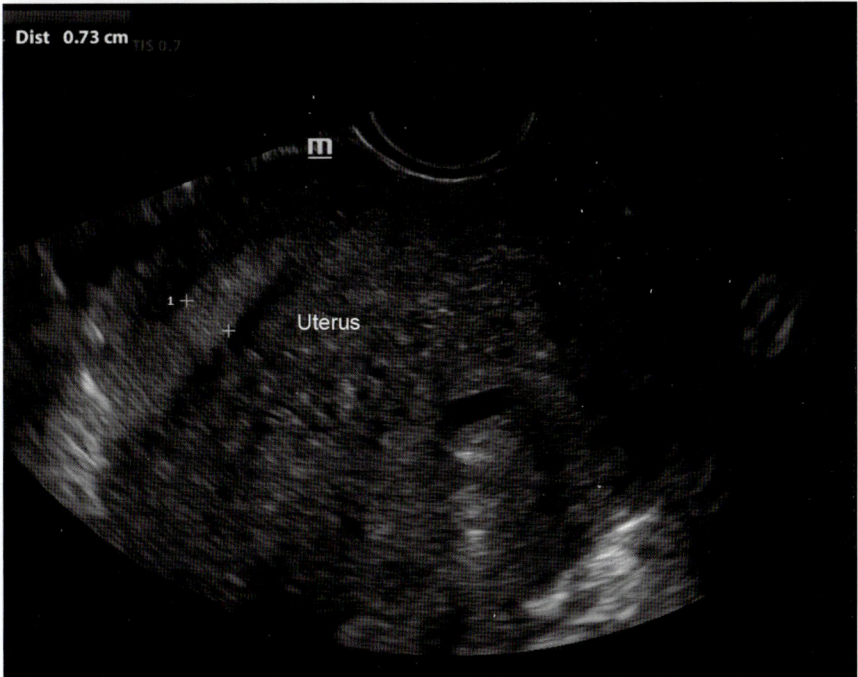

This is the ultrasound image of the uterus obtained from a 40-year-old multiparous woman.

5.1   Describe the abnormality seen in the image.   (2 marks)
5.2   What is your diagnosis?   (1 mark)
5.3   List 3 presenting symptoms of this condition.   (3 marks)
5.4   What is the best management option?   (2 marks)
5.5   What is the management option, if this woman is 35 years old and has one child?   (2 marks)

QUESTION 6

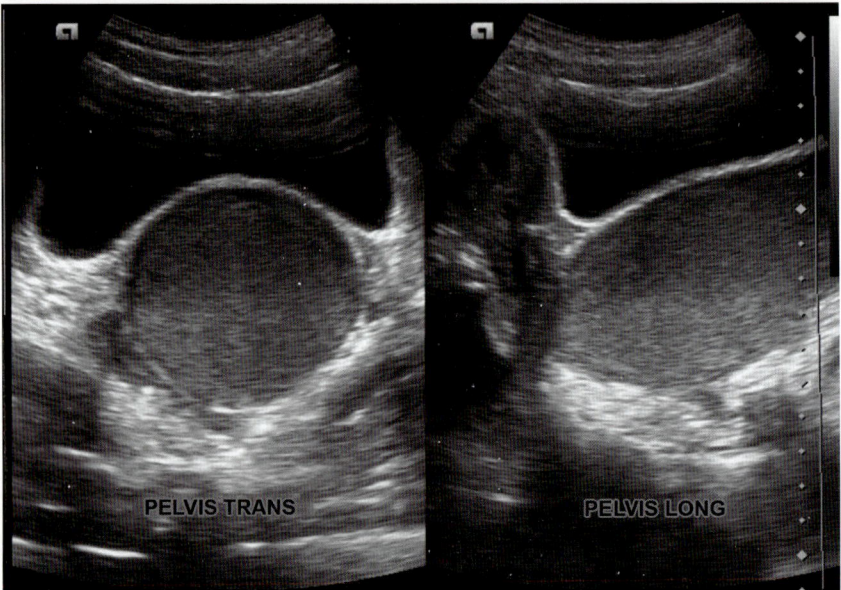

PELVIS TRANS   PELVIS LONG

This is the ultrasound image obtained from a 16-year-old girl who complains of primary amenorrhoea, abdominal pain and difficulty in passing urine.

6.1   Describe the findings and give your diagnosis.   (3 marks)
6.2   Mention the other clinical features of this condition.   (3 marks)
6.3   What is the best management option?   (4 marks)

QUESTION 7

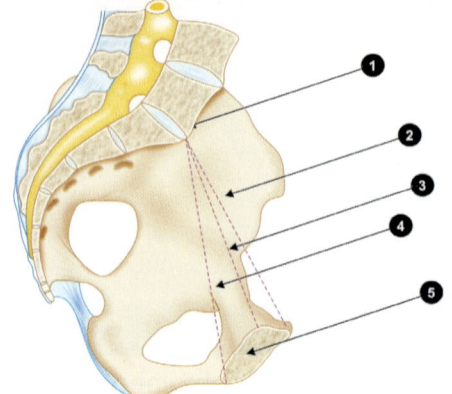

7.1   Name of the points 1, 2, 3, 4 and 5   (5 marks)

7.2   What are the measurements of 3 and 4 if the pelvis is adequate? (2 marks)
7.3   Explain why a pelvic assessment is not performed routinely before the onset
of labour.   (3 marks)

QUESTION 8

What is the best method of treatment for the following patients with abnormal
uterine bleeding?
8.1   A 16-year-old girl with irregular frequent menstrual bleeding.
8.2   A 40-year-old woman with heavy menstrual bleeding due to endometrial
hyperplasia without atypia.
8.3   A 35-year-old woman with two children who has irregular frequent menstrual
bleeding due to atypical endometrial hyperplasia.
8.4   A 20-year-old girl with recurrent periods of amenorrhoea followed by
prolonged bleeding.
8.5   A 30-year-old woman who has irregular vaginal bleeding following use of
DMPA for 1 year after the birth of her last child.
                                        (2 marks for each correct answer)

QUESTION 9

A multiparous woman is admitted with a history of mild lower abdominal pain at
a POA of 40 weeks.
9.1   How can you diagnose the onset of labour in this woman?   (3 marks)
9.2   List the steps you would follow before sending her to the labour ward.
                                                                    (5 marks)
9.3   What is your management option, if the woman is getting one contraction
per 15 minutes, lasting for 15 sec and the cervix is 50% effaced and dilated
to 3 cm? Give your reasons.   (2 marks)

QUESTION 10

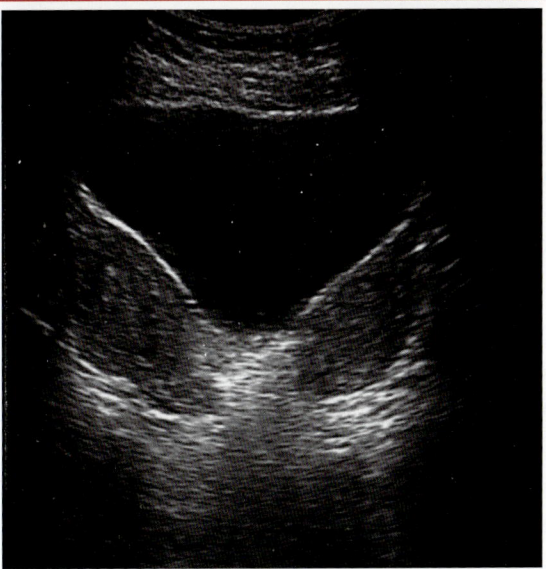

10.1 Name the abnormality shown in this ultrasound image. (1 mark)
10.2 List the symptoms which may be present during adolescence. (3 marks)
10.3 List the symptoms which may be present during the reproductive age.
(3 marks)
10.4 List the treatment options. (3 marks)

ANSWERS FOR EXAMINATION PAPER 13

Answer 1.1

She should start counting at a convenient time in the morning and mark the number of kicks during each time period. She should stop counting when she feels ten kicks. If she is unable to maintain a precise time period she can mark the kicks until she feels ten kicks. She should attend the hospital if she does not feel ten kicks in 12 hours.

Answer 1.2

- Listen to the fetal heart sounds using a hand Doppler machine.
- Perform a CTG.

Answer 1.3

An USS should be performed for umbilical artery Doppler studies, liquor volume and fetal biometry.

Answer 1.4

- Intrauterine growth restriction
- Pregnancy induced hypertension
- Diabetes mellitus.

Answer 1.5

Labour should be induced with vaginal prostaglandin if she does not have any risk factors. Fetal heart rate should be monitored carefully, preferably with continuous fetal heart rate monitoring.

Answer 2.1

- The woman will complain of lower abdominal pain which is increasing in frequency, intensity and duration with the passage of time.
- Abdominal examination will reveal palpable, painful, regular uterine contractions.
- A gentle vaginal examination should be performed to assess cervical dilatation.
- Regular uterine contractions can be seen on a CTG.

Answer 2.2

- Oral nifedepine
- Intravenous atosiban
- Intravenous ritodrine.

Answer 2.3

Oral nifedepine.
This drug is preferable because it is cheap, effective, can be given orally and has fewer side effects.

Answer 2.4

As the fetal heart rate tracing is normal and the contractions are few and of low intensity, she should be given oral nifedipine 20 mg twice daily. Two injections of 12.5 mg of betamethasone should be given 12 hours apart to bring about lung maturity. Nifedipine should be continued for 48 hours till the corticosteroids become effective.

Answer 2.5

It is better to perform a LSCS as the fetus is preterm and there are two decelerations in the strip in early labour. Also preterm fetuses are more sensitive to hypoxia.

Answer 3.1

- Pan systolic murmurs
- Diastolic murmurs

Answer 3.2

- Full blood count
- ECG
- Echocardiogram

Answer 3.3

NYHA cardiac grade 2.

Answer 3.4

- This woman can be managed as an out-patient as she is in NYHA cardiac grade 2.
- Advise regarding a balanced diet rich in iron, adequate rest and avoidance of respiratory tract infections. Prevent and treat anaemia.
- Treat dental caries under antibiotic cover.
- Frequent visits should be arranged to a specialised antenatal clinic and the cardiology clinic. A full cardiovascular assessment should be done at the clinic. A multidisciplinary team should be involved in the management
- Watch out for symptoms and signs of worsening of the cardiac condition such as increasing dyspnoea, palpitations, cough and paroxysmal nocturnal dyspnoea.
- A fetal echocardiogram should be done in the second trimester.

Answer 3.5

Normal vaginal delivery with spontaneous onset of labour is the best option.

Answer 4.1

- Oral contraceptive pills
- LNG-IUS.

Answer 4.2

- Copper IUCD
- LNG-IUS.

Answer 4.3
- Copper IUCD
- LNG-IUS.

Answer 4.4
- Insertion of a postpartum copper IUCD
- Insertion of a progesterone implant.

Answer 4.5
- Insertion of a postpartum copper IUCD at the time of caesarean section.
- Sterilization.

Answer 5.1
There is uterine enlargement with uniform hypertrophy of the myometrium. The endometrium appears normal. There are a few small cysts in the myometrium.

Answer 5.2
Adenomyosis.

Answer 5.3
- Heavy menstrual bleeding
- Secondary dysmenorrhea
- Deep dyspareunia.

Answer 5.4
Perform a total hysterectomy.

Answer 5.5
She can be treated with GnRH analogues 3.75 mg IM once a month for 3–6 months, but recurrence can occur.

Answer 6.1
The USS shows a normal uterus. The vagina is filled with an echogenic fluid which is most probably blood. The entire length of the vagina is not visible.

The diagnosis is cryptomenorrhoea with a haematocolpos due to an imperforate hymen or a low vaginal septum.

Answer 6.2
Primary amenorrhoea with:
- Monthly abdominal pain
- Normal height
- Normal secondary sexual characteristics
- Presence of a bluish bulging membrane at the vaginal introitus or the hymen and vaginal introitus may be normal with a thick septum within the vagina.

Answer 6.3
In the case of an imperforate hymen, perform a cruciate incision of the hymenal membrane and allow the blood to drain gradually.

If a vaginal septum is present excise it and restore continuity of the vagina and allow the blood to drain.

Answer 7.1

1. Sacral promontory
2. True conjugate
3. Obstetric conjugate
4. Diagonal conjugate
5. Pubic symphysis.

Answer 7.2

3. More than 10 cm
4. More than 11.5 cm.

Answer 7.3

The available space in the pelvis will increase during labour due to:
- Increase in the diameters of the pelvis due to stretching of the ligaments.
- Decrease in the fetal diameters as a result of complete flexion of the head in the presence of good contractions.
- Decrease in the fetal diameters as a result of grade 1 and grade 2 moulding.

Therefore, the pelvic capacity cannot be confirmed before the onset of labour. Hence pelvic assessment is not performed before the onset of labour in normal cases.

Answer 8.1

Combined oral contraceptive pills are given cyclically for 3–6 months together with oral iron.

Answer 8.2

Insert a LNG-IUS.

Answer 8.3

Perform total hysterectomy.

Answer 8.4

Combined oral contraceptive pills are given cyclically for 3–6 months together with oral iron. Weight reduction should be advised.

Answer 8.5

Commence combined oral contraceptive pills and stop DMPA injections.

Answer 9.1

Labour is diagnosed by signs and symptoms. The woman should have colicky lower abdominal pain and backache which increase in severity, frequency and duration with the passage of time. There should be palpable painful uterine contractions. Progressive cervical dilatation and effacement should be present. Regular contractions will be present in the CTG.

Answer 9.2

- Reassurance and explanation is essential.
- Peruse the antenatal records to exclude any complications.
- Perform a general, abdominal and a vaginal examination.
- Confirm onset of labour.
- Perform a CTG and an ultrasound scan.
- The perineum is shaved and a micro-enema is given.
- The jewelry and dentures should be removed.
- She should be dressed in clean hospital clothes and sent to the labour room.

Answer 9.3

Since she is a multiparous woman she may not be in labour or she may be in the early latent phase. She should be kept under observation in the antenatal ward. FHS should be charted half hourly and she should be reviewed after 4 hours.

Answer 10.1

Uterus didelphys.

Answer 10.2

The woman may not have any symptoms if both structures have cervices communicating with the vagina.

If one structure does not have a communicating cervix a haematometron can occur causing pain.

There may be dysmenorrhea and heavy menstrual bleeding.

Answer 10.3

Infertility.

Dyspareunia may occur if there is a double vagina; premature labour can occur if the uterine cavity containing the pregnancy happens to be small.

One uterus may obstruct the vaginal delivery of a pregnancy in the other horn.

Answer 10.4

No treatment is required in most cases of complete uterus didelphys.

Excision of the non-communicating horn should be done if a haematometron occurs.

Advice regarding the most suitable method of intercourse may be needed if dyspareunia occurs in the presence of a double vagina.

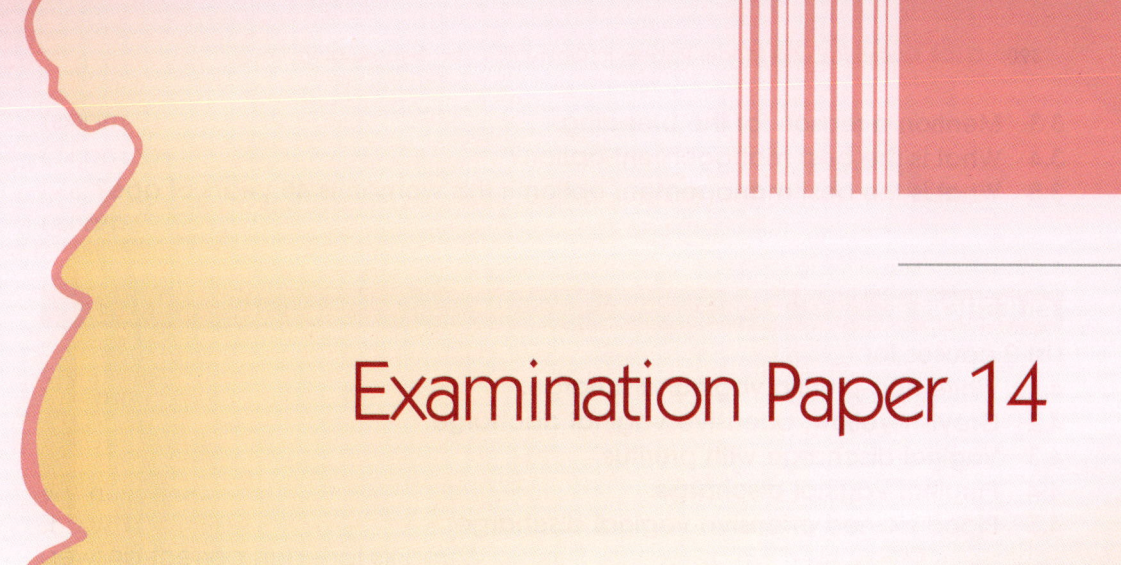

Examination Paper 14

QUESTION 1

A woman in her second pregnancy with a previous caesarean section attends the antenatal clinic at a POA of 37 weeks.

1.1 List 6 contraindications for VBAC (vaginal birth after caesarean section).

(3 marks)

1.2 List 4 precautions which should be taken during VBAC. Give your reasons.

(4 marks)

1.3 What are the earliest signs of scar dehiscence during labour? (2 marks)

1.4 List 2 advantages of VBAC which should be told to the woman when counselling regarding the mode of delivery. (0.5 × 2 = 1 mark)

QUESTION 2

2.1 List 3 causes of uterine enlargement which cause abdominally palpable masses. (3 marks)

2.2 List the physical signs which can be elicited during abdominal examination of an uterine mass. (4 marks)

2.3 Mention the method you would use to differentiate between an uterine and ovarian mass by vaginal examination. (3 marks)

QUESTION 3

A 55-year-old woman who is on continuous combined hormone replacement therapy complains of irregular spotting for 3 months. Abdominal and vaginal examinations are normal.

3.1 What is the first investigation you would perform? (2 marks)

3.2 If the above investigation is normal what is your first line management?

(2 marks)

A 35-year-old woman who is having a LNG-IUS complains of irregular spotting for 3 months. Abdominal and vaginal examinations and the transvaginal scan are normal.

3.3   Mention a reason for the bleeding.   (2 marks)
3.4   What is the best management option?   (2 marks)
3.5   What is the best management option if this woman is 45 years of age?
                                                                            (2 marks)

QUESTION 4

List 2 causes for:
4.1   White non-pruritic vaginal discharge.
4.2   Greyish-yellow, offensive vaginal discharge.
4.3   Vaginal discharge with pruritus.
4.4   Purulent vaginal discharge.
4.5   Blood stained offensive vaginal discharge.
                                            (2 marks for each correct answer)

QUESTION 5

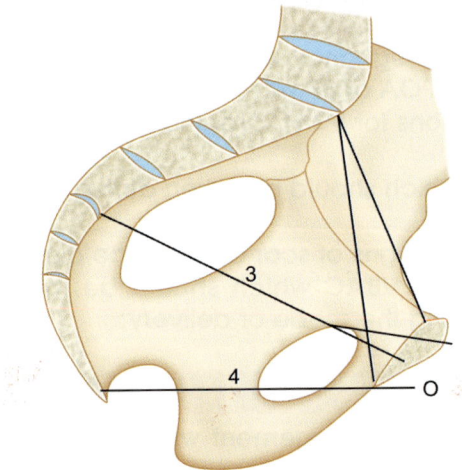

5.1   Name the pelvic planes shown by 3 and 4.
5.2   List two structural abnormalities felt during clinical pelvic assessment which
       can cause reduction in the length of 3.
5.3   What is the best management option if delay in the second stage occurs
       with reduction in the diameter of 3?
5.4   What is the pelvic type in which the diameter of 3 is reduced?
5.5   What is your management option if 4 is reduced?
                                            (2 marks for each correct answer)

QUESTION 6

Describe how you would administer oxytocin for induction or augmentation of
labour:
a. Using a gravity aided infusion set.
b. Using an infusion pump.   (5 marks for each correct answer)

QUESTION 7

7.1 What is the next management option for a 38-year-old woman with PCOS in whom routine ovulation induction with letrozole and hCG injection has failed after 6 cycles? (5 marks)

7.2 What is the next step if the woman fails to conceive with the treatment you have mentioned? (2 marks)

7.3 List 3 methods of confirming an adequate ovarian reserve in this woman. (3 marks)

QUESTION 8

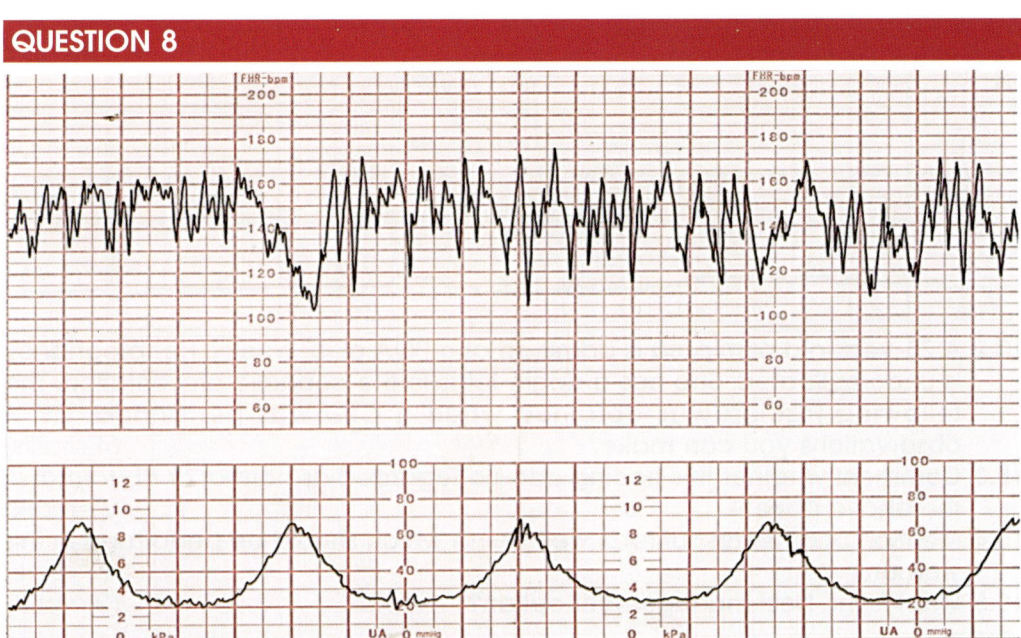

8.1 Name the fetal heart rate pattern shown in this CTG. Give your reasons. (2 marks)

8.2 During which stage of labour does this abnormality usually occur? (2 marks)

8.3 List 2 causes for this abnormality. (2 marks)

8.4 How will you manage this condition? (2 marks)

8.5 What is the significance of (a) presence of accelerations (b) absence of accelerations in a CTG? (2 marks)

QUESTION 9

9.1 List 4 contraindications for insertion of an IUCD. (4 marks)

9.2 What is your management if a woman becomes pregnant with an IUCD? (6 marks)

QUESTION 10

10.1 List 4 conditions in which the pregnancy should not be allowed to proceed beyond 40 weeks. (0.5 × 4 = 2 marks)

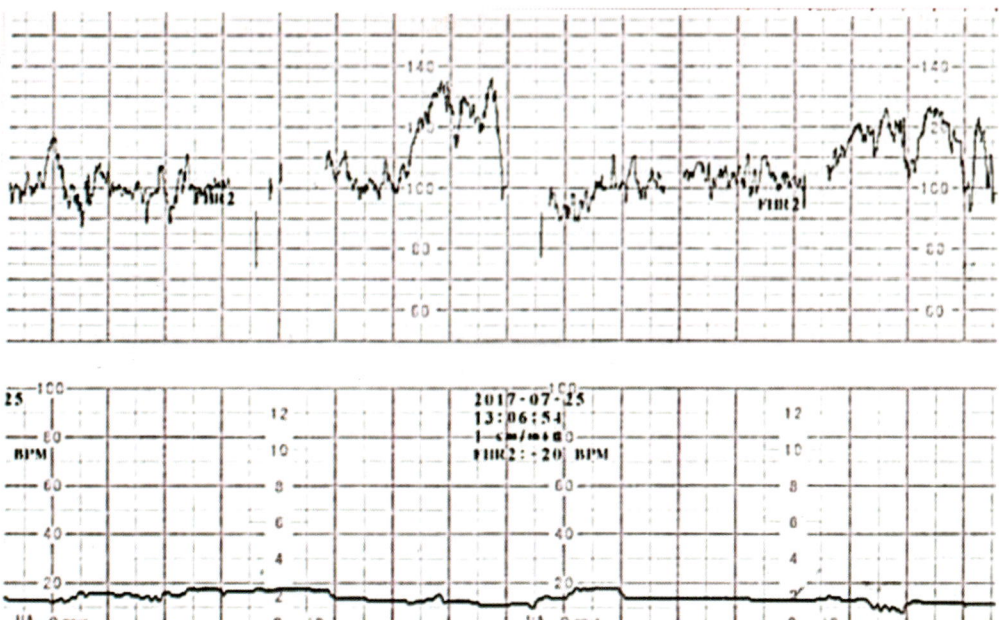

10.2 A 25-year-old primipara is admitted at a POA of 42 weeks. Her pregnancy is uncomplicated. She has a single fetus in the cephalic presentation. The following tracing was obtained when a CTG was performed. List 4 observations you can make. (4 marks)

10.3 Comment whether this tracing can be regarded as normal or abnormal in the above patient. (1 mark)

10.4 Mention another test of fetal well-being which should be performed in this woman. (1 mark)

10.5 What is the best management option? (2 marks)

ANSWERS FOR EXMANINATION PAPER 14

Answer 1.1

- Contraindications for vaginal delivery such as placenta praevia.
- Previous upper segment caesarean section or a lower segment caesarean section witha T-extension, tears or postpartum infection.
- Suspected cephalopelvic disproportion.
- Presence of an indication for early induction of labour.
- Twin pregnancy.
- Occurrence of malpresentations or malpositions.

Answer 1.2

- Labour should be conducted in a well-equipped hospital, with facilities for continuous intrapartum care and monitoring and resources for immediate caesarean section, blood transfusion and advanced neonatal resuscitation.
- Continuous electronic fetal heart rate monitoring should be carried out for the duration of labour as fetal distress is one of the earliest signs of scar dehiscence.
- A partograph should be maintained. Caesarean section should be performed if there is lack of progress as augmentation with oxytocin carries a risk of scar rupture.

- Second stage should be short as prolonged straining places a risk on the scar. Forceps or vacuum should be applied if the second stage is longer than half an hour.
- Rupture is most likely to occur during the second stage. Therefore, the patient should be carefully observed after the delivery for signs of intraperitoneal haemorrhage.

Answer 1.3
- Fetal distress
- Fresh vaginal bleeding.

Answer 1.4
- It will increase the chances of vaginal delivery during the next pregnancy.
- It will reduce the chances of formation of adhesions which can complicate future surgeries.

Answer 2.1
- Uterine fibroids
- Adenomyosis
- Pregnancy.

Answer 2.2
- Uterine masses are situated in the midline of the suprapubic area of the abdomen.
- They are firm in consistency except for a pregnant uterus which is soft.
- They are non-tender.
- They are mobile in the transverse plane with limited mobility in the vertical plane.
- It is not possible to reach below the mass.

Answer 2.3
- Insert 2 fingers of the right hand into the vagina.
- Place the left hand on the abdomen.
- Move the mass with the abdominal hand.
- Movement of the cervix can be felt by the fingers in the vagina if the mass is uterine.
- Movement of the cervix will not be felt if the mass is ovarian.

Answer 3.1
Perform a transvaginal ultrasound scan.

Answer 3.2
- The woman should be advised to take the pills regularly at the same time daily.
- She should be reviewed and a transvaginal scan should be performed in 3 months.

Answer 3.3
Break through bleeding due to release of small amounts of progesterone into the circulation.

Answer 3.4
Remove the LNG-IUS and advise to use combined oral contraceptive pills regularly.

Answer 3.5
Remove the LNG-IUS and insert a copper IUCD or perform sterilisation.

Answer 4.1
- Leucorrhoea
- Chlamydial infection.

Answer 4.2
- Trichomoniasis
- Bacterial vaginosis.

Answer 4.3
- Candidiasis
- Trichomoniasis.

Answer 4.4
- Gonorrhoea
- Acute or chronic pelvic inflammatory disease.

Answer 4.5
- Cervical polyp
- Cervical carcinoma.

Answer 5.1
3. Mid cavity
4. Outlet.

Answer 5.2
Presence of:
- A flat sacrum
- Prominent spines
- Reduced length of the sacrospinous ligaments.

Answer 5.3
Perform a caesarean section.

Answer 5.4
Android pelvis.

Answer 5.5
The posterior diameter of the outlet can be increased by performing an episiotomy.

Answer 6
Oxytocin is administered only after performing an amniotomy. Oxytocin is usually commenced if adequate contractions do not occur 2 hours after performing an amniotomy. Electronic fetal heart rate monitoring should be commenced.

a. Oxytocin is administered with 5 units in 500 ml of 0.9% sodium chloride solution. In situations where infusion pumps are not available, oxytocin may be administered starting at a drop rate of 15 per minute and increased at rates of 15 drops per minute every 30 minutes. If the CTG is normal, oxytocin may be continued in incremental doses until the woman is experiencing 4 or 5 contractions every 10 minutes, up to a maximum of 60 drops per minute.

b. If an infusion pump is used 10 units are included in 500 ml of 0.9% sodium chloride solution. The infusion is commenced at 1 MU per minute (3 ml/hr). The dose is doubled every hour till the contractions are satisfactory.

Answer 7.1

Treat with gonadotropin injections. Commence with 75 IU of FSH on the second day of the cycle. If the follicle does not reach 0.8 cm by the 7th day step up the dose by increments of 25–37.5 IU till a dose of 150 IU is reached. Give 5000 IU of hCG by IM injection when the follicle reaches 1.8 cm. If a long treatment schedule is used the initial dose is continued for 14 days.

Answer 7.2

In-vitro fertilization

Answer 7.3

If the woman has an adequate ovarian reserve:
- The total antral follicle count should be greater than 16.
- Anti-Mullerian hormone level should be greater than or equal to 25.0 pmol/L.
- Follicle-stimulating hormone level should be less than 4 IU/L.

Answer 8.1

Saltatory pattern.

There is wide variability of the fetal heart rate pattern with oscillations of the fetal heart rate above and below the baseline exceeding 25 bpm.

Answer 8.2

It usually occurs during the second stage of labour.

Answer 8.3

It is caused by:
- Fetal hypoxia due to maternal pushing
- Fetal hypoxia due to oxytocin infusion.

Answer 8.4

- Pushing should be stopped.
- The oxytocin drip should be stopped.
- If the condition does not improve immediate delivery is required.
- Since the patient is in the second stage forceps delivery can be performed if the other criteria are satisfied.

Answer 8.5
- Presence of accelerations indicate a neurologically responsive fetus without hypoxia or acidosis.
- Absence of accelerations is of uncertain significance.

Answer 9.1
- Pregnancy
- Acute pelvic inflammatory disease
- Uterine abnormalities such as bicornuate or septate uterus
- History of heavy menstrual bleeding or dysmenorrhea.

Answer 9.2
- Perform an USS to confirm a live intrauterine pregnancy, to exclude an ectopic pregnancy and to confirm the presence of the IUCD.
- Counsel regarding the possibility of miscarriage and infection.
- Remove the IUCD if the threads are visible. Advise to return if bleeding or infection occurs.
- If threads are not visible but the IUCD is seen on the scan reassure the patient and review if there is bleeding or discharge.
- Check for the IUCD at the time of delivery.
- Perform an USS after 6 weeks if the IUCD is not expelled at the time of delivery.

Answer 10.1
- Twin pregnancy
- Intrauterine growth restriction
- Pregnancy induced hypertension
- GDM/DM complicating pregnancy.

Answer 10.2
- There is baseline bradycardia
- There are accelerations
- The baseline variability is normal
- There are no decelerations.
- There are no uterine contractions.

Answer 10.3
Baseline bradycardia can be regarded as normal in a postmature patient if the baseline variability is normal, accelerations are present and there are no decelerations.

Answer 10.4
Ultrasound scanning for umbilical artery Doppler studies.

Answer 10.5
- Labour can be induced.
- Perform a vaginal examination to assess the Bishop score.
- Perform amniotomy if the Bishop score is more than 7 and commence an oxytocinin fusion after 2 hours. Insert dinoprostone 3 mg into the vagina if the Bishop score is less than 7.
- Continuous fetal heart rate monitoring is necessary.

Examination Paper 15

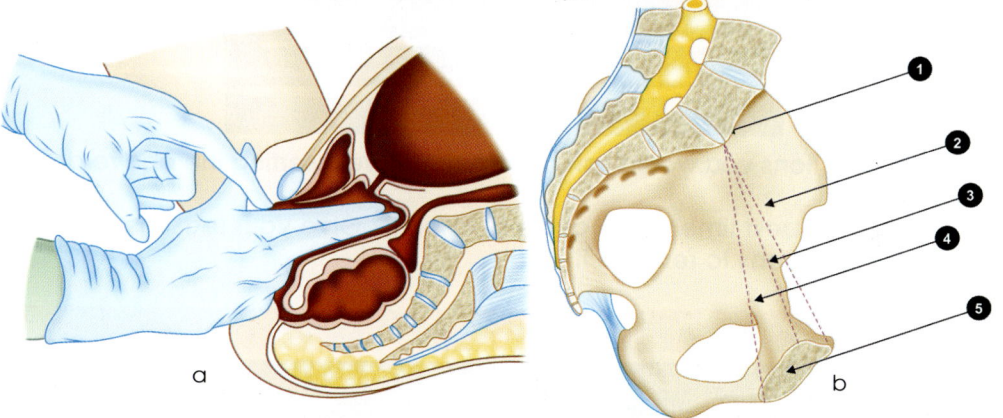

1.1 What is the measurement which is shown in (a) which is carried out in a pregnant woman during pelvic assessment? (2 marks)

1.2 Describe how the above measurement is taken. (4 marks)

1.3 How do you measure 3? (2 marks)

1.4 What is the best management option for a woman with a previous caesarean section if the length of 3 is 9 cm? (2 marks)

QUESTION 2

2.1 List (a) 5 advantages and (b) 2 disadvantages of VBAC which should be told when counselling a woman with a previous caesarean section regarding the mode of delivery. (7 marks)

2.2 List 3 factors which indicate the possibility of a successful VBAC. (3 marks)

QUESTION 3

3.1 What is the value of performing a speculum examination to diagnose the cause of vaginal discharge? (6 marks)

3.2 List 4 screening tests which are performed to exclude sexually transmitted infections in a woman with chronic pelvic inflammatory disease. (4 marks)

QUESTION 4

Describe the method you would adopt to prevent damage to the ureter when:

4.1 Suturing a deep angle tear of the uterus extending to the cervix sustained at caesarean section. (4 marks)

4.2 Ligating the internal iliac artery. (2 marks)

4.3 Performing a hysterectomy for multiple fibroids including a large cervical fibroid which is extending into the broad ligament. (4 marks)

QUESTION 5

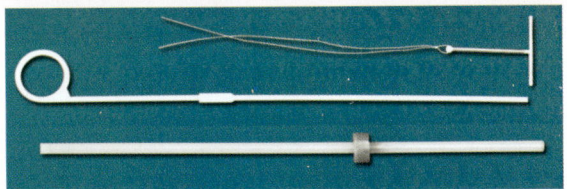

5.1 List 5 questions you would ask a woman before inserting the above device. (5 marks)

5.2 What is the best time of the cycle to insert it? Give your reasons. (1 mark)

5.3 List 4 indications to remove it. (4 marks)

QUESTION 6

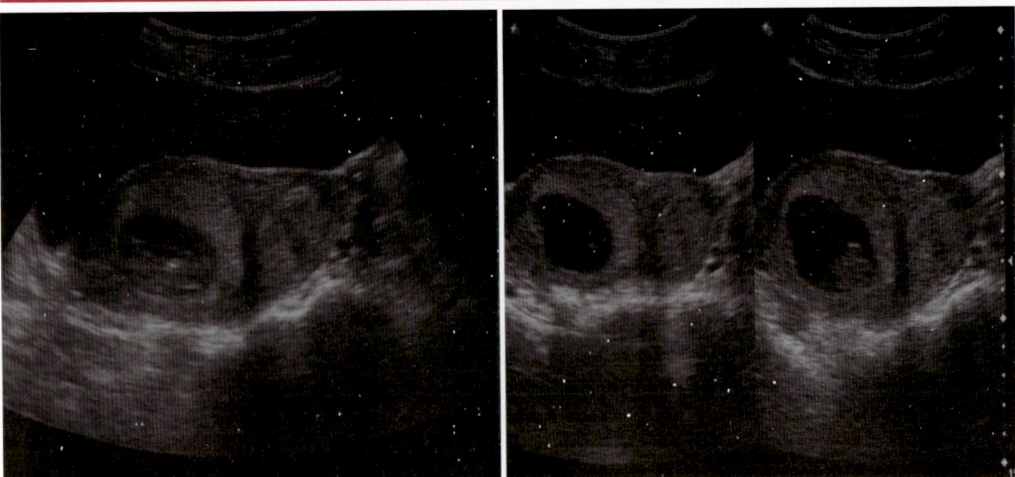

These ultrasound images were obtained from a woman who attended the antenatal clinic at a POA of 7 weeks.

6.1 What is your diagnosis? (1 mark)

6.2   What are the complications you would expect?   (5 marks)
6.3   How would you counsel this woman?   (4 marks)

QUESTION 7

How will you counsel a woman who has been diagnosed with a missed miscarriage at a POA of 8 weeks?   (10 marks)

QUESTION 8

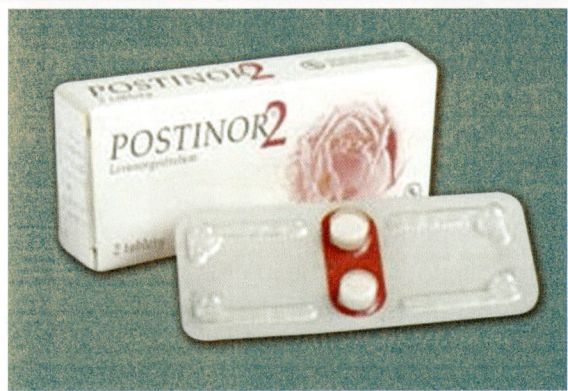

8.1   Mention the compound and the content in a single tablet of prostinor 2 and prostinor 1.   (3 marks)
8.2   Mention the indication, dose, frequency and the time of administration of prostinor.   (3 marks)
8.3   Mention the mode of action.   (2 marks)
8.4   Mention 2 methods of emergency contraception which can be given up to 5 days of intercourse.   (2 marks)

QUESTION 9

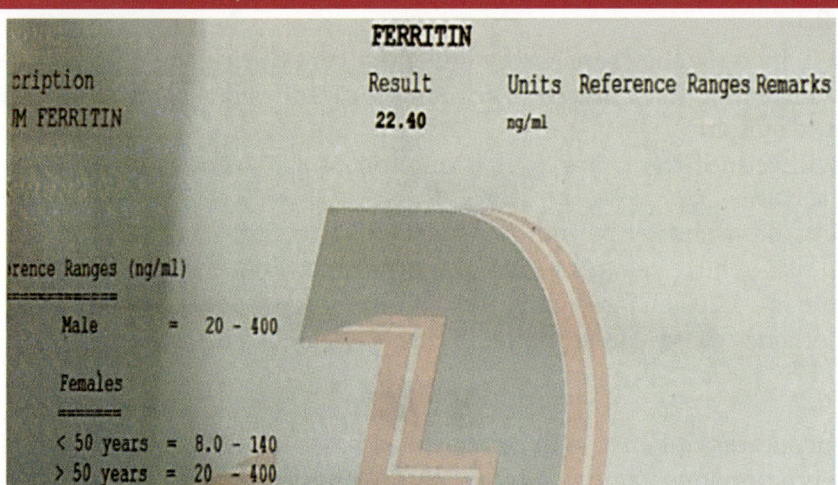

This investigation was performed in a woman at a POA of 16 weeks.
9.1   List 3 conditions which could cause the above abnormality.   (3 marks)

9.2   Mention how you would differentiate between these conditions. (3 marks)

9.3   What is the initial treatment of the conditions you have mentioned? (4 marks)

QUESTION 10

10.1 List 4 complications of an episiotomy. (4 marks)

10.2 List 4 important instructions you would give a woman regarding the care of an episiotomy. (4 marks)

10.3 List 4 conditions where it is mandatory to perform an episiotomy. (2 marks)

ANSWERS FOR EXAMINATION PAPER 15

Answer 1.1

Measurement of the diagonal conjugate of the pelvis.

Answer 1.2

- A vaginal examination is performed.
- The sacral promontory is not felt if the inlet is adequate.
- If the sacral promontory is felt, with the finger closely applied to the sacral promontory, the vaginal hand is elevated until it contacts the under surface of the symphysis pubis. This point is marked on the hand.
- The distance between the mark and the tip of the finger is measured in centimeters and is the diagonal conjugate.

Answer 1.3

The obstetric conjugate (3) is 1.5–2 cm less than the diagonal conjugate.

Answer 1.4

Perform a caesarean section as the pelvic inlet is inadequate.

Answer 2.1

a. • It will increase the chances of vaginal delivery during the next pregnancy.
   • It will reduce the chances of formation of adhesions which can complicate future surgeries.
   • It will reduce the chances of formation of a placenta previa with morbid adhesion.
   • VBAC has a shorter period of recovery.
   • The risk of birth related perinatal morbidity is low.
b. • There is a 1:200 chance of uterine rupture.
   • Emergency caesarean section will be necessary if VBAC fails.

Answer 2.2

Chance of successful VBAC will be increased if:

- There is a previous vaginal delivery before or after the caesarean section.
- There is a cephalic presentation with engagement of the head at term.
- Spontaneous onset of labour occurs between 38 and 41 weeks.

Answer 3.1

The following information obtained by performing a speculum examination will be helpful to diagnose the cause of the discharge.
- Inspect the discharge for colour, smell and the amount.
- Inspect the cervix for inflammation, ectropion, polyp, ulcer, discharge.
- Inspect the vaginal walls and obtain a high vaginal and an endocervical swab for:
  - Direct microscopy to diagnose motile protozoa in trichomoniasis, fungal hyphae in candidiasis and clue cells in bacterial vaginosis.
  - Gram stained smear to diagnose gram-positive yeasts in candidiasis, gram-negative intracellular diplococci in gonorrhoea (from an endocervical swab) and clue cells in bacterial vaginosis.
  - PCR test to diagnose chlamydia and gonorrhoea
  - Culture and ABST.
- Perform a cervical smear if cervical cancer screening has not been performed within 3 years.

Answer 3.2

Perform:
- PCR test on an endocervical swab for chlamydia and gonorrhea
- VDRL test
- ELISA test for HIV
- Hepatitis B surface antigen test.

Answer 4.1

- The uterus should be lifted out of the incision.
- The bladder should be pushed down below the tear as the ureter will go down with the bladder.
- Insert the first stitch at the lowest accessible point. Cut the ends of the thread long and apply the next stitch at a lower point by applying traction on these threads. Gradually reach the apex of the tear.
- It is better to trace the lower part of the ureter in deep lateral tears.

Answer 4.2

- The ureter should be identified at the point it is crossing the bifurcation of the common iliac artery.
- It should be pushed medially, away from the internal iliac artery.

Answer 4.3

The ureter is most likely to be damaged while removing the cervix as it may be very close to the cervical fibroid.
- Give GnRH 3.75 mg IM once a month for 3 months before performing the operation.
- At operation remove the cervical fibroid before proceeding with the hysterectomy.
- Identify the ureter before clamping the transverse cervical ligament.

Answer 5.1

Inquire whether she has:
- Heavy or frequent, irregular, menstrual bleeding.
- Dysmenorrhea.

- A past history of ectopic pregnancy.
- A period of amenorrhoea. Exclude pregnancy.
- A history suggestive of pelvic inflammatory disease such as abdominal pain, fever, purulent vaginal discharge or sexual promiscuity.

Answer 5.2

It should be inserted during the last day of menstrual bleeding or soon after menstruation because the cervical os will be more open and a pregnancy can be excluded.

Answer 5.3

Indications to remove it include:
- Pregnancy.
- Lapse of 10 years.
- Menopause
- Occurrence of complications such as abnormal menstrual bleeding, dysmenorrhea, abdominal pain or infection.
- Request by the patient.

Answer 6.1

Pregnancy in a septate bicornuate uterus.

Answer 6.2

- Miscarriage
- Rupture of the horn
- Placental abruption if the placenta forms on the septum
- Malpresentations
- Intrauterine growth restriction if the placenta forms on the septum
- Premature labour
- Intrauterine death.

Answer 6.3

She should be informed that:
- Her uterus is abnormal with 2 compartments and a dividing septum.
- Her pregnancy is in one compartment.
- Most probably her pregnancy will continue to term. However, the complications stated above can occur.
- It is better to deliver by caesarean section at 37 weeks as sudden intrauterine death can occur.

Answer 7

- Introduce yourself to the patient and reassure her. It is better if the partner is present.
- Explain that it is usually due to a lethal fetal abnormality due to a genetic defect in the sperm or the ovum.
- Inform her that it does not usually recur in subsequent pregnancies.
- Inquire regarding exposure to drugs, toxins, infections and radiation as occasionally these could be the cause.

Inform her that:

- Diet or exertion cannot cause a missed miscarriage.
- It is better to carry out expectant management for three weeks in the absence of bleeding or infection.
- Two doses of misoprostol will be inserted if expectant management is not successful.
- She can be observed for 1–2 weeks for expulsion to occur.
- Several scans will be done after the expulsion and an ERPC will be necessary if there is retained tissue.
- She should postpone the next pregnancy for 3 months.
- She should use 5 mg of folic acid daily.
- An early scan should be performed in the next pregnancy
- She can resume normal activity after resting for one week.

Answer 8.1

Prostinor contains levonorgestrel. Prostinor 1 has a single tablet containing 1.5 mg of levonorgestrel Prostinor 2 has two tablets each containing 0.75 mg of levonorgestrel.

Answer 8.2

It should be taken within 72 hours of unprotected intercourse. Prostinor two has 2 tablets. Take one immediately and the other after 12 hours. Prostinor one has only one tablet and is taken as a single dose.

Answer 8.3

It acts by preventing ovulation. It does not prevent implantation.

Answer 8.4

Ulipristal 30 mg or insertion of an IUCD.

Answer 9.1

- Iron deficiency anaemia
- Thalassemic trait
- Mixed deficiency anaemia.

Answer 9.2

- Perform a blood picture.
- Iron deficiency will cause a hypochromic microcytic blood picture with anisopoikilocytosis.
- Thalassemia will cause a hypochromic microcytic blood picture with target cells, basophilic stippling and irregularly contracted red cells. The diagnosis is confirmed by haemoglobin electrophoresis.
- Mixed deficiency anaemia will cause a microcytic and a macrocytic blood picture. The diagnosis may be confirmed by performing serum folate and Vit B_{12} levels.

Answer 9.3

- As the serum ferritin levels are low irrespective of the cause of the anaemia this woman will need dietary advice and iron therapy.

- She should be advised to eat food rich in iron such as green leaves, red meat and pulses.
- She should be commenced on oral iron tablets (60 mg of elemental iron twice daily) as the serum ferritin level is below 30 ng/ml.
- Treatment should be monitored by performing haemoglobin levels monthly.
- Folic acid 5 mg should be given daily if the woman has thalassaemia or mixed deficiency anaemia. Vitamin B_{12} injections should be given if there is mixed deficiency.
- If thalassemia is suspected haemoglobin electrophoresis should be carried out. If she is a thalassaemic trait carry-out haemoglobin electrophoresis in her husband. If he is not a thalassaemic trait there is no risk of the fetus having thalassaemia major.
- If the husband is also a thalassaemic trait amniocentesis should be done to exclude the occurrence of thalassaemia major in the fetus.

Answer 10.1

- Extension of the incision at the time of delivery
- Bleeding/formation of a haematoma
- Pain
- Wound infection and dehiscence
- Dyspareunia.

Answer 10.2

- The woman should be advised to wash the area with water twice a day. She should spray water softly to the wound with a bottle every time she urinates.
- The wound should be dried with clean gauze or cotton wool.
- Antiseptic solutions should not be used.
- She should change the pad frequently as the area should be kept clean and dry.
- She should eat plenty of fruits and vegetables to prevent constipation.
- If there is pain she can take mild analgesics such as paracetamol or NSAIDs. An ice pack may be placed if the pain is severe.
- She should be informed that the sutures are absorbable and will get absorbed or fall off gradually.
- She should be advised to consult a doctor if there is severe pain, discharge, redness of the area or fever.

Answer 10.3

- Twin delivery
- Breech delivery
- Instrumental delivery
- Face to pubes delivery

Reader's Notes

Reader's Notes